Cancer Survivorship

SOURCEBOOK

Second Edition

Health Reference Series

Second Edition

Cancer Survivorship SOURCEBOOK

Basic Consumer Health Information about the Physical, Educational, Emotional, Social, and Financial Needs of Cancer Patients from Diagnosis, through Cancer Treatment, and Beyond, Including Facts about Researching Specific Types of Cancer and Learning about Clinical Trials and Treatment Options, and Featuring Tips for Coping with the Side Effects of Cancer Treatments and Adjusting to Life after Cancer Treatment Concludes

Along with Suggestions for Caregivers, Friends, and Family Members of Cancer Patients, a Glossary of Cancer Care Terms, and Directories of Related Resources

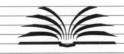

OMNIGRAPHICS

615 Griswold, Ste. 901, Detroit, MI 48226

Bibliographic Note
Because this page cannot legibly accommodate all the copyright notices, the Bibliographic
Note portion of the Preface constitutes an extension of the copyright notice.

* * *

Health Reference Series
Keith Jones, *Managing Editor*
***

OMNIGRAPHICS
A PART OF RELEVANT INFORMATION
***

Copyright © 2017 Omnigraphics
ISBN 978-0-7808-1549-0
E-ISBN 978-0-7808-1550-6

Library of Congress Cataloging-in-Publication Data

Names: Omnigraphics, Inc.

Title: Cancer survivorship sourcebook: basic consumer health information
about the physical, educational, emotional, social, and financial needs of cancer
patients from diagnosis, through cancer treatment, and beyond, including facts
about researching specific types of cancer and learning about clinical trials and
treatment options, and featuring tips for coping with the side effects of cancer
treatments and adjusting to life after cancer treatment concludes; along with
suggestions for caregivers, friends, and family members of cancer patients, a
glossary of cancer care terms, and directories of related resources.

Description: Second edition. | Detroit: Omnigraphics, [2017] | Series: Health
reference series | Includes bibliographical references and index.

Identifiers: LCCN 2016059223 (print) | LCCN 2017001751 (ebook) | ISBN
9780780815490 (hardcover: alk. paper) | ISBN 9780780815506 (ebook) | ISBN
9780780815506 (eBook)

Subjects: LCSH: Cancer--Popular works. | Cancer--Patients--Care. | Cancer--
Patients--Life skills guides.

Classification: LCC RC263.C296 2017 (print) | LCC RC263 (ebook) | DDC
362.19699/4--dc23

LC record available at https://lccn.loc.gov/2016059223

Table of Contents

Part III: Clinical Trials and Cancer Research Updates

Part IV: Coping with Side Effects and Complications of Cancer Treatment

Part V: Emotional, Cognitive, and Mental Health Issues in Cancer Care

Part VI: Maintaining Wellness during and after Cancer Treatment

Part VII: Information for Friends, Family Members, and Caregivers

Part VIII: Additional Help and Information

Preface

About This Book

There are more than 15.5 million cancer survivors alive in the United States today, and that number will grow to more than 20 million by 2026—a number made possible through better and earlier detection of cancer, advances in medical technologies, and improved treatments. Statistics also suggest that approximately 67% of people diagnosed with cancer will live at least five years after their diagnosis, and nearly 17% of those will live at least twenty years. Cancer survivorship presents multiple challenges, however. Cancer survivors often lack the information they need to make treatment choices, maintain optimal physical and mental health during and after treatment, prevent disability and late effects associated with cancer, and handle economic issues related to cancer care.

Cancer Survivorship Sourcebook, Second Edition, provides information for cancer patients and their family members, friends, and caregivers. It includes tips for researching specific types of cancer, treatment advances, and clinical trials, and it offers suggestions for coping with the side effects and complications of cancer treatments. Facts about emotional, cognitive, and mental health issues in cancer care are included, and a special section focuses on the challenges of maintaining wellness during and after cancer treatment. A glossary of cancer care terms is also provided, along with a directory of resources for cancer patients and information about financial assistance for cancer care.

Readers seeking information about the major forms and stages of cancers affecting specific organs and body systems may wish to consult *Cancer Sourcebook*, Seventh Edition, a separate volume within the *Health Reference Series*. In addition, some specific forms of cancer are discussed in a more in-depth manner in other *Health Reference Series* books:

- Breast cancer: *Breast Cancer Sourcebook*, Fifth Edition

- Gynecological cancers: *Cancer Sourcebook for Women*, Fifth Edition

How to Use This Book

This book is divided into parts and chapters. Parts focus on broad areas of interest. Chapters are devoted to single topics within a part.

Part I: If Your Doctor Says It's Cancer begins with information on the process of finding a qualified healthcare provider and getting a second opinion. Cancer screening, diagnostic procedures, and understanding the diagnosis are also discussed. It also provides facts about the tests that are used to diagnose cancer and to monitor the effectiveness of cancer treatments.

Part II: Making Treatment and Cancer Care Decisions gives insight to help understand your cancer prognosis and provides an overview of commonly used cancer treatments, medications, and complementary and alternative medicine (CAM) practices. It also discusses the use of palliative and hospice care, and describes the transitions that may occur during care if cancer treatments are not effective in halting the advance of the disease.

Part III: Clinical Trials and Cancer Research Updates provides information for cancer patients who are considering participating in cancer-related research studies. It explains the procedures commonly used in clinical trials and explains how to locate one. It also offers updated information about recent research results, new treatments, and current research initiatives that offer hope for the future.

Part IV: Coping with Side Effects and Complications of Cancer Treatment discusses side effects that often accompany commonly used cancer treatments. It explains why treatments can cause such physical effects as nausea, vomiting, weight loss, hair loss, and fatigue. It also includes practical suggestions for dealing with these types of effects and other medical complications of cancer treatment.

Part V: Emotional, Cognitive, and Mental Health Issues in Cancer Care provides facts about the non-physical effects and complications of cancer and its treatment. These include changes in self-image that result from illness or from body-altering surgical procedures and the ways people adjust to new circumstances. It also describes mental health disorders that may accompany cancer treatment, including depression, anxiety disorders, posttraumatic stress disorder, and substance abuse.

Part VI: Maintaining Wellness during and after Cancer Treatment describes various steps cancer survivors can take to achieve optimal health while they are receiving cancer treatments and after their treatments have been completed. These include eating a healthy diet, participating in rehabilitative programs, exercising, and smoking cessation. Additional chapters address concerns related to resuming "normal" life once cancer treatment is over and appropriate follow-up care. The part also deals with cancer recurrence and its effects.

Part VII: Information for Friends, Family Members, and Caregivers gives an overview of family issues after treatment, offers guidelines for dealing with family matters, life planning, and practical aspects of cancer caregiving. Individual chapters address specific concerns of loved ones, parents, children, and siblings.

Part VIII: Additional Help and Information includes a glossary of cancer care terms and a glossary of terms commonly used by health insurance companies and in medical billing. It also offers directories of resources able to provide services and support to cancer patients and their families.

Bibliographic Note

This volume contains documents and excerpts from publications issued by the following U.S. government agencies: Centers for Disease Control and Prevention (CDC); National Cancer Institute (NCI); National Institute of Nursing Research (NINR); Office of Disease Prevention and Health Promotion (ODPHP); U.S. Department of Agriculture (USDA); and U.S. Food and Drug Administration (FDA).

It may also contain original material produced by Omnigraphics and reviewed by medical consultants.

About the Health Reference Series

The *Health Reference Series* is designed to provide basic medical information for patients, families, caregivers, and the general public. Each volume takes a particular topic and provides comprehensive coverage. This is especially important for people who may be dealing with a newly diagnosed disease or a chronic disorder in themselves or in a family member. People looking for preventive guidance, information about disease warning signs, medical statistics, and risk factors for health problems will also find answers to their questions in the *Health Reference Series*. The *Series*, however, is not intended to serve as a tool for diagnosing illness, in prescribing treatments, or as a substitute for the physician/patient relationship. All people concerned about medical symptoms or the possibility of disease are encouraged to seek professional care from an appropriate health care provider.

A Note about Spelling and Style

Health Reference Series editors use *Stedman's Medical Dictionary* as an authority for questions related to the spelling of medical terms and the *Chicago Manual of Style* for questions related to grammatical structures, punctuation, and other editorial concerns. Consistent adherence is not always possible, however, because the individual volumes within the *Series* include many documents from a wide variety of different producers, and the editor's primary goal is to present material from each source as accurately as is possible. This sometimes means that information in different chapters or sections may follow other guidelines and alternate spelling authorities.

Medical Review

Omnigraphics contracts with a team of qualified, senior medical professionals who serve as medical consultants for the *Health Reference Series*. As necessary, medical consultants review reprinted and originally written material for currency and accuracy. Citations including the phrase, "Reviewed (month, year)" indicate material reviewed by this team. Medical consultation services are provided to the *Health Reference Series* editors by:

Dr. Senthil Selvan, MBBS, DCH, MD
Dr. K. Sivanandham, MBBS, DCH, MS (Research), PhD

Our Advisory Board

We would like to thank the following board members for providing initial guidance on the development of this series:

- Dr. Lynda Baker, Associate Professor of Library and Information Science, Wayne State University, Detroit, MI

- Nancy Bulgarelli, William Beaumont Hospital Library, Royal Oak, MI

- Karen Imarisio, Bloomfield Township Public Library, Bloomfield Township, MI

- Karen Morgan, Mardigian Library, University of Michigan-Dearborn, Dearborn, MI

- Rosemary Orlando, St. Clair Shores Public Library, St. Clair Shores, MI

Health Reference Series *Update Policy*

The inaugural book in the *Health Reference Series* was the first edition of *Cancer Sourcebook* published in 1989. Since then, the *Series* has been enthusiastically received by librarians and in the medical community. In order to maintain the standard of providing high-quality health information for the layperson the editorial staff at Omnigraphics felt it was necessary to implement a policy of updating volumes when warranted.

Medical researchers have been making tremendous strides, and it is the purpose of the *Health Reference Series* to stay current with the most recent advances. Each decision to update a volume is made on an individual basis. Some of the considerations include how much new information is available and the feedback we receive from people who use the books. If there is a topic you would like to see added to the update list, or an area of medical concern you feel has not been adequately addressed, please write to:

Managing Editor
Health Reference Series
Omnigraphics
615 Griswold, Ste. 901
Detroit, MI 48226

Part One

If Your Doctor Says It's Cancer

Chapter 1

Finding a Cancer Doctor

What Is Cancer?

Cancer is the name given to a collection of related diseases. In all types of cancer, some of the body's cells begin to divide without stopping and spread into surrounding tissues.

Cancer can start almost anywhere in the human body, which is made up of trillions of cells. Normally, human cells grow and divide to form new cells as the body needs them. When cells grow old or become damaged, they die, and new cells take their place. When cancer develops, however, this orderly process breaks down. As cells become more and more abnormal, old or damaged cells survive when they should die, and new cells form when they are not needed. These extra cells can divide without stopping and may form growths called tumors.

Many cancers form solid tumors, which are masses of tissue. Cancers of the blood, such as leukemias, generally do not form solid tumors.

This chapter contains text excerpted from the following sources: Text under the heading "What Is Cancer?" is excerpted from "Understanding Cancer," National Cancer Institute (NCI), February 9, 2015; Text under the heading "Cancer Is Preventable" is excerpted from "Cancer," Office of Disease Prevention and Health Promotion (ODPHP), U.S. Department of Health and Human Services (HHS), September 27, 2016; Text beginning with the heading "Finding a Doctor" is excerpted from "How to Find a Doctor or Treatment Facility If You Have Cancer," National Cancer Institute (NCI), June 5, 2013. Reviewed February 2017; Text under the heading "Questions to Ask Your Doctor" is excerpted from "Questions to Ask Your Doctor about Your Diagnosis," National Cancer Institute (NCI), April 2, 2015.

Cancerous tumors are malignant, which means they can spread into, or invade nearby tissues. In addition, as these tumors grow, some cancer cells can break off and travel to distant places in the body through the blood or the lymph system and form new tumors far from the original tumor. Unlike malignant tumors, benign tumors do not spread into, or invade nearby tissues. Benign tumors can sometimes be quite large, however. When removed, they usually don't grow back, whereas malignant tumors sometimes do. Unlike most benign tumors elsewhere in the body, benign brain tumors can be life threatening.

Cancer Is Preventable

Many cancers are preventable by reducing risk factors such as:

- Use of tobacco products

- Physical inactivity and poor nutrition

- Obesity

- Ultraviolet light exposure

Other cancers can be prevented by getting vaccinated against human papillomavirus (HPV) and hepatitis B virus.

Screening is effective in identifying some types of cancers in early, often highly treatable stages, including:

- Breast cancer (using mammography)

- Cervical cancer (using Pap test alone or combined Pap test and HPV test)

- Colorectal cancer (using fecal occult blood testing, sigmoidoscopy, or colonoscopy)

In the past decade, overweight, and obesity have emerged as new risk factors for developing certain cancers, including colorectal, breast, uterine corpus (endometrial), and kidney cancers. The impact of the current weight trends on cancer incidence will not be fully known for several decades. Continued focus on preventing weight gain will lead to lower rates of cancer and many chronic diseases.

Finding a Doctor

One way to find a doctor who specializes in cancer care is to ask for a referral from your primary care physician. You may know a specialist yourself, or through the experience of a family member, coworker, or friend.

The following resources may also be able to provide you with names of doctors who specialize in treating specific diseases or conditions. However, these resources may not have information about the quality of care that the doctors provide.

- Your local hospital or its patient referral service may be able to provide you with a list of specialists who practice at that hospital.

- Your nearest National Cancer Institute (NCI)-designated cancer center can provide information about doctors who practice at that center. The NCI-Designated Cancer Centers Find a Cancer Center page (www.cancer.gov/research/nci-role/cancer-centers/find) provides contact information to help healthcare providers and cancer patients with referrals to NCI-designated cancer centers located throughout the United States.

- The ABMS has a list of doctors who have met certain education and training requirements and have passed specialty examinations. Is Your Doctor Board Certified (www.certificationmatters. org) lists doctors' names along with their specialty and their educational background. Users must register to use this online self-serve resource, which allows users to conduct searches by a physician's name or area of certification and a state name. The directory is available in most libraries.

- The American Medical Association (AMA) database provides basic information on licensed physicians in the United States. Users can search for physicians by name or by medical specialty.

- The American Society of Clinical Oncology (ASCO) provides an online list of doctors who are members of ASCO. The member database has the names and affiliations of nearly 30,000 oncologists worldwide. It can be searched by doctor's name, institution, location, oncology specialty, and/or type of board certification.

- The American College of Surgeons (ACS) membership database is an online list of surgeons who are members of the ACS. The list can be searched by doctor's name, geographic location, or medical specialty. The ACS can be contacted by telephone at 1-800-621-4111.

- The American Osteopathic Association (AOA) Find a Doctor (doctorsthatdo.org) database provides an online list of practicing osteopathic physicians who are AOA members. The information can be searched by doctor's name, geographic location, or medical specialty. The AOA can be contacted by telephone at 1-800-621-1773.

- Local medical societies may maintain lists of doctors in each specialty.

- Public and medical libraries may have print directories of doctors' names listed geographically by specialty.

- Your local Yellow Pages or Yellow Book may have doctors listed by specialty under "Physicians."

If you are a member of a health insurance plan, your choice may be limited to doctors who participate in your plan. Your insurance company can provide you with a list of participating primary care doctors and specialists. It is important to ask whether the doctor you are considering is accepting new patients through your health plan. You also have the option of seeing a doctor outside your health plan and paying the costs yourself. If you have the option to change health insurance plans, you may first wish to consider which doctor or doctors you would like to use, and then choose a plan that includes your chosen physician(s).

If you are using a federal or state health insurance program such as Medicare or Medicaid, you may want to ask whether the doctor you are considering is accepting patients who use these programs.

You will have many factors to consider when choosing a doctor. To make an informed decision, you may wish to speak with several doctors before choosing one. When you meet with each doctor, you might want to consider the following:

- Does the doctor have the education and training to meet my needs?

- Does the doctor use the hospital that I have chosen?

- Does the doctor listen to me and treat me with respect?

- Does the doctor explain things clearly and encourage me to ask questions?

- What are the doctor's office hours?

- Who covers for the doctor when he or she is unavailable? Will that person have access to my medical records?

- How long does it take to get an appointment with the doctor?

If you are choosing a surgeon, you may wish to ask additional questions about the surgeon's background and experience with specific procedures. These questions may include:

- Is the surgeon board certified?

- Has the surgeon been evaluated by a national professional association of surgeons, such as the ACS?

- At which treatment facility or facilities does the surgeon practice?

- How often does the surgeon perform the type of surgery I need?

- How many of these procedures has the surgeon performed? What was the success rate?

It is important for you to feel comfortable with the specialist that you choose because you will be working closely with that person to make decisions about your cancer treatment. Trust your own observations and feelings when deciding on a doctor for your medical care.

Choosing Trained and Certified Doctors

When choosing a doctor for your cancer care, you may find it helpful to know some of the terms used to describe a doctor's training and credentials. Most physicians who treat people with cancer are medical doctors (they have an M.D. degree) or osteopathic doctors (they have a D.O. degree). The basic training for both types of physicians includes 4 years of premedical education at a college or university, 4 years of medical school to earn an M.D. or D.O. degree, and postgraduate medical education through internships and residences. This training usually lasts 3 to 7 years. Physicians must pass an exam to become licensed (legally permitted) to practice medicine in their state. Each state or territory has its own procedures and general standards for licensing physicians.

Specialists are physicians who have completed their residency training in a specific area, such as internal medicine. Independent specialty boards certify physicians after they have fulfilled certain requirements. These requirements include meeting specific education and training criteria, being licensed to practice medicine, and passing an examination given by the specialty board. Doctors who have met all of the requirements are given the status of "Diplomate" and are board certified as specialists. Doctors who are board eligible have obtained the required education and training but have not completed the specialty board examination.

After being trained and certified as a specialist, a physician may choose to become a subspecialist. A subspecialist has at least 1 additional year of full-time education in a particular area of a specialty. This training is designed to increase the physician's expertise in a specific field. Specialists can be board certified in their subspecialty as well.

The following are some specialties and subspecialties that pertain to cancer treatment:

- **Medical Oncology** is a subspecialty of internal medicine. Doctors who specialize in internal medicine treat a wide range of medical problems. Medical oncologists treat cancer and manage the patient's course of treatment. A medical oncologist may also consult with other physicians about the patient's care or refer the patient to other specialists.

- **Hematology** is a subspecialty of internal medicine. Hematologists focus on diseases of the blood and related tissues, including the bone marrow, spleen, and lymph nodes.

- **Radiation Oncology** is a subspecialty of radiology. Radiology is the use of X-rays and other forms of radiation to diagnose and treat disease. Radiation oncologists specialize in the use of radiation to treat cancer.

- **Surgery** is a specialty that pertains to the treatment of disease by surgical operation. General surgeons perform operations on almost any area of the body. Physicians can also choose to specialize in a certain type of surgery; for example, thoracic surgeons are specialists who perform operations specifically in the chest area, including the lungs and the esophagus.

The American Board of Medical Specialties (ABMS) is a not-for-profit organization that assists medical specialty boards with the development and use of standards for evaluation and certification of physicians. Information about other specialties that treat cancer is available from the ABMS website (www.abms.org).

Almost all board-certified specialists are members of their medical specialty society. Physicians can attain Fellowship status in a specialty society, such as the American College of Surgeons (ACS), if they demonstrate outstanding achievement in their profession. Criteria for Fellowship status may include the number of years of membership in the specialty society, years practicing in the specialty, and professional recognition by peers.

How Can I Find Treatment Facilities?

Choosing a treatment facility is another important consideration for getting the best medical care possible. Although you may not be able to choose which hospital treats you in an emergency, you can choose a facility for scheduled and ongoing care. If you have already found a doctor for your cancer treatment, you may need to choose a facility based on where your doctor practices. Your doctor may be able to recommend a facility that provides quality care to meet your needs. You may wish to ask the following questions when considering a treatment facility:

- Has the facility had experience and success in treating my condition?

- Has the facility been rated by state, consumer, or other groups for its quality of care?

- How does the facility check on and work to improve its quality of care?

- Has the facility been approved by a nationally recognized accrediting body, such as the ACS Commission on Cancer and/or The Joint Commission (www.jointcommission.org)?

- Does the facility explain patients' rights and responsibilities? Are copies of this information available to patients?

- Does the treatment facility offer support services, such as social workers and resources, to help me find financial assistance if I need it?

- Is the facility conveniently located?

If you are a member of a health insurance plan, your choice of treatment facilities may be limited to those that participate in your plan. Your insurance company can provide you with a list of approved facilities. Although the costs of cancer treatment can be very high, you do have the option of paying out-of-pocket if you want to use a treatment facility that is not covered by your insurance plan. If you are considering paying for treatment yourself, you may wish to discuss the possible costs with your doctor beforehand. You may also want to speak with the person who does the billing for the treatment facility. Nurses and social workers may also be able to provide you with more information about coverage, eligibility, and insurance issues.

The following resources may help you find a hospital or treatment facility for your care:

- The NCI-Designated Cancer Centers Find a Cancer Center page (www.cancer.gov/research/nci-role/cancer-centers/find) provides contact information for NCI-designated cancer centers located throughout the country.

- The ACS's Commission on Cancer (CoC) accredits cancer programs at hospitals and other treatment facilities. More than 1,430 programs in the United States have been designated by the CoC as Approved Cancer Programs. The ACS website offers a searchable database of these programs. The CoC can be contacted by telephone at 312-202-5085 or by e-mail at CoC@facs. org.

- The Joint Commission is an independent not-for-profit organization that evaluates and accredits healthcare organizations and programs in the United States. It also offers information for the general public about choosing a treatment facility. The Joint Commission can be contacted by telephone at 630-792-5000.

The Joint Commission offers an online quality check service (www. qualitycheck.org) that patients can use to determine whether a specific facility has been accredited by the Joint Commission and to view the organization's performance reports.

Questions to Ask Your Doctor

Learning that you have cancer can be a shock and you may feel overwhelmed at first. When you meet with your doctor, you will hear a lot of information. These questions may help you learn more about your cancer and what you can expect next.

- What type of cancer do I have?

- What is the stage of my cancer?

- Has it spread to other areas of my body?

- Will I need more tests before treatment begins? Which ones?

- Will I need a specialist(s) for my cancer treatment?

- Will you help me find a doctor to give me another opinion on the best treatment plan for me?

- How serious is my cancer?

- What are my chances of survival?

Chapter 2

Getting a Second Opinion

After your doctor gives you advice about the diagnosis and treatment plan, you may want to get another doctor's opinion before you begin treatment. This is known as getting a second opinion. You can do this by asking another specialist to review all of the materials related to your case. The doctor who gives the second opinion can confirm or suggest modifications to your doctor's proposed treatment plan, provide reassurance that you have explored all of your options, and answer any questions you may have.

Getting a second opinion is done frequently, and most physicians welcome another doctor's views. In fact, your doctor may be able to recommend a specialist for this consultation. However, some people find it uncomfortable to request a second opinion. When discussing this issue with your doctor, it may be helpful to express satisfaction with your doctor's decision and care and to mention that you want your decision about treatment to be as thoroughly informed as possible. You may also wish to bring a family member along for support when asking for a second opinion. It is best to involve your doctor in the process of getting a second opinion, because your doctor will need to make your medical records (such as your test results and X-rays) available to the specialist who is giving the second opinion.

Some healthcare plans require a second opinion, particularly if a doctor recommends surgery. Other healthcare plans will pay for a second opinion if the patient requests it. If your plan does not cover

This chapter includes text excerpted from "How to Find a Doctor or Treatment Facility If You Have Cancer," National Cancer Institute (NCI), June 5, 2013. Reviewed February 2017.

a second opinion, you can still obtain one if you are willing to cover the cost.

If your doctor is unable to recommend a specialist for a second opinion, or if you prefer to choose one on your own, the following resources can help:

- Many of the resources listed above for finding a doctor can also help you find a specialist for a consultation.

- The National Institutes of Health (NIH) Clinical Center in Bethesda, Maryland, is the research hospital for the NIH, including National Cancer Institute (NCI). Several branches of the NCI provide second opinion services.

- The R. A. Bloch Cancer Foundation, Inc., can refer cancer patients to institutions that are willing to provide multidisciplinary second opinions. A list of these institutions is available on the organization's website (blochcancer.org/resources/multi-disciplinary-second-opinion-centers). You can also contact the R. A. Bloch Cancer Foundation, Inc., by telephone at 816–854–5050 or 1–800–433–0464.

How Can People Who Live Outside the United States Get a Second Opinion in the United States?

Some people living outside the United States may wish to obtain a second opinion or have their cancer treatment in this country. Many facilities in the United States offer these services to international cancer patients. These facilities may also provide support services, such as language interpretation, assistance with travel, and guidance in finding accommodations near the treatment facility for patients and their families.

If you live outside the United States and would like to obtain cancer treatment in this country, you should contact cancer treatment facilities directly to find out whether they have an international patient office.

The NCI-Designated Cancer Centers *Find a Cancer Center* page (www.cancer.gov/research/nci-role/cancer-centers/find) offers contact information for NCI-designated cancer centers throughout the United States.

Citizens of other countries who are planning to travel to the United States for cancer treatment generally must first obtain a nonimmigrant visa for medical treatment from the U.S. Embassy or Consulate in their home country. Visa applicants must demonstrate that the purpose of their trip is to enter the United States for medical treatment; that they plan to remain for a specific, limited period; that they have funds to cover expenses in the United States; that they have a residence and social and economic ties outside the United States; and that they intend to return to their home country.

To determine the specific fees and documentation required for the nonimmigrant visa and to learn more about the application process, contact the U.S. Embassy or Consulate in your home country. A list of links to the websites of U.S. Embassies and Consulates worldwide can be found on the U.S. Department of State's website (www.usembassy.gov).

Chapter 3

Cancer Screening

What Is Cancer Screening?

Screening tests can help find cancer at an early stage, before symptoms appear. When abnormal tissue or cancer is found early, it may be easier to treat or cure. By the time symptoms appear, the cancer may have grown and spread. This can make the cancer harder to treat or cure. It is important to remember that when your doctor suggests a screening test, it does not always mean he or she thinks you have cancer. Screening tests are done when you have no cancer symptoms.

Kinds of Screening Tests

Screening tests include the following:

- **Physical exam and history**. An exam of the body to check general signs of health, including checking for signs of disease, such as lumps or anything else that seems unusual. A history of the patient's health habits and past illnesses and treatments will also be taken.

- **Laboratory tests**. Medical procedures that test samples of tissue, blood, urine, or other substances in the body.

- **Imaging procedures**. Procedures that make pictures of areas inside the body.

This chapter includes text excerpted from "Cancer Screening Overview (PDQ®)–Patient Version," National Cancer Institute (NCI), April 6, 2016.

- **Genetic tests**. Tests that look for certain gene mutations (changes) that are linked to some types of cancer.

Screening Tests Have Risks

Not all screening tests are helpful and most have risks. It is important to know the risks of the test and whether it has been proven to decrease the chance of dying from cancer.

- **Some screening tests can cause serious problems.** Some screening procedures can cause bleeding or other problems. For example, colon cancer screening with sigmoidoscopy or colonoscopy can cause tears in the lining of the colon.

- **False-positive test results are possible.** Screening test results may appear to be abnormal even though there is no cancer. A false-positive test result (one that shows there is cancer when there really isn't) can cause anxiety and is usually followed by more tests and procedures, which also have risks.

- **False-negative test results are possible.** Screening test results may appear to be normal even though there is cancer. A person who receives a false-negative test result (one that shows there is no cancer when there really is) may delay seeking medical care even if there are symptoms.

- **Finding the cancer may not improve the person's health or help the person live longer.** Some cancers never cause symptoms or become life-threatening, but if found by a screening test, the cancer may be treated. There is no way to know if treating the cancer would help the person live longer than if no treatment were given. In both teenagers and adults, there is an increased risk of suicide in the first year after being diagnosed with cancer. Also, treatments for cancer have side effects.

For some cancers, finding and treating the cancer early does not improve the chance of a cure or help the person live longer.

What Are the Goals of Screening Tests?

Screening tests have many goals. A screening test that works the way it should and is helpful does the following:

- Finds cancer before symptoms appear.

- Screens for cancer that is easier to treat and cure when found early.

- Has few false-negative test results and false-positive test results.

- Decreases the chance of dying from cancer.

Screening tests are not meant to diagnose cancer. Screening tests usually do not diagnose cancer. If a screening test result is abnormal, more tests may be done to check for cancer. For example, a screening mammogram may find a lump in the breast. A lump may be cancer or something else. More tests need to be done to find out if the lump is cancer. These are called diagnostic tests. Diagnostic tests may include a biopsy, in which cells or tissues are removed so a pathologist can check them under a microscope for signs of cancer.

Who Needs to Be Screened?

Certain screening tests may be suggested only for people who have a high risk for certain cancers. Anything that increases the chance of cancer is called a cancer risk factor. Having a risk factor does not mean that you will get cancer; not having risk factors doesn't mean that you will not get cancer.

Some screening tests are used only for people who have known risk factors for certain types of cancer. People known to have a higher risk of cancer than others include those who:

- Have had cancer in the past; or

- Have two or more first-degree relatives (a parent, brother, or sister) who have had cancer; or

- Have certain gene mutations (changes) that have been linked to cancer.

People who have a high risk of cancer may need to be screened more often or at an earlier age than other people. Cancer screening research includes finding out who has an increased risk of cancer. Scientists are trying to better understand who is likely to get certain types of cancer. They study the things we do and the things around us to see if they cause cancer. This information helps doctors figure out who should be screened for cancer, which screening tests should be used, and how often the tests should be done.

How Is Cancer Risk Measured?

Cancer risk is measured in different ways. The findings from surveys and studies about cancer risk are studied and the results are explained in different ways. Some of the ways risk is explained include absolute risk, relative risk, and odds ratios.

- **Absolute risk**. This is the risk a person has of developing a disease, in a given population (for example, the entire U.S. population) over a certain period of time. Researchers estimate the absolute risk by studying a large number of people that are part of a certain population (for example, women in a given age group). Researchers count the number of people in the group who get a certain disease over a certain period of time. For example, a group of 100,000 women between the ages of 20 and 29 are observed for one year, and 4 of them get breast cancer during that time. This means that the one-year absolute risk of breast cancer for a woman in this age group is 4 in 100,000, or 4 chances in 100,000.

- **Relative risk**. This is often used in research studies to find out whether a trait or a factor can be linked to the risk of a disease. Researchers compare two groups of people who are a lot alike. However, the people in one of the groups must have the trait or factor being studied (they have been "exposed"). The people in the other group do not have it (they have not been exposed). To figure out relative risk, the percentage of people in the exposed group who have the disease is divided by the percentage of people in the unexposed group who have the disease.

Relative risks can be:

- Larger than 1: The trait or factor is linked to an increase in risk.

- Equal to 1: The trait or factor is not linked to risk.

- Less than 1: The trait or factor is linked to a decrease in risk. Relative risks are also called risk ratios.

- **Odds ratio.** In some types of studies, researchers don't have enough information to figure out relative risks. They use something called an odds ratio instead. An odds ratio can be an estimate of relative risk.

One type of study that uses an odds ratio instead of relative risk is called a case-control study. In a case-control study, two groups of people are compared. However, the individuals in each group are chosen based on whether or not they have a certain disease. Researchers look at the odds that the people in each group were exposed to something (a trait or factor) that might have caused the disease. Odds describes the number of times the trait or factor was present or happened, divided by the number of times it wasn't present or didn't happen. To get an odds ratio, the odds for one group are divided by the odds for the other group.

Odds ratios can be:

- Larger than 1: The trait or factor is linked to an increase in risk.

- Equal to 1: The trait or factor is not linked to risk.

- Less than 1: The trait or factor is linked to a decrease in risk.

Looking at traits and exposures in people with and without cancer can help find possible risk factors. Knowing who is at an increased risk for certain types of cancer can help doctors decide when and how often they should be screened.

Does Screening Help People Live Longer?

Finding some cancers at an early stage (before symptoms appear) may help decrease the chance of dying from those cancers. For many cancers, the chance of recovery depends on the stage (the amount or spread of cancer in the body) of the cancer when it was diagnosed. Cancers that are diagnosed at earlier stages are often easier to treat or cure.

Studies of cancer screening compare the death rate of people screened for a certain cancer with the death rate from that cancer in people who were not screened. Some screening tests have been shown to be helpful both in finding cancers early and in decreasing the chance of dying from those cancers. These include mammograms for breast cancer and sigmoidoscopy and fecal occult blood testing for colorectal cancer. Other tests are used because they have been shown to find a certain type of cancer in some people before symptoms appear, but they have not been proven to decrease the risk of dying from that cancer. If a cancer is fast-growing and spreads quickly, finding it early may not help the person survive the cancer.

Screening studies are done to see whether deaths from cancer decrease when people are screened. When collecting information on how long cancer patients live, some studies define survival as living five years after the diagnosis. This is often used to measure how well cancer treatments work. However, to see if screening tests are useful, studies usually look at whether deaths from the cancer decrease in people who were screened. Over time, signs that a cancer screening test is working include:

- An increase in the number of early-stage cancers found.
- A decrease in the number of late-stage cancers found.
- A decrease in the number of deaths from cancer.

The number of deaths from cancer is lower today than it was in the past. It is not always clear if this is because screening tests found the cancers earlier or because cancer treatments have gotten better, or both. The Surveillance, Epidemiology, and End Results (SEER) Program of the National Cancer Institute (NCI) collects and reports information on survival times of people with cancer in the United States. This information is studied to see if finding cancer early affects how long these people live.

Certain factors may cause survival times to look like they are getting better when they are not. These factors include lead-time bias and overdiagnosis.

- **Lead-time bias.** Survival time for cancer patients is usually measured from the day the cancer is diagnosed until the day they die. Patients are often diagnosed after they have signs and symptoms of cancer. If a screening test leads to a diagnosis before a patient has any symptoms, the patient's survival time is increased because the date of diagnosis is earlier. This increase in survival time makes it seem as though screened patients are living longer when that may not be happening. This is called lead-time bias. It could be that the only reason the survival time appears to be longer is that the date of diagnosis is earlier for the screened patients. But the screened patients may die at the same time they would have without the screening test.

- **Overdiagnosis.** Sometimes, screening tests find cancers that don't matter because they would have gone away on their own or never caused any symptoms. These cancers would never have been found if not for the screening test. Finding these cancers is called overdiagnosis. Overdiagnosis can make it seem like more people are surviving cancer longer, but in reality, these are people who would not have died from cancer anyway.

Chapter 4

Tests Used to Diagnose and Monitor Cancer

Chapter Contents

Section 4.1

Lab Tests and Other Procedures Used to Diagnose and Monitor Cancer

This section includes text excerpted from "Diagnosis and Staging,"
National Cancer Institute (NCI), March 9, 2015.

If you have a symptom or your screening test result suggests cancer, the doctor must find out whether it is due to cancer or some other cause. The doctor may ask about your personal and family medical history and do a physical exam. The doctor also may order lab tests, scans, or other tests or procedures.

Lab Tests

High or low levels of certain substances in your body can be a sign of cancer. So, lab tests of the blood, urine, or other body fluids that measure these substances can help doctors make a diagnosis. However, abnormal lab results are not a sure sign of cancer. Lab tests are an important tool, but doctors cannot rely on them alone to diagnose cancer.

*Types of Lab Tests**

The following are some of the tests that are used for cancer diagnosis and monitoring:

Blood Chemistry Test

What it measures: The amounts of certain substances that are released into the blood by the organs and tissues of the body, such as metabolites, electrolytes, fats, and proteins, including enzymes. Blood chemistry tests usually include tests for blood urea nitrogen (BUN) and creatinine.

How it is used: Diagnosis and monitoring of patients during and after treatment. High or low levels of some substances can be signs of disease or side effects of treatment.

Cancer Gene Mutation Testing

What it measures: The presence or absence of specific inherited mutations in genes that are known to play a role in cancer development. Examples include tests to look for *BRCA1* and *BRCA2* gene mutations, which play a role in development of breast, ovarian, and other cancers.

How it is used: Assessment of cancer risk.

Complete Blood Count (CBC)

What it measures: Numbers of the different types of blood cells, including red blood cells, white blood cells, and platelets, in a sample of blood. This test also measures the amount of hemoglobin (the protein that carries oxygen) in the blood, the percentage of the total blood volume that is taken up by red blood cells (hematocrit), the size of the red blood cells, and the amount of hemoglobin in red blood cells.

How it is used: Diagnosis, particularly in leukemias, and monitoring during and after treatment.

Cytogenetic Analysis

What it measures: Changes in the number and/or structure of chromosomes in a patient's white blood cells or bone marrow cells.

How it is used: Diagnosis, deciding on appropriate treatment.

Immunophenotyping

What it measures: Identifies cells based on the types of antigens present on the cell surface.

How it is used: Diagnosis, staging, and monitoring of cancers of the blood system and other hematologic disorders, including leukemias, lymphomas, myelodysplastic syndromes, and myeloproliferative disorders. It is most often done on blood or bone marrow samples, but it may also be done on other bodily fluids or biopsy tissue samples.

Sputum Cytology (Also Called Sputum Culture)

What it measures: The presence of abnormal cells in sputum (mucus and other matter brought up from the lungs by coughing).

How it is used: Diagnosis of lung cancer.

Urinalysis

What it measures: The color of urine and its contents, such as sugar, protein, red blood cells, and white blood cells.

How it is used: Detection and diagnosis of kidney cancer and urothelial cancers.

Urine Cytology

What it measures: The presence of abnormal cells shed from the urinary tract into urine to detect disease.

How it is used: Detection and diagnosis of bladder cancer and other urothelial cancers, monitoring patients for cancer recurrence.

*Text excerpted from "Understanding Laboratory Tests," National Cancer Institute (NCI), December 11, 2013.

Imaging Procedures

Imaging procedures create pictures of areas inside your body that help the doctor see whether a tumor is present. These pictures can be made in several ways:

- **Computerized tomography (CT) Scan:** An X-ray machine linked to a computer takes a series of detailed pictures of your organs. You may receive a dye or other contrast material to highlight areas inside the body. Contrast material helps make these pictures easier to read.

- **Nuclear scan:** For this scan, you receive an injection of a small amount of radioactive material, which is sometimes called a tracer. It flows through your bloodstream and collects in certain bones or organs. A machine called a scanner detects and measures the radioactivity. The scanner creates pictures of bones or organs on a computer screen or on film. Your body gets rid of the radioactive substance quickly. This type of scan may also be called radionuclide scan.

- **Ultrasound:** An ultrasound device sends out sound waves that people cannot hear. The waves bounce off tissues inside your body like an echo. A computer uses these echoes to create a picture of areas inside your body. This picture is called a sonogram.

- **Magnetic resonance imaging (MRI):** A strong magnet linked to a computer is used to make detailed pictures of areas in your body. Your doctor can view these pictures on a monitor and print them on film.

- **Positron emission tomography (PET) scan:** For this scan, you receive an injection of a tracer. Then, a machine makes 3-D pictures that show where the tracer collects in the body. These scans show how organs and tissues are working.

- **X-rays:** X-rays use low doses of radiation to create pictures of the inside of your body.

Biopsy

In most cases, doctors need to do a biopsy to make a diagnosis of cancer. A biopsy is a procedure in which the doctor removes a sample of tissue. A pathologist then looks at the tissue under a microscope to see if it is cancer. The sample may be removed in several ways:

- **With a needle:** The doctor uses a needle to withdraw tissue or fluid.

- **With an endoscope:** The doctor looks at areas inside the body using a thin, lighted tube called an endoscope. The scope is inserted through a natural opening, such as the mouth. Then, the doctor uses a special tool to remove tissue or cells through the tube.

- **With surgery:** Surgery may be excisional or incisional.

  - In an excisional biopsy, the surgeon removes the entire tumor. Often some of the normal tissue around the tumor also is removed.

  - In an incisional biopsy, the surgeon removes just part of the tumor.

Section 4.2

Tumor Marker

This section includes text excerpted from
"Tumor Marker," National Cancer
Institute (NCI), November 4, 2015.

What Are Tumor Markers?

Tumor markers are substances that are produced by cancer or by other cells of the body in response to cancer or certain benign (noncancerous) conditions. Most tumor markers are made by normal cells as well as by cancer cells; however, they are produced at much higher levels in cancerous conditions. These substances can be found in the blood, urine, stool, tumor tissue, or other tissues or bodily fluids of some patients with cancer. Most tumor markers are proteins. However, more recently, patterns of gene expression and changes to DNA have also begun to be used as tumor markers.

Many different tumor markers have been characterized and are in clinical use. Some are associated with only one type of cancer, whereas others are associated with two or more cancer types. No "universal" tumor marker that can detect any type of cancer has been found.

There are some limitations to the use of tumor markers. Sometimes, noncancerous conditions can cause the levels of certain tumor markers to increase. In addition, not everyone with a particular type of cancer will have a higher level of a tumor marker associated with that cancer. Moreover, tumor markers have not been identified for every type of cancer.

How Are Tumor Markers Used in Cancer Care?

Tumor markers are used to help detect, diagnose, and manage some types of cancer. Although an elevated level of a tumor marker may suggest the presence of cancer, this alone is not enough to diagnose cancer. Therefore, measurements of tumor markers are usually combined with other tests, such as biopsies, to diagnose cancer.

Tumor marker levels may be measured before treatment to help doctors plan the appropriate therapy. In some types of cancer, the level of a tumor marker reflects the stage (extent) of the disease and/or the patient's prognosis (likely outcome or course of disease).

Tumor markers may also be measured periodically during cancer therapy. A decrease in the level of a tumor marker or a return to the marker's normal level may indicate that the cancer is responding to treatment, whereas no change or an increase may indicate that the cancer is not responding.

Tumor markers may also be measured after treatment has ended to check for recurrence (the return of cancer).

How Are Tumor Markers Measured?

A doctor takes a sample of tumor tissue or bodily fluid and sends it to a laboratory, where various methods are used to measure the level of the tumor marker.

If the tumor marker is being used to determine whether treatment is working or whether there is a recurrence, the marker's level will be measured in multiple samples taken over time. Usually these "serial measurements," which show whether the level of a marker is increasing, staying the same, or decreasing, are more meaningful than a single measurement.

Does National Cancer Institute (NCI) Have Guidelines for the Use of Tumor Markers?

National Cancer Institute (NCI) does not have such guidelines. However, some national and international organizations do have guidelines for the use of tumor markers for some types of cancer:

- The American Society of Clinical Oncology (ASCO) has published clinical practice guidelines on a variety of topics, including tumor markers for breast cancer, colorectal cancer, lung cancer, and others.

- The National Academy of Clinical Biochemistry (NACB) publishes laboratory medicine practice guidelines, including *Use of Tumor Markers in Clinical Practice: Quality Requirements,* which focuses on the appropriate use of tumor markers for specific cancers.

What Tumor Markers Are Currently Being Used, and for Which Cancer Types?

A number of tumor markers are currently being used for a wide range of cancer types. Although most of these can be tested in laboratories that meet standards set by the Clinical Laboratory Improvement Amendments, some cannot be and may therefore be considered experimental. Tumor markers that are currently in common use are listed below.

Table 4.1. Tumor Markers for Cancer

Tumor Marker	Cancer Type	Tissue Analyzed	How Used
ALK gene rearrangements and overexpression	Non-small cell lung cancer and anaplastic large cell lymphoma	Tumor	To help determine treatment and prognosis
Alpha-fetoprotein (AFP)	Liver cancer and germ cell tumors	Blood	To help diagnose liver cancer and follow response to treatment; to assess stage, prognosis, and response to treatment of germ cell tumors
Beta-2-microglobulin (B2M)	Multiple myeloma, chronic lymphocytic leukemia, and some lymphomas	Blood, urine, or cerebrospinal fluid	To determine prognosis and follow response to treatment
Beta-human chorionic gonadotropin (Beta-hCG)	Choriocarcinoma and germ cell tumors	Urine or blood	To assess stage, prognosis, and response to treatment
BRCA1 and *BRCA2* gene mutations	Ovarian cancer	Blood	To determine whether treatment with a particular type of targeted therapy is appropriate

Table 4.1. Continued

Tumor Marker	Cancer Type	Tissue Analyzed	How Used
BCR-ABL fusion gene (Philadelphia chromosome)	Chronic myeloid leukemia, acute lymphoblastic leukemia, and acute myelogenous leukemia	Blood and/or bone marrow	To confirm diagnosis, predict response to targeted therapy, and monitor disease status
BRAF V600 mutations	Cutaneous melanoma and colorectal cancer	Tumor	To select patients who are most likely to benefit from treatment with certain targeted therapies
C-kit/CD117	Gastrointestinal stromal tumor and mucosal melanoma	Tumor	To help in diagnosing and determining treatment
CA15-3/CA27.29	Breast cancer	Blood	To assess whether treatment is working or disease has recurred
CA19-9	Pancreatic cancer, gallbladder cancer, bile duct cancer, and gastric cancer	Blood	To assess whether treatment is working
CA-125	Ovarian cancer	Blood	To help in diagnosis, assessment of response to treatment, and evaluation of recurrence
Calcitonin	Medullary thyroid cancer	Blood	To aid in diagnosis, check whether treatment is working, and assess recurrence

Table 4.1. Continued

Tumor Marker	Cancer Type	Tissue Analyzed	How Used
Carcinoembryonic antigen (CEA)	Colorectal cancer and some other cancers	Blood	To keep track of how well cancer treatments are working or check if cancer has come back
CD20	Non-Hodgkin lymphoma	Blood	To determine whether treatment with a targeted therapy is appropriate
Chromogranin A (CgA)	Neuroendocrine tumors	Blood	To help in diagnosis, assessment of treatment response, and evaluation of recurrence
Chromosomes 3, 7, 17, and 9p21	Bladder cancer	Urine	To help in monitoring for tumor recurrence
Circulating tumor cells of epithelial origin (CELLSEARCH®)	Metastatic breast, prostate, and colorectal cancers	Blood	To inform clinical decision making, and to assess prognosis
Cytokeratin fragment 21-1	Lung cancer	Blood	To help in monitoring for recurrence
EGFR gene mutation analysis	Non-small cell lung cancer	Tumor	To help determine treatment and prognosis
Estrogen receptor (ER)/progesterone receptor (PR)	Breast cancer	Tumor	To determine whether treatment with hormone therapy and some targeted therapies is appropriate
Fibrin/fibrinogen	Bladder cancer	Urine	To monitor progression and response to treatment

Table 4.1. Continued

Tumor Marker	Cancer Type	Tissue Analyzed	How Used
HE4	Ovarian cancer	Blood	To plan cancer treatment, assess disease progression, and monitor for recurrence
HER2/neu gene amplification or protein overexpression	Breast cancer, gastric cancer, and gastroesophageal junction adenocarcinoma	Tumor	To determine whether treatment with certain targeted therapies is appropriate
Immunoglobulins	Multiple myeloma and Waldenström macroglobulinemia	Blood and urine	To help diagnose disease, assess response to treatment, and look for recurrence
KRAS gene mutation analysis	Colorectal cancer and non-small cell lung cancer	Tumor	To determine whether treatment with a particular type of targeted therapy is appropriate
Lactate dehydrogenase	Germ cell tumors, lymphoma, leukemia, melanoma, and neuroblastoma	Blood	To assess stage, prognosis, and response to treatment
Neuron-specific enolase (NSE)	Small cell lung cancer and neuroblastoma	Blood	To help in diagnosis and to assess response to treatment
Nuclear matrix protein 22	Bladder cancer	Urine	To monitor response to treatment
Programmed death ligand 1 (PD-L1)	Non-small cell lung cancer	Tumor	To determine whether treatment with a particular type of targeted therapy is appropriate

Table 4.1. Continued

Tumor Marker	Cancer Type	Tissue Analyzed	How Used
Prostate-specific antigen (PSA)	Prostate cancer	Blood	To help in diagnosis, assess response to treatment, and look for recurrence
Thyroglobulin	Thyroid cancer	Blood	To evaluate response to treatment and look for recurrence
Urokinase plasminogen activator (uPA) and plasminogen activator inhibitor (PAI-1)	Breast cancer	Tumor	To determine aggressiveness of cancer and guide treatment
5-Protein signature (OVA1®)	Ovarian cancer	Blood	To pre-operatively assess pelvic mass for suspected ovarian cancer
21-Gene signature (Oncotype DX®)	Breast cancer	Tumor	To evaluate risk of recurrence
70-Gene signature (Mammaprint®)	Breast cancer	Tumor	To evaluate risk of recurrence

Can Tumor Markers Be Used in Cancer Screening?

Because tumor markers can be used to assess the response of a tumor to treatment and for prognosis, researchers have hoped that they might also be useful in screening tests that aim to detect cancer early, before there are any symptoms. For a screening test to be useful, it should have very high sensitivity (ability to correctly identify people who have the disease) and specificity (ability to correctly identify people who do not have the disease). If a test is highly sensitive, it will identify most people with the disease—that is, it will result in very few false-negative results. If a test is highly specific, only a small number of people will test positive for the disease who do not have it—in other words, it will result in very few false-positive results.

Although tumor markers are extremely useful in determining whether a tumor is responding to treatment or assessing whether it has recurred, no tumor marker identified to date is sufficiently sensitive or specific to be used on its own to screen for cancer.

For example, the prostate-specific antigen (PSA) test, which measures the level of PSA in the blood, is often used to screen men for prostate cancer. However, an increased PSA level can be caused by benign prostate conditions as well as by prostate cancer, and most men with an elevated PSA level do not have prostate cancer. Initial results from two large randomized controlled trials, the NCI-sponsored Prostate, Lung, Colorectal, and Ovarian Cancer Screening Trial (PLCO), and the European Randomized Study of Screening for Prostate Cancer showed that PSA testing at best leads to only a small reduction in the number of prostate cancer deaths. Moreover, it is not clear whether the benefits of PSA screening outweigh the harms of follow-up diagnostic tests and treatments for cancers that in many cases would never have threatened a man's life.

Similarly, results from the PLCO trial showed that CA-125, a tumor marker that is sometimes elevated in the blood of women with ovarian cancer but can also be elevated in women with benign conditions, is not sufficiently sensitive or specific to be used together with transvaginal ultrasound to screen for ovarian cancer in women at average risk of the disease. An analysis of 28 potential markers for ovarian cancer in blood from women who later went on to develop ovarian cancer found that none of these markers performed even as well as CA-125 at detecting the disease in women at average risk.

Chapter 5

Understanding Your Cancer Diagnosis

Chapter Contents

Section 5.1

Tumor Grades and Stages

This section contains text excerpted from the following sources:
Text under the heading "Tumor Grade: Questions and Answers"
is excerpted from "Tumor," National Cancer Institute (NCI),
May 3, 2013. Reviewed February 2017; Text under the heading
"Staging: Questions and Answers" is excerpted from "Staging,"
National Cancer Institute (NCI), March 9, 2015.

Tumor Grade: Questions and Answers

What Is Tumor Grade?

Tumor grade is the description of a tumor based on how abnormal
the tumor cells and the tumor tissue look under a microscope. It is an
indicator of how quickly a tumor is likely to grow and spread. If the
cells of the tumor and the organization of the tumor's tissue are close
to those of normal cells and tissue, the tumor is called "well-differen-
tiated." These tumors tend to grow and spread at a slower rate than
tumors that are "undifferentiated" or "poorly differentiated," which
have abnormal-looking cells and may lack normal tissue structures.
Based on these and other differences in microscopic appearance, doctors assign a numerical "grade" to most cancers. The factors used to
determine tumor grade can vary between different types of cancer.

Tumor grade is not the same as the stage of a cancer. Cancer stage
refers to the size and/or extent (reach) of the original (primary) tumor
and whether or not cancer cells have spread in the body. Cancer stage
is based on factors such as the location of the primary tumor, tumor
size, regional lymph node involvement (the spread of cancer to nearby
lymph nodes), and the number of tumors present.

How Is Tumor Grade Determined?

If a tumor is suspected to be malignant, a doctor removes all or part
of it during a procedure called a biopsy. A pathologist (a doctor who
identifies diseases by studying cells and tissues under a microscope)
then examines the biopsied tissue to determine whether the tumor

is benign or malignant. The pathologist also determines the tumor's grade and identifies other characteristics of the tumor.

How Are Tumor Grades Classified?

Grading systems differ depending on the type of cancer. In general, tumors are graded as 1, 2, 3, or 4, depending on the amount of abnormality. In Grade 1 tumors, the tumor cells and the organization of the tumor tissue appear close to normal. These tumors tend to grow and spread slowly. In contrast, the cells and tissue of Grade 3 and Grade 4 tumors do not look like normal cells and tissue. Grade 3 and Grade 4 tumors tend to grow rapidly and spread faster than tumors with a lower grade.

If a grading system for a tumor type is not specified, the following system is generally used:

- GX: Grade cannot be assessed (undetermined grade)

- G1: Well differentiated (low grade)

- G2: Moderately differentiated (intermediate grade)

- G3: Poorly differentiated (high grade)

- G4: Undifferentiated (high grade)

What Are Some of the Cancer Type-Specific Grading Systems?

Breast and prostate cancers are the most common types of cancer that have their own grading systems.

Breast cancer. Doctors most often use the Nottingham grading system (also called the Elston-Ellis modification of the Scarff-Bloom-Richardson grading system) for breast cancer. This system grades breast tumors based on the following features:

- Tubule formation: how much of the tumor tissue has normal breast (milk) duct structures

- Nuclear grade: an evaluation of the size and shape of the nucleus in the tumor cells

- Mitotic rate: how many dividing cells are present, which is a measure of how fast the tumor cells are growing and dividing

Each of the categories gets a score between 1 and 3; a score of "1" means the cells and tumor tissue look the most like normal cells and tissue, and a score of "3" means the cells and tissue look the most abnormal. The scores for the three categories are then added, yielding a total score of 3 to 9. Three grades are possible:

- Total score = 3–5: G1 (Low grade or well differentiated)

- Total score = 6–7: G2 (Intermediate grade or moderately differentiated)

- Total score = 8–9: G3 (High grade or poorly differentiated)

Prostate cancer. The Gleason scoring system is used to grade prostate cancer. The Gleason score is based on biopsy samples taken from the prostate. The pathologist checks the samples to see how similar the tumor tissue looks to normal prostate tissue. Both a primary and a secondary pattern of tissue organization are identified. The primary pattern represents the most common tissue pattern seen in the tumor, and the secondary pattern represents the next most common pattern. Each pattern is given a grade from 1 to 5, with 1 looking the most like normal prostate tissue and 5 looking the most abnormal. The two grades are then added to give a Gleason score. The American Joint Committee on Cancer (AJCC) recommends grouping Gleason scores into the following categories:

- Gleason X: Gleason score cannot be determined

- Gleason 2–6: The tumor tissue is well differentiated

- Gleason 7: The tumor tissue is moderately differentiated

- Gleason 8–10: The tumor tissue is poorly differentiated or undifferentiated

How Does Tumor Grade Affect a Patient's Treatment Options?

Doctors use tumor grade and other factors, such as cancer stage and a patient's age and general health, to develop a treatment plan and to determine a patient's prognosis (the likely outcome or course of a disease; the chance of recovery or recurrence). Generally, a lower grade indicates a better prognosis. A higher-grade cancer may grow and spread more quickly and may require immediate or more aggressive treatment.

The importance of tumor grade in planning treatment and determining a patient's prognosis is greater for certain types of cancer, such as soft tissue sarcoma, primary brain tumors, and breast and prostate cancer.

Patients should talk with their doctor for more information about tumor grade and how it relates to their treatment and prognosis.

Staging: Questions and Answers

What Is a Stage?

Stage refers to the extent of your cancer, such as how large the tumor is, and if it has spread. Knowing the stage of your cancer helps your doctor:

- Understand how serious your cancer is and your chances of survival
- Plan the best treatment for you
- Identify clinical trials that may be treatment options for you

A cancer is always referred to by the stage it was given at diagnosis, even if it gets worse or spreads. New information about how a cancer has changed over time gets added onto the original stage. So, the stage doesn't change, even though the cancer might.

How Is Stage Determined?

To learn the stage of your disease, your doctor may order X-rays, lab tests, and other tests or procedures.

What Are the Common Elements of Staging Systems?

There are many staging systems. Some, such as the TNM staging system, are used for many types of cancer. Others are specific to a particular type of cancer. Most staging systems include information about:

- Where the tumor is located in the body
- The cell type (such as, adenocarcinoma or squamous cell carcinoma)
- The size of the tumor
- Whether the cancer has spread to nearby lymph nodes
- Whether the cancer has spread to a different part of the body
- Tumor grade, which refers to how abnormal the cancer cells look and how likely the tumor is to grow and spread

41

What Is the TNM Staging System?

The TNM system is the most widely used cancer staging system. Most hospitals and medical centers use the TNM system as their main method for cancer reporting. You are likely to see your cancer described by this staging system in your pathology report, unless you have a cancer for which a different staging system is used. Examples of cancers with different staging systems include brain and spinal cord tumors and blood cancers.

In the TNM system:

- The T refers to the size and extent of the main tumor. The main tumor is usually called the primary tumor.

- The N refers to the number of nearby lymph nodes that have cancer.

- The M refers to whether the cancer has metastasized. This means that the cancer has spread from the primary tumor to other parts of the body.

When your cancer is described by the TNM system, there will be numbers after each letter that give more details about the cancer—for example, T1N0MX or T3N1M0. The following explains what the letters and numbers mean:

Primary tumor (T)

- TX: Main tumor cannot be measured.

- T0: Main tumor cannot be found.

- T1, T2, T3, T4: Refers to the size and/or extent of the main tumor. The higher the number after the T, the larger the tumor or the more it has grown into nearby tissues. T's may be further divided to provide more detail, such as T3a and T3b.

Regional lymph nodes (N)

- NX: Cancer in nearby lymph nodes cannot be measured.

- N0: There is no cancer in nearby lymph nodes.

- N1, N2, N3: Refers to the number and location of lymph nodes that contain cancer. The higher the number after the N, the more lymph nodes that contain cancer.

Distant metastasis (M)

- MX: Metastasis cannot be measured.

- M0: Cancer has not spread to other parts of the body.

- M1: Cancer has spread to other parts of the body.

What Are the Other Ways to Describe Stage?

The TNM system helps describe cancer in great detail. But, for many cancers, the TNM combinations are grouped into five less-detailed stages. When talking about your cancer, your doctor or nurse may describe it as one of these stages:

Table 5.1. Stages and What It Means

Stage	What It Means
Stage 0	Abnormal cells are present but have not spread to nearby tissue. Also called carcinoma in situ, or CIS. CIS is not cancer, but it may become cancer.
Stage I, Stage II, and Stage III	Cancer is present. The higher the number, the larger the cancer tumor and the more it has spread into nearby tissues.
Stage IV	The cancer has spread to distant parts of the body.

Another staging system that is used for all types of cancer groups the cancer into one of five main categories. This staging system is more often used by cancer registries than by doctors. But, you may still hear your doctor or nurse describe your cancer in one of the following ways:

- **In situ**: Abnormal cells are present but have not spread to nearby tissue.

- **Localized**: Cancer is limited to the place where it started, with no sign that it has spread.

- **Regional**: Cancer has spread to nearby lymph nodes, tissues, or organs.

- **Distant**: Cancer has spread to distant parts of the body.

- **Unknown**: There is not enough information to figure out the stage.

Section 5.2

Pathology Reports

This section includes text excerpted from
"Pathology Reports," National Cancer Institute (NCI),
September 23, 2010. Reviewed February 2017.

What Is a Pathology Report?

A pathology report is a document that contains the diagnosis determined by examining cells and tissues under a microscope. The report may also contain information about the size, shape, and appearance of a specimen as it looks to the naked eye. This information is known as the gross description.

A pathologist is a doctor who does this examination and writes the pathology report. Pathology reports play an important role in cancer diagnosis and staging (describing the extent of cancer within the body, especially whether it has spread), which helps determine treatment options.

How Is Tissue Obtained for Examination by the Pathologist?

In most cases, a doctor needs to do a biopsy or surgery to remove cells or tissues for examination under a microscope.

Some common ways a biopsy can be done are as follows:

- A needle is used to withdraw tissue or fluid.

- An endoscope (a thin, lighted tube) is used to look at areas inside the body and remove cells or tissues.

- Surgery is used to remove part of the tumor or the entire tumor. If the entire tumor is removed, typically some normal tissue around the tumor is also removed.

Tissue removed during a biopsy is sent to a pathology laboratory, where it is sliced into thin sections for viewing under a microscope. This is known as histologic (tissue) examination and is usually the best way to tell if cancer is present. The pathologist may also examine cytologic (cell) material. Cytologic material is present in urine, cerebrospinal fluid (the fluid around the brain and spinal cord), sputum (mucus from the lungs), peritoneal (abdominal cavity) fluid, pleural (chest cavity) fluid, cervical/vaginal smears, and in fluid removed during a biopsy.

How Is Tissue Processed after a Biopsy or Surgery? What Is a Frozen Section?

The tissue removed during a biopsy or surgery must be cut into thin sections, placed on slides, and stained with dyes before it can be examined under a microscope. Two methods are used to make the tissue firm enough to cut into thin sections: frozen sections and paraffin-embedded (permanent) sections. All tissue samples are prepared as permanent sections, but sometimes frozen sections are also prepared.

Permanent sections are prepared by placing the tissue in fixative (usually formalin) to preserve the tissue, processing it through additional solutions, and then placing it in paraffin wax. After the wax has hardened, the tissue is cut into very thin slices, which are placed on slides and stained. The process normally takes several days. A permanent section provides the best quality for examination by the pathologist and produces more accurate results than a frozen section.

Frozen sections are prepared by freezing and slicing the tissue sample. They can be done in about 15 to 20 minutes while the patient is in the operating room. Frozen sections are done when an immediate answer is needed; for example, to determine whether the tissue is cancerous so as to guide the surgeon during the course of an operation.

How Long after the Tissue Sample Is Taken Will the Pathology Report Be Ready?

The pathologist sends a pathology report to the doctor within 10 days after the biopsy or surgery is performed. Pathology reports are written in technical medical language. Patients may want to ask their doctors to give them a copy of the pathology report and to explain the report to them. Patients also may wish to keep a copy of their pathology report in their own records.

What Information Does a Pathology Report Usually Include?

The pathology report may include the following information:

- Patient information: Name, birth date, biopsy date.

- Gross description: Color, weight, and size of tissue as seen by the naked eye.

- Microscopic description: How the sample looks under the microscope and how it compares with normal cells.

- Diagnosis: Type of tumor/cancer and grade (how abnormal the cells look under the microscope and how quickly the tumor is likely to grow and spread).

- Tumor size: Measured in centimeters.

- Tumor margins: There are three possible findings when the biopsy sample is the entire tumor:

- Positive margins mean that cancer cells are found at the edge of the material removed.

- Negative, not involved, clear, or free margins mean that no cancer cells are found at the outer edge.

- Close margins are neither negative nor positive.

- Other information: Usually notes about samples that have been sent for other tests or a second opinion.

- Pathologist's signature and name and address of the laboratory.

What Might the Pathology Report Say about the Physical and Chemical Characteristics of the Tissue?

After identifying the tissue as cancerous, the pathologist may perform additional tests to get more information about the tumor that cannot be determined by looking at the tissue with routine stains, such as hematoxylin and eosin (also known as H&E), under a microscope. The pathology report will include the results of these tests. For example, the pathology report may include information obtained from immunochemical stains (IHC). IHC uses antibodies to identify specific antigens on the surface of cancer cells. IHC can often be used to:

- Determine where the cancer started

- Distinguish among different cancer types, such as carcinoma, melanoma, and lymphoma

- Help diagnose and classify leukemias and lymphomas

The pathology report may also include the results of flow cytometry. Flow cytometry is a method of measuring properties of cells in a sample, including the number of cells, percentage of live cells, cell size and shape, and presence of tumor markers on the cell surface. Tumor markers are substances produced by tumor cells or by other cells in the body in response to cancer or certain noncancerous conditions.) Flow cytometry can be used in the diagnosis, classification, and management of cancers such as acute leukemia, chronic lymphoproliferative disorders, and non-Hodgkin lymphoma.

Finally, the pathology report may include the results of molecular diagnostic and cytogenetic studies. Such studies investigate the presence or absence of malignant cells, and genetic or molecular abnormalities in specimens.

What Information about the Genetics of the Cells Might Be Included in the Pathology Report?

Cytogenetics uses tissue culture and specialized techniques to provide genetic information about cells, particularly genetic alterations. Some genetic alterations are markers or indicators of specific cancer. For example, the Philadelphia chromosome is associated with chronic myelogenous leukemia (CML). Some alterations can provide information about prognosis, which helps the doctor make treatment recommendations. Some tests that might be performed on a tissue sample include:

- Fluorescence in situ hybridization (FISH): Determines the positions of particular genes. It can be used to identify chromosomal abnormalities and to map genes.

- Polymerase chain reaction (PCR): A method of making many copies of particular deoxyribonucleic acid (DNA) sequences of relevance to the diagnosis.

- Real-time PCR or quantitative PCR: A method of measuring how many copies of a particular DNA sequence are present.

- Reverse-transcriptase polymerase chain reaction (RT-PCR): A method of making many copies of a specific ribonucleic acid (RNA) sequence.

- Southern blot hybridization: Detects specific DNA fragments.

- Western blot hybridization: Identifies and analyzes proteins or peptides.

Can Individuals Get a Second Opinion about their Pathology Results?

Although most cancers can be easily diagnosed, sometimes patients or their doctors may want to get a second opinion about the pathology results. Patients interested in getting a second opinion should talk with their doctor. They will need to obtain the slides and/or paraffin block from the pathologist who examined the sample or from the hospital where the biopsy or surgery was done.

Many institutions provide second opinions on pathology specimens. National Cancer Institute (NCI)-designated cancer centers or academic institutions are reasonable places to consider. Patients should contact the facility in advance to determine if this service is available, the cost, and shipping instructions.

Part Two

Making Treatment and Cancer Care Decisions

Chapter 6

Learning about Your Cancer and Treatment Choices

Understanding Cancer Treatment Options

The treatment for cancer depends on the type of cancer and the stage of the disease (how severe the cancer is, and whether it has spread). Doctors may also consider the patient's age and general health. Often, the goal of treatment is to cure the cancer. In other cases, the goal is to control the disease or to reduce symptoms for as long as possible. The treatment plan for a person may change over time.

Most treatment plans include surgery, radiation therapy, or chemotherapy. Other plans involve biological therapy or hormonal therapy.

- **Surgery.** An operation where doctors cut out tissue with cancer cells.

- **Chemotherapy.** Using special medicines to shrink or kill cancer cells. The drugs can be pills you take or medicines given in your veins, or sometimes both.

This chapter contains text excerpted from the following sources: Text beginning with the heading "Understanding Cancer Treatment Options" is excerpted from "Cancer Survivorship," Centers for Disease Control and Prevention (CDC), March 7, 2016; Text under the heading "Questions to Ask Your Doctor about Your Treatment" is excerpted from "Questions to Ask Your Doctor about Your Treatment," National Cancer Institute (NCI), February 14, 2012. Reviewed February 2017.

- **Hormonal therapy.** Blocks cancer cells from getting the hormones they need to grow.

- **Biological therapy.** Works with your body's immune system to help it fight cancer cells or to control side effects from other cancer treatments. Side effects are how your body reacts to drugs or other treatments.

- **Radiation therapy.** Using high-energy rays (similar to X-rays) to kill cancer cells.

Some cancers respond best to a single type of treatment. Other cancers may respond best to a combination of treatments.

Doctors may recommend a stem cell transplant, also known as a bone marrow transplant, for patients who get very high doses of chemotherapy or radiation therapy. This is because high-dose therapies destroy both cancer cells and normal blood cells. A stem cell transplant can help the body to make healthy blood cells to replace the ones lost due to the cancer treatment. It's a complicated procedure with many side effects and risks.

Talk to Your Doctor about the Right Treatment for You

Choosing the treatment that is right for you may be hard. Talk to your cancer doctor about the treatment options available for your type and stage of cancer. Your doctor can explain the risks and benefits of each treatment and their side effects.

Sometimes people get an opinion from more than one cancer doctor. This is called a "second opinion." Getting a second opinion may help you choose the treatment that is right for you.

Clinical Trials

Cancer survivors might also talk to their doctor about clinical trials. Clinical trials are health-related studies that research medical strategies, treatments, or devices to see if they are safe and effective for people who have cancer or other illnesses. A clinical trial may test:

- A medical product, like a drug or device.

- A medical procedure.

- Instructions on how to change behavior, such as how to change your diet.

Complementary and Alternative Medicine (CAM)

Complementary and alternative medicine (CAM) are medicines and health practices that are not standard cancer treatments. Complementary medicine is used in addition to standard treatments, and alternative medicine is used instead of standard treatments. Meditation, yoga, and supplements like vitamins and herbs are some examples. Many kinds of complementary and alternative medicine have not been tested scientifically, so information is not available about their safety and effectiveness. Talk to your doctor about the risks and benefits before you start any kind of complementary or alternative medicine.

Questions to Ask Your Doctor about Your Treatment

You may want to ask your doctor some of the following questions before you decide on your cancer treatment.

Questions about Cancer Treatment

- What are the ways to treat my type and stage of cancer?
- What are the benefits and risks of each of these treatments?
- What treatment do you recommend? Why do you think it is best for me?
- When will I need to start treatment?
- Will I need to be in the hospital for treatment? If so, for how long?
- What is my chance of recovery with this treatment?
- How will we know if the treatment is working?
- Would a clinical trial (research study) be right for me?
- How do I find out about studies for my type and stage of cancer?

Questions about Finding a Specialist and Getting a Second Opinion

- Will I need a specialist(s) for my cancer treatment?
- Will you help me find a doctor to give me another opinion on the best treatment plan for me?

Questions about Surgery

- Is surgery an option for me? If so, what kind of surgery do you suggest?
- How long will I stay in the hospital?
- If I have pain, how will it be controlled?

Questions about Other Types of Treatment

- Where will I go for treatment?
- How is the treatment given?
- How long will each treatment session take?
- How many treatment sessions will I have?
- Should a family member or friend come with me to my treatment sessions?

Questions about Side Effects

- What are the possible side effects of the treatment?
- What side effects may happen during or between my treatment sessions?
- Are there any side effects that I should call you about right away?
- Are there any lasting effects of the treatment?
- Will this treatment affect my ability to have children?
- How can I prevent or treat side effects?

Questions about Medicines and Other Products You Might Be Taking

- Do I need to tell you about the medicines I am taking now?
- Should I tell you about dietary supplements (such as vitamins, minerals, herbs, or fish oil) that I am taking?
- Could any drugs or supplements change the way that cancer treatment works?

Chapter 7

Understanding Cancer Prognosis

If you have cancer, you may have questions about how serious your cancer is and your chances of survival. The estimate of how the disease will go for you is called prognosis. It can be hard to understand what prognosis means and also hard to talk about, even for doctors.

Many Factors Can Affect Your Prognosis

Some of the factors that affect prognosis include:

- The type of cancer and where it is in your body

- The stage of the cancer, which refers to the size of the cancer and if it has spread to other parts of your body

- The cancer's grade, which refers to how abnormal the cancer cells look under a microscope. Grade provides clues about how quickly the cancer is likely to grow and spread.

- Certain traits of the cancer cells

- Your age and how healthy you were before cancer

- How you respond to treatment

This chapter includes text excerpted from "Understanding Cancer Prognosis," National Cancer Institute (NCI), November 24, 2014.

Seeking Information about Your Prognosis Is a Personal Decision

When you have cancer, you and your loved ones face many unknowns. Understanding your cancer and knowing what to expect can help you and your loved ones make decisions. Some of the decisions you may face include:

- Which treatment is best for you

- If you want treatment

- How to best take care of yourself and manage treatment side effects

- How to deal with financial and legal matters

Many people want to know their prognosis. They find it easier to cope when they know more about their cancer. You may ask your doctor about survival statistics or search for this information on your own. Or, you may find statistics confusing and frightening, and think they are too impersonal to be of value to you. It is up to you to decide how much information you want.

If you do decide you want to know more, the doctor who knows the most about your situation is in the best position to discuss your prognosis and explain what the statistics may mean.

Understanding Statistics about Survival

Doctors estimate prognosis by using statistics that researchers have collected over many years about people with the same type of cancer. Several types of statistics may be used to estimate prognosis. The most commonly used statistics include:

- **Cancer-specific survival.** This is the percentage of patients with a specific type and stage of cancer who have not died from their cancer during a certain period of time after diagnosis. The period of time may be 1 year, 2 years, 5 years, etc., with 5 years being the time period most often used. Cancer-specific survival is also called disease-specific survival. In most cases, cancer-specific survival is based on causes of death listed in medical records.

- **Relative survival.** This statistic is another method used to estimate cancer-specific survival that does not use information about the cause of death. It is the percentage of cancer patients who have survived for a certain period of time after diagnosis compared to people who do not have cancer.

- **Overall survival.** This is the percentage of people with a specific type and stage of cancer who have not died from any cause during a certain period of time after diagnosis.

- **Disease-free survival.** This statistic is the percentage of patients who have no signs of cancer during a certain period of time after treatment. Other names for this statistic are recurrence-free or progression-free survival.

Because statistics are based on large groups of people, they cannot be used to predict exactly what will happen to you. Everyone is different. Treatments and how people respond to treatment can differ greatly. Also, it takes years to see the benefit of new treatments and ways of finding cancer. So, the statistics your doctor uses to make a prognosis may not be based on treatments being used today.

Still, your doctor may tell you that you have a good prognosis if statistics suggest that your cancer is likely to respond well to treatment. Or, he may tell you that you have a poor prognosis if the cancer is harder to control. Whatever your doctor tells you, keep in mind that a prognosis is an educated guess. Your doctor cannot be certain how it will go for you.

If You Decide Not to Have Treatment

If you decide not to have treatment, the doctor who knows your situation best is in the best position to discuss your prognosis.

Survival statistics most often come from studies that compare treatments with each other, rather than treatment with no treatment. So, it may not be easy for your doctor to give you an accurate prognosis.

Understanding the Difference between Cure and Remission

Cure means that there are no traces of your cancer after treatment and the cancer will never come back.

Remission means that the signs and symptoms of your cancer are reduced. Remission can be partial or complete. In a complete remission, all signs and symptoms of cancer have disappeared.

If you remain in complete remission for five years or more, some doctors may say that you are cured. Still, some cancer cells can remain in your body for many years after treatment. These cells may cause the cancer to come back one day. For cancers that return, most do so within the first 5 years after treatment. But, there is a chance that cancer will come back later. For this reason, doctors cannot say for sure that you are cured. The most they can say is that there are no signs of cancer at this time.

Because of the chance that cancer can come back, your doctor will monitor you for many years and do tests to look for signs of cancer's return. They will also look for signs of late side effects from the cancer treatments you received.

Chapter 8

Using Trusted Resources for Decision Making

Health information, whether in print or online, should come from a trusted, credible source. Government agencies, hospitals, universities, and medical journals and books that provide evidence-based information are sources you can trust. Too often, other sources can provide misleading or incorrect information. If a source makes claims that are too good to be true, remember—they usually are.

There are many websites, books, and magazines that provide health information to the public, but not all of them are trustworthy. Use the resources provided below to safeguard yourself when reviewing sources of health information.

Websites

Online sources of health information should make it easy for people to learn who is responsible for posting the information. They should make clear the original source of the information, along with the medical credentials of the people who prepare or review the posted material.

Use the following questions to determine the credibility of health information published online.

This chapter includes text excerpted from "Using Trusted Resources," National Cancer Institute (NCI), March 10, 2015.

Who Manages This Information?

The person or group that has published health information online should be identified somewhere.

Who Is Paying for the Project, and What Is Their Purpose?

You should be able to find this information in the "About Us" section.

What Is the Original Source of the Information That They Have Posted?

If the information was originally published in a research journal or a book, they should say which one(s) so that you can find it.

How Is Information Reviewed before It Gets Posted?

Most health information publications have someone with medical or research credentials (e.g., someone who has earned an M.D., D.O., or Ph.D.) review the information before it gets posted, to make sure it is correct.

How Current Is the Information?

Online health information sources should show you when the information was posted or last reviewed.

If They Are Asking for Personal Information, How Will They Use That Information and How Will They Protect Your Privacy?

This is very important. Do not share personal information until you understand the policies under which it will be used and you are comfortable with any risk involved in sharing your information online.

Books

A number of books have been written about cancer, cancer treatment, and complementary and alternative medicine (CAM). Some books contain trustworthy content, while others do not.

It's important to know that information is always changing and that new research results are reported every day. Be aware that if a book is written by only one person, you may only be getting that one person's view.

If you go to the library, ask the staff for suggestions. Or if you live near a college or university, there may be a medical library available. Local bookstores may also have people on staff who can help you. If you find a book online, look very carefully at the author's credentials, background, and expertise. Questions you may want to ask yourself are:

- Is the author an expert on this subject?

- Do you know anyone else who has read the book?

- Has the book been reviewed by other experts?

- Was it published in the past five years?

- Does the book offer different points of view, or does it seem to hold one opinion?

- Has the author researched the topic in full?

- Are the references listed in the back?

Magazines

If you want to look for articles you can trust, search online medical journal databases or ask your librarian to help you look for medical journals, books, and other research that has been done by experts.

Articles in popular magazines are usually not written by experts. Rather, the authors speak with experts, gather information, and then write the article. If claims are made in a magazine, remember:

- The authors may not have expert knowledge in this area.

- They may not say where they found their information.

- The articles have not been reviewed by experts.

- The publisher may have ties to advertisers or other organizations. Therefore, the article may be one-sided in the information or view(s) it presents.

When you read these articles, you can use the same process that the magazine writer uses:

- Speak with experts.

- Ask lots of questions.

- Then decide if the therapy is right for you.

Where to Get More Help

Cancer Treatment Scams

A page (www.consumer.ftc.gov/articles/0104-cancer-treatment-scams) from the Federal Trade Commission (FTC) that advises people to ask their healthcare provider about products that claim to cure or treat cancer and offers tips for spotting treatment scams.

For Consumers: Protecting Yourself

A page (www.fda.gov/ForConsumers/ProtectYourself/default.htm) from the Food and Drug Administration (FDA) that includes links to several resources that have tips about buying medicines and other products online.

Evaluating Cancer Information on the Internet

Developed by the American Society of Clinical Oncology (ASCO), Cancer.Net provides information, including common misconceptions about cancer and tips to evaluate the credibility of online cancer information.

Rumors, Myths, and Truths

The American Cancer Society (ACS) (www.cancer.org) offers a variety of services and programs for patients and their families, including educational programs and links to information about possible cancer hoaxes.

Chapter 9

Types of Cancer Treatment

Chapter Contents

Section 9.1

Surgery

This section includes text excerpted from "Surgery,"
National Cancer Institute (NCI), April 29, 2015.

Surgery, when used to treat cancer, is a procedure in which a surgeon removes cancer from your body. Surgeons are medical doctors with special training in surgery.

How Surgery Is Performed

Surgeons often use small, thin knives, called scalpels, and other sharp tools to cut your body during surgery. Surgery often requires cuts through skin, muscles, and sometimes bone. After surgery, these cuts can be painful and take some time to recover from.

Anesthesia keeps you from feeling pain during surgery. Anesthesia refers to drugs or other substances that cause you to lose feeling or awareness. There are three types of anesthesia:

- Local anesthesia causes loss of feeling in one small area of the body.

- Regional anesthesia causes loss of feeling in a part of the body, such as an arm or leg.

- General anesthesia causes loss of feeling and a complete loss of awareness that seems like a very deep sleep.

There are other ways of performing surgery that do not involve cuts with scalpels. Some of these include:

- **Cryosurgery.** Cryosurgery is a type of treatment in which extreme cold produced by liquid nitrogen or argon gas is used to destroy abnormal tissue. Cryosurgery may be used to treat early-stage skin cancer, retinoblastoma, and precancerous growths on the skin and cervix. Cryosurgery is also called cryotherapy.

- **Lasers.** This is a type of treatment in which powerful beams of light are used to cut through tissue. Lasers can focus very

accurately on tiny areas, so they can be used for precise surgeries. Lasers can also be used to shrink or destroy tumors or
growths that might turn into cancer. Lasers are most often used
to treat tumors on the surface of the body or on the inside lining
of internal organs. Examples include basal cell carcinoma, cervical changes that might turn into cancer, and cervical, vaginal,
esophageal, and non-small cell lung cancer.

- **Hyperthermia.** Hyperthermia is a type of treatment in which
  small areas of body tissue are exposed to high temperatures. The
  high heat can damage and kill cancer cells or make them more
  sensitive to radiation and certain chemotherapy drugs. Radiofre-
  quency ablation is one type of hyperthermia that uses high-energy radio waves to generate heat. Hyperthermia is not widely
  available and is being studied in clinical trials.

- **Photodynamic Therapy.** Photodynamic therapy is a type of
  treatment that uses drugs which react to a certain type of light.
  When the tumor is exposed to this light, these drugs become
  active and kill nearby cancer cells. Photodynamic therapy is
  used most often to treat or relieve symptoms caused by skin cancer, mycosis fungoides, and non-small cell lung cancer.

Types of Surgery

There are many types of surgery. The types differ based on the
purpose of the surgery, the part of the body that requires surgery, the
amount of tissue to be removed, and, in some cases, what the patient
prefers.

Surgery may be open or minimally invasive.

- In open surgery, the surgeon makes one large cut to remove
  the tumor, some healthy tissue, and maybe some nearby lymph
  nodes.

- In minimally invasive surgery, the surgeon makes a few small
  cuts instead of one large one. She inserts a long, thin tube with a
  tiny camera into one of the small cuts. This tube is called a lapa-
  roscope. The camera projects images from the inside of the body
  onto a monitor, which allows the surgeon to see what she is doing.
  She uses special surgery tools that are inserted through the other
  small cuts to remove the tumor and some healthy tissue.

Because minimally invasive surgery requires smaller cuts, it takes
less time to recover from than open surgery.

Who Has Surgery

Many people with cancer are treated with surgery. Surgery works best for solid tumors that are contained in one area. It is a local treatment, meaning that it treats only the part of your body with the cancer. It is not used for leukemia (a type of blood cancer) or for cancers that have spread.

Sometimes surgery will be the only treatment you need. But most often, you will also have other cancer treatments.

How Surgery Works against Cancer

Depending on your type of cancer and how advanced it is, surgery can be used to:

- **Remove the entire tumor.** Surgery removes cancer that is contained in one area.

- **Debulk a tumor.** Surgery removes some, but not all, of a cancer tumor. Debulking is used when removing an entire tumor might damage an organ or the body. Removing part of a tumor can help other treatments work better.

- **Ease cancer symptoms.** Surgery is used to remove tumors that are causing pain or pressure.

Risks of Surgery

Surgeons are highly trained and will do everything they can to prevent problems during surgery. Even so, sometimes problems do occur. Common problems are:

- **Pain.** After surgery, most people will have pain in the part of the body that was operated on. How much pain you feel will depend on the extent of the surgery, the part of your body where you had surgery, and how you feel pain. Your doctor or nurse can help you manage pain after surgery. Talk with your doctor or nurse before surgery about ways to control pain. After surgery, tell them if your pain is not controlled.

- **Infection.** Infection is another problem that can happen after surgery. To help prevent infection, follow your nurse's instructions about caring for the area where you had surgery. If you do develop an infection, your doctor can prescribe a medicine (called an antibiotic) to treat it. Other risks of surgery include bleeding, damage to nearby tissues, and reactions to the anesthesia. Talk to your doctor about possible risks for the type of surgery you will have.

Section 9.2

Radiation Therapy

This section includes text excerpted from "Radiation Therapy," National Cancer Institute (NCI), April 29, 2015.

Radiation therapy (also called radiotherapy) is a cancer treatment that uses high doses of radiation to kill cancer cells and shrink tumors. At low doses, radiation is used in X-rays to see inside your body, as with X-rays of your teeth or broken bones.

How Radiation Therapy Works against Cancer

At high doses, radiation kills cancer cells or slows their growth. Radiation therapy is used to:

- **Treat cancer.** Radiation can be used to cure cancer, to prevent it from returning, or to stop or slow its growth.

- **Ease cancer symptoms.** Radiation may be used to shrink a tumor to treat pain and other problems caused by the tumor. Or, it can lessen problems that may be caused by a growing tumor, such as trouble breathing or loss of bowel and bladder control.

Radiation therapy does not kill cancer cells right away. It takes days or weeks of treatment before cancer cells start to die. Then, cancer cells keep dying for weeks or months after radiation therapy ends.

Types of Radiation Therapy

There are two main types of radiation therapy, external beam and internal.

External Beam Radiation Therapy

External beam radiation therapy comes from a machine that aims radiation at your cancer. The machine is large and may be noisy. It does not touch you, but can move around you, sending radiation to a part of your body from many directions.

External beam radiation therapy treats a specific part of your body. For example, if you have cancer in your lung, you will have radiation only to your chest, not to your whole body.

Internal Radiation Therapy

Internal radiation therapy is a treatment in which a source of radiation is put inside your body. The radiation source can be solid or liquid.

Internal radiation therapy with a solid source is called brachytherapy. In this type of treatment, radiation in the form of seeds, ribbons, or capsules is placed in your body in or near the cancer.

You receive liquid radiation through an IV line. Liquid radiation travels throughout your body, seeking out and killing cancer cells.

Who Receives Radiation Therapy

External beam radiation therapy is used to treat many types of cancer. For some people, radiation may be the only treatment you need. But, most often, you will have radiation therapy and other cancer treatments, such as surgery and chemotherapy.

Brachytherapy is used to treat cancers of the head and neck, breast, cervix, prostate, and eye.

Liquid forms of internal radiation are most often used to treat thyroid cancer.

How Radiation Is Used with Other Cancer Treatments

Radiation may be given before, during, or after surgery. Doctors may use radiation:

- Before surgery, to shrink the size of the cancer.

- During surgery, so that it goes straight to the cancer without passing through the skin. Radiation therapy used this way is called intraoperative radiation.

- After surgery, to kill any cancer cells that may remain.

Radiation may also be given before, during, or after other cancer treatments to shrink the cancer or to kill any cancer cells that might remain.

Radiation Therapy Can Cause Side Effects

Radiation not only kills or slows the growth of cancer cells, it can also affect nearby healthy cells. Damage to healthy cells can cause side effects. External radiation and brachytherapy cause side effects only in the part of the body being treated.

The most common side effect of radiation therapy is fatigue, which is feeling exhausted and worn out. Fatigue can happen all at once or little by little. People feel fatigue in different ways. You may feel more or less fatigue than someone else who is also getting radiation therapy.

You can prepare for fatigue by:

- Asking someone to drive you to and from radiation therapy

- Planning time to rest

- Asking for help with meals and child care

Healthy cells that are damaged during radiation treatment almost always recover after it is over. But sometimes people may have side effects that are severe or do not improve. Other side effects may show up months or years after radiation therapy is over. These are called late effects.

Doctors try to protect healthy cells during treatment by:

- **Using as low a dose of radiation as possible.** The radiation dose is balanced between being high enough to kill cancer cells, yet low enough to limit damage to healthy cells.

- **Spreading out treatment over time.** You may get radiation therapy once a day, or in smaller doses twice a day for several weeks. Spreading out the radiation dose allows normal cells to recover while cancer cells die.

- **Aiming radiation at a precise part of your body.** With external radiation therapy, for example, your doctor is able to aim high doses of radiation at your cancer while reducing the amount of radiation that reaches nearby healthy tissue. These treatments use a computer to deliver precise radiation doses to a tumor or to specific areas within the tumor.

Section 9.3

Chemotherapy

This section includes text excerpted from "Chemotherapy,"
National Cancer Institute (NCI), April 29, 2015.

Chemotherapy (also called chemo) is a type of cancer treatment
that uses drugs to kill cancer cells.

How Chemotherapy Works against Cancer

Chemotherapy works by stopping or slowing the growth of cancer
cells, which grow and divide quickly. Chemotherapy is used to:

- **Treat cancer.** Chemotherapy can be used to cure cancer, lessen
  the chance it will return, or stop or slow its growth.

- **Ease cancer symptoms.** Chemotherapy can be used to shrink
  tumors that are causing pain and other problems.

Who Receives Chemotherapy

Chemotherapy is used to treat many types of cancer. For some people, chemotherapy may be the only treatment you receive. But most
often, you will have chemotherapy and other cancer treatments. The
types of treatment that you need depends on the type of cancer you
have, if it has spread and where, and if you have other health problems.

How Chemotherapy Is Used with Other Cancer Treatments

When used with other treatments, chemotherapy can:

- Make a tumor smaller before surgery or radiation therapy. This
  is called neoadjuvant chemotherapy.

- Destroy cancer cells that may remain after treatment with surgery or radiation therapy. This is called adjuvant chemotherapy.

- Help other treatments work better.

- Kill cancer cells that have returned or spread to other parts of your body.

Chemotherapy Can Cause Side Effects

Chemotherapy not only kills fast-growing cancer cells, but also kills or slows the growth of healthy cells that grow and divide quickly. Examples are cells that line your mouth and intestines and those that cause your hair to grow. Damage to healthy cells may cause side effects, such as mouth sores, nausea, and hair loss. Side effects often get better or go away after you have finished chemotherapy.

The most common side effect is fatigue, which is feeling exhausted and worn out. You can prepare for fatigue by:

- Asking someone to drive you to and from chemotherapy

- Planning time to rest on the day of and day after chemotherapy

- Asking for help with meals and child care on the day of and at least one day after chemotherapy

There are many ways you can help manage chemotherapy side effects.

Section 9.4

Immunotherapy

This section includes text excerpted from "Immunotherapy," National Cancer Institute (NCI), April 29, 2015.

Immunotherapy is a type of cancer treatment that helps your immune system fight cancer. The immune system helps your body fight infections and other diseases. It is made up of white blood cells and organs and tissues of the lymph system.

Immunotherapy is a type of biological therapy. Biological therapy is a type of treatment that uses substances made from living organisms to treat cancer.

71

Types of Immunotherapy

Many different types of immunotherapy are used to treat cancer. They include:

- **Monoclonal antibodies,** which are drugs that are designed to bind to specific targets in the body. They can cause an immune response that destroys cancer cells. Other types of monoclonal antibodies can "mark" cancer cells so it is easier for the immune system to find and destroy them. These types of monoclonal antibodies may also be referred to as targeted therapy.

- **Adoptive cell transfer,** which is a treatment that attempts to boost the natural ability of your T cells to fight cancer. T cells are a type of white blood cell and part of the immune system. Researchers take T cells from the tumor. They then isolate the T cells that are most active against your cancer or modify the genes in them to make them better able to find and destroy your cancer cells. Researchers then grow large batches of these T cells in the lab. You may have treatments to reduce your immune cells. After these treatments, the T cells that were grown in the lab will be given back to you via a needle in your vein. The process of growing your T cells in the lab can take 2 to 8 weeks, depending on how fast they grow.

- **Cytokines,** which are proteins that are made by your body's cells. They play important roles in the body's normal immune responses and also in the immune system's ability to respond to cancer. The two main types of cytokines used to treat cancer are called interferons and interleukins.

- **Treatment Vaccines,** which work against cancer by boosting your immune system's response to cancer cells. Treatment vaccines are different from the ones that help prevent disease.

- **BCG**, which stands for Bacillus Calmette-Guérin, is an immunotherapy that is used to treat bladder cancer. It is a weakened form of the bacteria that causes tuberculosis. When inserted directly into the bladder with a catheter, BCG causes an immune response against cancer cells. It is also being studied in other types of cancer.

Who Receives Immunotherapy

Immunotherapy is not yet as widely used as surgery, chemotherapy, and radiation therapy. However, immunotherapies have been approved to treat people with many types of cancer.

Many other immunotherapies are being studied in clinical trials, which are research studies involving people.

How Immunotherapy Works against Cancer

One reason that cancer cells thrive is because they are able to hide from your immune system. Certain immunotherapies can mark cancer cells so it is easier for the immune system to find and destroy them. Other immunotherapies boost your immune system to work better against cancer.

Immunotherapy Can Cause Side Effects

Immunotherapy can cause side effects. The side effects you may have depend on the type of immunotherapy you receive and how your body reacts to it.

The most common side effects are skin reactions at the needle site. These side effects include:

- Pain
- Swelling
- Soreness
- Redness
- Itchiness
- Rash

You may have flu-like symptoms, which include:

- Fever
- Chills
- Weakness
- Dizziness
- Nausea or vomiting
- Muscle or joint aches
- Fatigue
- Headache
- Trouble breathing
- Low or high blood pressure

Other side effects might include:

- Swelling
- Weight gain from retaining fluid
- Heart palpitations
- Sinus congestion
- Diarrhea
- Risk of infection

Immunotherapies may also cause severe or even fatal allergic reactions. However, these reactions are rare.

How Immunotherapy Is Given

Different forms of immunotherapy may be given in different ways. These include:

- **Intravenous (IV).** The immunotherapy goes directly into a vein.

- **Oral.** The immunotherapy comes in pills or capsules that you swallow.

- **Topical.** The immunotherapy comes in a cream that you rub onto your skin. This type of immunotherapy can be used for very early skin cancer.

- **Intravesical.** The immunotherapy goes directly into the bladder.

Section 9.5

Targeted Therapy

This section includes text excerpted from "Targeted Therapy," National Cancer Institute (NCI), August 15, 2014.

What Is Targeted Therapy?

Targeted therapy is the foundation of precision medicine. It is a type of cancer treatment that targets the changes in cancer cells that help them grow, divide, and spread. As researchers learn more about the cell changes that drive cancer, they are better able to design promising therapies that target these changes or block their effects.

Types of Targeted Therapy

Most targeted therapies are either small-molecule drugs or monoclonal antibodies.

1. **Small-molecule** drugs are small enough to enter cells easily, so they are used for targets that are inside cells.

2. **Monoclonal antibodies** are drugs that are not able to enter cells easily. Instead, they attach to specific targets on the outer surface of cancer cells.

Who Receives Targeted Therapy

For some types of cancer, most patients with that cancer will have a target for a certain drug, so they can be treated with that drug. But, most of the time, your tumor will need to be tested to see if it contains targets for which we have drugs.

To have your tumor tested for targets, you may need to have a biopsy. A biopsy is a procedure in which your doctor removes a piece of the tumor for testing. There are some risks to having a biopsy. These risks vary depending on the size of the tumor and where it is located. Your doctor will explain the risks of having a biopsy for your type of tumor.

How Targeted Therapy Works against Cancer

Most targeted therapies help treat cancer by interfering with specific proteins that help tumors grow and spread throughout the body. They treat cancer in many different ways. They can:

- **Help the immune system destroy cancer cells.** One reason that cancer cells thrive is because they are able to hide from your immune system. Certain targeted therapies can mark cancer cells so it is easier for the immune system to find and destroy them. Other targeted therapies help boost your immune system to work better against cancer.

- **Stop cancer cells from growing.** Healthy cells in your body usually divide to make new cells only when they receive strong signals to do so. These signals bind to proteins on the cell surface, telling the cells to divide. This process helps new cells form only as your body needs them. But, some cancer cells have changes in the proteins on their surface that tell them to divide whether or not signals are present. Some targeted therapies interfere with these proteins, preventing them from telling the cells to divide. This process helps slow cancer's uncontrolled growth.

- **Stop signals that help form blood vessels.** Tumors need to form new blood vessels to grow beyond a certain size. These new blood vessels form in response to signals from the tumor.

Some targeted therapies are designed to interfere with these signals to prevent a blood supply from forming. Without a blood supply, tumors stay small. Or, if a tumor already has a blood supply, these treatments can cause blood vessels to die, which causes the tumor to shrink.

- **Deliver cell-killing substances to cancer cells.** Some monoclonal antibodies are combined with toxins, chemotherapy drugs, and radiation. Once these monoclonal antibodies attach to targets on the surface of cancer cells, the cells take up the cell-killing substances, causing them to die. Cells that don't have the target will not be harmed.

- **Cause cancer cell death.** Healthy cells die in an orderly manner when they become damaged or are no longer needed. But, cancer cells have ways of avoiding this dying process. Some targeted therapies can cause cancer cells to go through this process of cell death.

- **Starve cancer of the hormones it needs to grow.** Some breast and prostate cancers require certain hormones to grow. Hormone therapies are a type of targeted therapy that can work in two ways. Some hormone therapies prevent your body from making specific hormones. Others prevent the hormones from acting on your cells, including cancer cells.

Drawbacks of Targeted Therapy

Targeted therapies do have some drawbacks. These include:

- Cancer cells can become resistant to them. For this reason, targeted therapies may work best when used with other targeted therapies or with other cancer treatments, such as chemotherapy and radiation.

- Drugs for some targets are hard to develop. Reasons include the target's structure, the target's function in the cell, or both.

Targeted Therapy Can Cause Side Effects

Targeted therapy can cause side effects. The side effects you may have depend on the type of targeted therapy you receive and how your body reacts to the therapy.

The most common side effects of targeted therapy include diarrhea and liver problems. Other side effects might include problems with blood clotting and wound healing, high blood pressure, fatigue, mouth sores, nail changes, the loss of hair color, and skin problems. Skin problems might include rash or dry skin. Very rarely, a hole might form through the wall of the esophagus, stomach, small intestine, large bowel, rectum, or gallbladder.

There are medicines for many of these side effects. These medicines may prevent the side effects from happening or treat them once they occur.

Most side effects of targeted therapy go away after treatment ends.

Section 9.6

Hormone Therapy

This section includes text excerpted from "Hormone Therapy,"
National Cancer Institute (NCI), April 29, 2015.

Hormone therapy is a cancer treatment that slows or stops the growth of cancer that uses hormones to grow. Hormone therapy is also called hormonal therapy, hormone treatment, or endocrine therapy.

How Hormone Therapy Works against Cancer

Hormone therapy is used to:

- **Treat cancer.** Hormone therapy can lessen the chance that cancer will return or stop or slow its growth.

- **Ease cancer symptoms.** Hormone therapy may be used to reduce or prevent symptoms in men with prostate cancer who are not able to have surgery or radiation therapy.

Types of Hormone Therapy

Hormone therapy falls into two broad groups, those that block the body's ability to produce hormones and those that interfere with how hormones behave in the body.

Who Receives Hormone Therapy

Hormone therapy is used to treat prostate and breast cancers that use hormones to grow. Hormone therapy is most often used along with other cancer treatments. The types of treatment that you need depend on the type of cancer, if it has spread and how far, if it uses hormones to grow, and if you have other health problems.

How Hormone Therapy Is Used with Other Cancer Treatments

When used with other treatments, hormone therapy can:

- Make a tumor smaller before surgery or radiation therapy. This is called neo-adjuvant therapy.

- Lower the risk that cancer will come back after the main treatment. This is called adjuvant therapy.

- Destroy cancer cells that have returned or spread to other parts of your body.

Hormone Therapy Can Cause Side Effects

Because hormone therapy blocks your body's ability to produce hormones or interferes with how hormones behave, it can cause unwanted side effects. The side effects you have will depend on the type of hormone therapy you receive and how your body responds to it. People respond differently to the same treatment, so not everyone gets the same side effects. Some side effects also differ if you are a man or a woman.

Some common side effects for men who receive hormone therapy for prostate cancer include:

- Hot flashes

- Loss of interest in or ability to have sex

- Weakened bones

- Diarrhea

- Nausea

- Enlarged and tender breasts

- Fatigue

Some common side effects for women who receive hormone therapy for breast cancer include:

- Hot flashes

- Vaginal dryness

- Changes in your periods if you have not yet reached menopause

- Loss of interest in sex

- Nausea

- Mood changes

- Fatigue

Section 9.7

Precision Medicine

This section includes text excerpted from "Understanding Precision Medicine in Cancer Treatment," National Cancer Institute (NCI), November 16, 2015.

Precision medicine is an approach to patient care that allows doctors to select treatments that are most likely to help patients based on a genetic understanding of their disease. This may also be called personalized medicine. The idea of precision medicine is not new, but recent advances in science and technology have helped speed up the pace of this area of research.

When you are diagnosed with cancer, you usually receive the same treatment as others who have same type and stage of cancer. Even so, different people may respond differently, and, until recently, doctors didn't know why. After decades of research, scientists now understand that patients' tumors have genetic changes that cause cancer to grow and spread. They have also learned that the changes that occur in one person's cancer may not occur in others who have the same type of cancer. And, the same cancer-causing changes may be found in different types of cancer.

The Promise of Precision Medicine

The hope of precision medicine is that treatments will one day be tailored to the changes in each person's cancer. Scientists see a future when patients will receive drugs that their tumors are most likely to respond to and will be spared from receiving drugs that are not likely to help. Research studies are going on now to test whether treating patients with drugs that target the cancer-causing genetic changes in their tumors, no matter where the cancer develops in the body, will help them. Many of these drugs are known as targeted therapies.

Though experts believe that precision medicine can become an additional option for people with cancer, it is not likely to replace the cancer treatments already available. Currently, if you need treatment for cancer, you may receive a combination of treatments, including surgery, chemotherapy, radiation therapy, and immunotherapy. Which treatments you receive will depend on the type of cancer, its size, and whether it has spread. With precision medicine, if your cancer has a genetic change that can be targeted with a known drug, you may also receive that drug.

There are drugs that have been proven effective against specific genetic changes in certain cancers and approved by the U.S. Food and Drug Administration (FDA). Approved treatments should be available wherever you have cancer treatment.

Precision Medicine as a Treatment Option

Even though researchers are making progress every day, treatment using precision medicine is not yet part of routine care for most patients. Many new drugs used in precision medicine are being tested right now in clinical trials. Some clinical trials are accepting patients with specific types and stages of cancer. Others accept patients with a variety of cancer types and stages. To be eligible for precision medicine trials, your tumor must have a genetic change that can be targeted by a drug being tested.

Not Every Person with Cancer Will Have Their Cancer Tested for Genetic Changes

If there is a targeted drug approved for your type of cancer, you will likely be tested for a genetic change that might be driving it. For instance, people with melanoma, some leukemias, and breast, lung, colon, and rectal cancers usually have their cancers tested for certain genetic changes when they are diagnosed. Since additional genetic changes that can drive cancer may occur over time, you might also have your cancer tested if it comes back or gets worse.

If there is not an approved targeted drug for your type of cancer, you still may be tested for genetic changes. For instance, your cancer may be tested to see if you can join a precision medicine clinical trial.

How Genetic Changes in Your Cancer Are Identified

To figure out which genetic changes are in your cancer, you may need to have a biopsy. A biopsy is a procedure in which your doctor removes a sample of the cancer. This sample will be sent to a special lab, where a machine called a DNA sequencer looks for genetic changes that may be causing the cancer to grow. The process of looking for genetic changes in cancer may be called DNA sequencing, genomic testing, molecular profiling, or tumor profiling.

Chapter 10

Understanding Cancer Medications

Chapter Contents

Section 10.1

Drugs Approved for Different Types of Cancer

This section includes text excerpted from "Drugs Approved for Different Types of Cancer," National Cancer Institute (NCI), January 16, 2015.

This section includes a selected list of drugs approved for specific types of cancer. It is not the comprehensive list for all drugs. To see the most current list of all available, U.S. Department of Food and Drug Administration (FDA) approved cancer drugs visit www.cancer.gov/about-cancer/treatment/drugs/cancer-type.

Anal Cancer

- **Gardasil (Recombinant HPV Quadrivalent Vaccine).** It is approved to prevent some conditions caused by certain types of Human papillomavirus (HPV). It is used in males or females aged 9 to 26 years to prevent anal cancer.

- **Gardasil 9 (Recombinant HPV Nonavalent Vaccine).** It is approved to prevent some conditions caused by certain types of HPV. The vaccine protects against nine different types of HPV. It is used in females aged 9 to 26 years and males aged 9 to 15 years to prevent anal cancer.

Bladder Cancer

- **Cisplatin.** Cisplatin is approved to be used alone or with other drugs to treat bladder cancer that cannot be treated with surgery or radiation therapy.

- **Thiotepa.** Thiotepa is approved to treat bladder cancer. It is also being studied in the treatment of other types of cancer and as part of a regimen to prepare patients for bone marrow and stem cell transplants.

Bone Cancer

- **Cosmegen** (Dactinomycin). Dactinomycin is approved to be used alone or with other drugs to treat bone cancer.

- **Denosumab**. Denosumab is approved to treat:
  - Giant cell tumor of the bone. It is used in adults and in adolescents whose bones have finished growing. This use is approved for the Xgeva brand of Denosumab.
  - Denosumab is approved to prevent and treat:
  - Broken bones and other bone problems caused by solid tumors that have metastasized (spread) to bone. This use is approved for the Xgeva brand of denosumab.
  - Osteoporosis in postmenopausal women who have a high risk of breaking bones. This use is approved for the Prolia brand of denosumab.

Denosumab is also approved to increase bone mass in patients who are at high risk of breaking bones.

Brain Tumors

- **Afinitor (Everolimus)**. Everolimus is approved to treat brain tumors. The use of everolimus to treat cancer is approved for the Afinitor brand. Everolimus is also approved to treat transplant rejection. This use is approved for the Zortress brand.

- **Lomustine**. Lomustine is approved to be used alone or with other drugs to treat brain tumors.

- **Temozolomide**(Methazolastone / Temodar). Temozolomide is approved to treat the following types of brain tumors in adults:
  - Anaplastic astrocytoma.
  - Glioblastoma multiforme (GBM).

Breast Cancer

- **Ado-Trastuzumab Emtansine (Kadcyla)**. Ado-trastuzumab emtansine is approved to treat breast cancer that is HER2 positive and has metastasized (spread to other parts of the body).

It is used in patients who have already been treated with tras-tuzumab and a taxane. It is also used in these patients if cancer recurs (comes back) after adjuvant therapy.

- **Ixabepilone (Ixempra)**. Ixabepilone is approved to be used alone or with capecitabine to treat breast cancer that is locally advanced or has metastasized (spread to other parts of the body). It is used in patients who have not gotten better with other chemotherapy.

Cervical Cancer

- **Bevacizumab**. Bevacizumab is approved to be used alone or with other drugs to treat cervical cancer that has not gotten better with other treatment, has metastasized (spread to other parts of the body), or has recurred.

- **Bleomycin**. Bleomycin is approved to be used alone or with other drugs as palliative treatment of cervical cancer. It is also approved to treat malignant pleural effusion and keep it from recurring.

Colon Cancer

- **Cetuximab**. Cetuximab is approved to be used alone or with other drugs to treat colorectal cancer that has metastasized (spread to other parts of the body).

- **Leucovorin Calcium**. Leucovorin calcium is approved to be used alone or with other drugs to treat colorectal cancer. It is used with fluorouracil as palliative treatment in patients with advanced disease.

Rectal Cancer

- **Ramucirumab**. Ramucirumab is approved to be used alone or with other drugs to treat

  - Adenocarcinoma of the stomach or gastroesophageal junction that is advanced or has metastasized (spread to other parts of the body). It is used in patients whose disease has gotten worse after treatment with certain chemotherapy. It is used alone or with paclitaxel.

  - Colorectal cancer that has metastasized. It is used with FOLFIRI in patients whose disease has gotten worse during or after treatment with certain anticancer drugs.

- Non-small cell lung cancer that has metastasized. It is used with docetaxel in patients whose disease has gotten worse after treatment with certain chemotherapy. For patients whose cancer has a mutation in the epidermal growth factor receptor (*EGFR*) gene or anaplastic lymphoma kinase (*ALK*) gene, ramucirumab is used if their disease has gotten worse after treatment with FDA-approved therapy for these mutations.

- **Xeloda** (Capecitabine). Capecitabine is approved to be used alone or with other drugs to treat colorectal cancer. It is used to treat stage III colorectal cancer in patients who have had surgery to remove cancer. It is also used as first-line treatment of patients with metastatic colorectal cancer.

Gastroenteropancreatic Neuroendocrine Tumors

- **Afinitor** (Everolimus). Everolimus is approved to treat:

  - Pancreatic cancer, gastrointestinal cancer, and lung cancer (certain types). It is used in adults with progressive neuroendocrine tumors that cannot be removed by surgery, are locally advanced, or have metastasized (spread to other parts of the body).

  - Renal cell carcinoma (a type of kidney cancer) that is advanced, in adults who have not gotten better with other chemotherapy.

  - Subependymal giant cell astrocytoma in adults and children who have tuberous sclerosis and are not able to have surgery. Everolimus is available as tablets (Afinitor) or tablets for oral suspension (Afinitor Disperz). Only Afinitor Disperz is used in children.

- **Lanreotide Acetate**. Lanreotide acetate is approved to treat gastroenteropancreatic neuroendocrine tumors. It is used for some tumors that cannot be removed by surgery, are locally advanced, or have metastasized (spread to other parts of the body).

Endometrial Cancer

Megestrol Acetate. Megestrol acetate in tablet form is approved for palliative treatment of advanced disease in endometrial cancer.

Esophageal Cancer

- **Ramucirumab**. Ramucirumab is approved to be used alone or with other drugs to treat:

  - Adenocarcinoma of the stomach or gastroesophageal junction that is advanced or has metastasized (spread to other parts of the body). It is used in patients whose disease has gotten worse after treatment with certain chemotherapy. It is used alone or with paclitaxel.

  - Colorectal cancer that has metastasized. It is used with FOLFIRI in patients whose disease has gotten worse during or after treatment with certain anticancer drugs.

  - Non-small cell lung cancer that has metastasized. It is used with docetaxel in patients whose disease has gotten worse after treatment with certain chemotherapy. For patients whose cancer has a mutation in the epidermal growth factor receptor (*EGFR*) gene or anaplastic lymphoma kinase (*ALK*) gene, ramucirumab is used if their disease has gotten worse after treatment with FDA-approved therapy for these mutations.

- **Trastuzumab**. Trastuzumab is approved to be used alone or with other drugs to treat:

  - Adenocarcinoma of the stomach or gastroesophageal junction. It is used for HER2 positive (HER2+) disease that has metastasized (spread to other parts of the body) in patients who have not already been treated for metastatic cancer.

  - Breast cancer that is HER2+.

Gastrointestinal Stromal Tumors

- **Imatinib Mesylate**. Imatinib mesylate is approved to treat:

  - Gastrointestinal stromal tumor (GIST).

  - Myelodysplastic/myeloproliferative neoplasms.

  - Systemic mastocytosis.

- **Sunitinib Malate**. Sunitinib malate is approved to treat gastrointestinal stromal tumor (a type of stomach cancer). It is used in patients whose condition has become worse while taking another drug called imatinib mesylate or who are not able to take imatinib mesylate.

Gestational Trophoblastic Disease

- **Dactinomycin.** Dactinomycin is approved to be used alone or with other drugs to treat:

  - Ewing sarcoma.

  - Gestational trophoblastic disease.

  - Rhabdomyosarcoma in children.

  - Solid tumors. It is used as palliative and/or adjuvant therapy for disease that has recurred.

  - Testicular cancer. It is used for nonseminomas that have metastasized (spread to other parts of the body).

  - Wilms tumor.

- **Velsar (Vinblastine Sulfate).** Vinblastine sulfate is approved to treat:

  - Mycosis fungoides.

  - Non-Hodgkin lymphoma (NHL).

  - Testicular cancer.

Head and Neck Cancer

- **Bleomycin.** Bleomycin is approved to be used alone or with other drugs as palliative treatment of:

  - Squamous cell carcinoma of the cervix.

  - Squamous cell carcinoma of the head and neck (SCCHN).

  - Squamous cell carcinoma of the vulva.

  Bleomycin is also approved to treat malignant pleural effusion and keep it from recurring.

- **Nivolumab.** Nivolumab is approved to be used alone or with other drugs to treat:

  - Classical Hodgkin lymphoma that has gotten worse after an autologous stem cell transplant and treatment with brentuximab vedotin.

  - Melanoma that cannot be removed by surgery or that has metastasized (spread to other parts of the body).

- It is used with ipilimumab in patients whose cancer does not have a certain *BRAF* gene mutation.

- It is used alone in patients whose disease got worse after being treated with ipilimumab and, if their cancer had a certain *BRAF* gene mutation, with a drug called a BRAF inhibitor.

- Squamous cell carcinoma of the head and neck that has metastasized or recurred (come back) in patients whose disease got worse during or after treatment with platinum chemotherapy.

Hodgkin Lymphoma

- **Carmubris (Carmustine)**. Carmustine is approved to be used alone or with other drugs to treat:

  - It is used with other drugs in patients whose disease has not gotten better with other treatment or has recurred (come back).

  - It is used with prednisone.

  - It is used with other drugs in patients whose disease has not gotten better with other treatment or has recurred (come back).

  Carmustine is also being studied in the treatment of other types of cancer. It is also available in a different form called carmustine implant.

- **Procarbazine Hydrochloride**. Procarbazine hydrochloride is approved to be used with other drugs to treat hodgkin lymphoma that is advanced.

Kaposi Sarcoma

- **Paclitaxel**. Paclitaxel is approved to be used alone or with other drugs to treat:

  - AIDS-related Kaposi sarcoma.

  - Breast cancer.

  - Non-small cell lung cancer.

  - Ovarian cancer.

Paclitaxel is also available in a different form called paclitaxel albumin-stabilized nanoparticle formulation.

- **Vinblastine Sulfate**. Vinblastine sulfate is approved to treat:
  - Kaposi sarcoma.
  - Mycosis fungoides.
  - Non-Hodgkin lymphoma (NHL).

Kidney (Renal Cell) Cancer

- **Cabozantinib-S-Malate**. Cabozantinib-s-malate is approved to treat:
  - Medullary thyroid cancer that is progressive and has metastasized (spread to other parts of the body). This use is approved for the Cometriq brand of cabozantinib-s-malate.
  - Renal cell carcinoma (a type of kidney cancer) that is advanced. It is used in patients who have already received angiogenesis inhibitor therapy. This use is approved for the Cabometyx brand of cabozantinib-s-malate.
- **Opdivo (Nivolumab)**. Nivolumab is approved to be used alone or with other drugs to treat:
  - Classical Hodgkin lymphoma that has gotten worse after an autologous stem cell transplant and treatment with brentuximab vedotin.
  - Melanoma that cannot be removed by surgery or that has metastasized (spread to other parts of the body).
  - It is used with ipilimumab in patients whose cancer does not have a certain *BRAF* gene mutation.
  - It is used alone in patients whose disease got worse after being treated with ipilimumab and, if their cancer had a certain *BRAF* gene mutation, with a drug called a BRAF inhibitor.
  - Renal cell carcinoma (a type of kidney cancer) that is advanced. It is used in patients who have already received angiogenesis inhibitor therapy.

Acute Lymphoblastic Leukemia (ALL)

- **Folex (Methotrexate).** Methotrexate is approved to be used alone or with other drugs to treat:

  - Acute lymphoblastic leukemia that has spread to the central nervous system, or to prevent it from spreading there.

  - Mycosis fungoides (a type of cutaneous T-cell lymphoma) that is advanced.

  - Non-Hodgkin lymphoma that is advanced.

  - Osteosarcoma that has not spread to other parts of the body. It is used following surgery to remove the primary tumor.

- **Purixan (Mercaptopurine).** Mercaptopurine is approved to be used with other drugs to treat acute lymphoblastic leukemia (ALL). It is used as maintenance therapy in adults and children.

Acute Myeloid Leukemia (AML)

- **Daunorubicin Hydrochloride.** Daunorubicin hydrochloride is approved to be used with other drugs as remission induction therapy to treat:

  - Acute lymphoblastic leukemia in adults and children.

  - Acute myeloid leukemia in adults.

- **Thioguanine.** Thioguanine is approved to be used as remission induction therapy and remission consolidation therapy to treat acute myeloid leukemia (AML).

Chronic Lymphocytic Leukemia

- **Arzerra (Ofatumumab).** Ofatumumab is approved to be used alone or with other drugs to treat chronic lymphocytic leukemia (CLL).

  - It is used alone as extended treatment in patients with recurrent or progressive disease who are in complete or partial response after at least two other types of treatment.

  - It is used alone in patients who have not gotten better with other drugs.

- It is used with chlorambucil in patients who have never been treated and cannot receive certain chemotherapy.

- **Gazyva (Obinutuzumab)**. Obinutuzumab is approved to be used with other drugs to treat chronic lymphocytic leukemia (CLL). It is used with chlorambucil in patients who have not already been treated for CLL.

Chronic Myelogenous Leukemia (CML)

- **Busulfex (Busulfan)**. Busulfan is approved to treat:

  - Chronic myelogenous leukemia (CML). It is used as palliative treatment. It is also used with other drugs to prepare patients with CML for a stem cell transplant.

- **Hydrea (Hydroxyurea)**. Hydroxyurea is approved to treat chronic myelogenous leukemia that is refractory (does not respond to treatment). The use of hydroxyurea to treat cancer is approved for the Hydrea brand. Hydroxyurea is also approved to treat sickle cell anemia. This use is approved for the Droxia brand.

Meningeal Leukemia

Cytosar-U (Cytarabine). Cytarabine is approved to be used with other drugs to treat acute myeloid leukemia (AML) and chronic myelogenous leukemia (CML). Cytarabine is also approved to be used alone to prevent and treat meningeal leukemia (leukemia that has spread to the meninges). It is given as intrathecal therapy. Cytarabine is also available in a different form called cytarabine liposome.

Liver Cancer

- **Nexavar (Sorafenib Tosylate)**. Sorafenib tosylate is approved to treat:

  - Hepatocellular carcinoma (a type of liver cancer) that cannot be removed by surgery.

  - Renal cell carcinoma (a type of kidney cancer) that is advanced.

Thyroid cancer in certain patients with progressive, recurrent, or metastatic disease that does not respond to treatment with radioactive iodine.

Non-Small Cell Lung Cancer

- **Xalkori (Crizotinib).** Crizotinib is approved to treat:
  - Non-small cell lung cancer that has metastasized (spread to other parts of the body). It is used in patients whose cancer has a certain type of chromosome mutation that affects the anaplastic lymphoma kinase (*ALK*) gene or the *ROS1* gene.
  - Crizotinib is also being studied in the treatment of other types of cancer.

- **Zykadia (Ceritinib).** Ceritinib is approved to treat non-small cell lung cancer that has metastasized (spread to other parts of the body). It is used in patients whose cancer has a mutation in the anaplastic lymphoma kinase (*ALK*) gene and who cannot be treated with crizotinib or have gotten worse while taking it.

Malignant Mesothelioma

- **Alimta (Pemetrexed Disodium).** Pemetrexed disodium is approved to be used alone or with other drugs to treat:
  - Malignant pleural mesothelioma in patients who cannot be treated with surgery.
  - Non-small cell lung cancer (certain types) in patients whose disease is locally advanced or has metastasized (spread to other parts of the body).

Melanoma

- **Yervoy (Ipilimumab).** Ipilimumab is approved to treat:
  - Melanoma.
  - It is used as adjuvant therapy in patients with melanoma in the skin and lymph nodes who have already had surgery.
  - It is used in patients whose disease cannot be removed by surgery or has metastasized (spread to other parts of the body).

- **Zelboraf (Vemurafenib).** Vemurafenib is approved to treat:
  - Melanoma that cannot be removed by surgery or has metastasized (spread to other parts of the body). It is used in patients whose cancer has a certain mutation in the *BRAF* gene.

Multicentric Castleman Disease

Siltuximab. Siltuximab is approved to treat multicentric Castleman disease in patients who do not have human immunodeficiency virus (HIV) or human herpesvirus 8 (HHV8).

Multiple Myeloma and Other Plasma Cell Neoplasms

- **Kyprolis (Carfilzomib).** Carfilzomib is approved to be used alone or with other drugs to treat:

  - Multiple myeloma.

  - It is used with lenalidomide and dexamethasone in patients whose disease has recurred (come back) and who have already received one to three other types of treatment.

  - It is used alone in patients whose disease has gotten worse during or after treatment with bortezomib and immunomodulator therapy.

- **Velcade (Bortezomib).** Bortezomib is approved to treat:

  - Multiple myeloma.

  - Mantle cell lymphoma in patients who have already received at least one other type of treatment.

Myeloproliferative Neoplasms

- **Gleevec (Imatinib Mesylate).** Imatinib mesylate is approved to treat:

  - Chronic eosinophilic leukemia or hypereosinophilic syndrome.

  - Chronic myelogenous leukemia that is Philadelphia chromosome positive.

  - Dermatofibrosarcoma protuberans.

  - Gastrointestinal stromal tumor (GIST).

  - Myelodysplastic/myeloproliferative neoplasms.

  - Systemic mastocytosis.

- **Jakafi (Ruxolitinib Phosphate)**. Ruxolitinib phosphate is approved to treat:

  - Myelofibrosis (a bone marrow disease) that is intermediate or high-risk.

  - Polycythemia vera in patients who cannot be treated with or have not gotten better with hydroxyurea.

Neuroblastoma

- **Unituxin (Dinutuximab)**. Dinutuximab is approved to be used with granulocyte-macrophage colony-stimulating factor (GM-CSF), aldesleukin (IL-2), and 13-cis retinoic acid to treat neuroblastoma that is high risk. It is used in children who had at least a partial response to other drugs and other types of treatment.

- **Vincasar PFS (Vincristine Sulfate)**. Vincristine sulfate is approved to treat:

  - Acute leukemia.

  - Hodgkin lymphoma

  Vincristine sulfate is also available in a different form called vincristine sulfate liposome.

Non-Hodgkin Lymphoma

- **Gazyva (Obinutuzumab)**. Obinutuzumab is approved to be used with other drugs to treat chronic lymphocytic leukemia (CLL). It is used with chlorambucil in patients who have not already been treated for CLL.

- **Prednisone**. Prednisone is approved to be used to reduce inflammation and suppress (lower) the body's immune response.

  Prednisone is used alone or with other drugs to prevent or treat the following conditions related to cancer:

- Anemia

- Drug hypersensitivity (allergic reactions)

- Hypercalcemia (high blood levels of calcium)

- Thrombocytopenia (low platelet levels)

Ovarian, Fallopian Tube, or Primary Peritoneal Cancer

- **Alkeran (Melphalan).** Melphalan is approved for palliative treatment of:

  - Multiple myeloma.

  - Ovarian epithelial cancer that cannot be removed by surgery.

  Melphalan is also available in an injectable form for patients who cannot take melphalan by mouth.

- **Taxol (Paclitaxel).** Paclitaxel is approved to be used alone or with other drugs to treat:

  - AIDS-related Kaposi sarcoma

  - Breast cancer

  - Non-small cell lung cancer

  - Ovarian cancer

  Paclitaxel is also available in a different form called paclitaxel albumin-stabilized nanoparticle formulation.

Pancreatic Cancer

- **Irinotecan Hydrochloride Liposome.** Irinotecan hydrochloride liposome is approved to be used with fluorouracil and leucovorin to treat:

  - Pancreatic cancer that has metastasized (spread to other parts of the body). It is used in patients whose disease has gotten worse after treatment with gemcitabine.

  - Irinotecan hydrochloride liposome is a form of irinotecan hydrochloride contained inside liposomes (very tiny particles of fat). This form may work better than other forms of irinotecan hydrochloride and have fewer side effects. Also, because its effects last longer in the body, it doesn't need to be given as often.

- **Sunitinib Malate.** Sunitinib malate is approved to treat:

  - Gastrointestinal stromal tumor (a type of stomach cancer). It is used in patients whose condition has become worse while taking another drug called imatinib mesylate or who are not able to take imatinib mesylate.

- Pancreatic cancer. It is used in patients with progressive neuroendocrine tumors that cannot be removed by surgery, are locally advanced, or have metastasized (spread to other parts of the body).

- Renal cell carcinoma (a type of kidney cancer) that has metastasized.

Gastroenteropancreatic Neuroendocrine Tumors

- **Somatuline Depot (Lanreotide Acetate).** Lanreotide acetate is approved to treat:

  - Gastroenteropancreatic neuroendocrine tumors. It is used for some tumors that cannot be removed by surgery, are locally advanced, or have metastasized.

Penile Cancer

- **Blenoxane (Bleomycin).** Bleomycin is approved to be used alone or with other drugs as palliative treatment of:

  - Penile cancer

  - Squamous cell carcinoma of the cervix

  - Squamous cell carcinoma of the head and neck (SCCHN)

  - Squamous cell carcinoma of the vulva

  - Testicular cancer

  Bleomycin is also approved to treat malignant pleural effusion and keep it from recurring.

Prostate Cancer

- **Jevtana (Cabazitaxel).** Cabazitaxel is approved to be used with prednisone to treat prostate cancer that has metastasized (spread to other parts of the body) in men whose cancer is hormone-refractory (does not respond to hormone treatment) and who have already been treated with other chemotherapy.

- **Nilandron (Nilutamide).** Nilutamide is approved to treat prostate cancer that has metastasized (spread to other parts of the body). It is used in patients who have had surgery to remove the testicles (orchiectomy).

Retinoblastoma

- **Neosar (Cyclophosphamide).** Cyclophosphamide is approved to be used alone or with other drugs to treat retinoblastoma.

Rhabdomyosarcoma

- **Dactinomycin.** Dactinomycin is approved to be used alone or with other drugs to treat rhabdomyosarcoma in children.

- **Vincasar PFS (Vincristine Sulfate).** Vincristine sulfate is approved to treat rhabdomyosarcoma. Vincristine sulfate is also available in a different form called vincristine sulfate liposome.

Basal Cell Carcinoma

- **Imiquimod.** Imiquimod is approved to treat:
  - Basal cell carcinoma that is superficial
  - Actinic keratosis
  - Genital warts

- **Odomzo (Sonidegib).** Sonidegib is approved to treat basal cell carcinoma that is locally advanced. It is used in patients whose disease has recurred (come back) after surgery or radiation therapy or who cannot be treated with surgery or radiation therapy.

Melanoma

- **Yervoy (Ipilimumab).** Ipilimumab is approved to treat:
  - Melanoma.
  - It is used as adjuvant therapy in patients with melanoma in the skin and lymph nodes who have already had surgery.
  - It is used in patients whose disease cannot be removed by surgery or has metastasized (spread to other parts of the body).

- **Zelboraf (Vemurafenib).** Vemurafenib is approved to treat melanoma that cannot be removed by surgery or has metastasized (spread to other parts of the body). It is used in patients whose cancer has a certain mutation in the *BRAF* gene.

Soft Tissue Sarcoma

- **Halaven (Eribulin Mesylate).** Eribulin mesylate is approved to treat:

  - Breast cancer that has metastasized (spread to other parts of the body). It is used in patients who have already been treated with an anthracycline and a taxane.

  - Liposarcoma (a type of soft tissue sarcoma) that cannot be removed by surgery or has metastasized. It is used in patients who have already been treated with anthracycline chemotherapy.

- **Yondelis (Trabectedin).** Trabectedin is approved to treat liposarcoma and leiomyosarcoma (types of soft tissue sarcoma) that cannot be removed by surgery or have metastasized (spread to other parts of the body). It is used in patients who have already been treated with anthracycline chemotherapy.

Stomach (Gastric) Cancer

- **Cyramza (Ramucirumab).** Ramucirumab is approved to be used alone or with other drugs to treat:

  - Adenocarcinoma of the stomach or gastroesophageal junction that is advanced or has metastasized (spread to other parts of the body). It is used in patients whose disease has gotten worse after treatment with certain chemotherapy. It is used alone or with paclitaxel.

  - Colorectal cancer that has metastasized. It is used with FOLFIRI in patients whose disease has gotten worse during or after treatment with certain anticancer drugs.

  - Non-small cell lung cancer that has metastasized. It is used with docetaxel in patients whose disease has gotten worse after treatment with certain chemotherapy. For patients whose cancer has a mutation in the epidermal growth factor receptor (*EGFR*) gene or anaplastic lymphoma kinase (*ALK*) gene, ramucirumab is used if their disease has gotten worse after treatment with FDA-approved therapy for these mutations.

- **Herceptin (Trastuzumab).** Trastuzumab is approved to be used alone or with other drugs to treat:

  - Adenocarcinoma of the stomach or gastroesophageal junction. It is used for HER2 positive (HER2+) disease that has metastasized (spread to other parts of the body) in patients who have not already been treated for metastatic cancer.

  - Breast cancer that is HER2+.

Testicular Cancer

- **Cyfos (Ifosfamide).** Ifosfamide is approved to be used with other drugs to treat testicular germ cell tumors that are malignant. It is used in patients who have already been treated with two other types of chemotherapy.

- **Etoposide Phosphate.** Etoposide phosphate is approved to be used with other drugs to treat:

  - Small cell lung cancer.

  - Testicular cancer. It is used in patients who have already been treated with surgery, radiation therapy, or other chemotherapy and have not gotten better.

Thyroid Cancer

- **Nexavar (Sorafenib Tosylate).** Sorafenib tosylate is approved to treat:

  - Hepatocellular carcinoma (a type of liver cancer) that cannot be removed by surgery.

  - Renal cell carcinoma (a type of kidney cancer) that is advanced.

  - Thyroid cancer in certain patients with progressive, recurrent, or metastatic disease that does not respond to treatment with radioactive iodine.

- **Vandetanib.** Vandetanib is approved to treat medullary thyroid cancer that cannot be removed by surgery and is locally advanced or has metastasized.

Vaginal Cancer

- **Recombinant Human Papillomavirus (HPV) Quadrivalent Vaccine.** Recombinant human papillomavirus (HPV) quadrivalent vaccine is approved to prevent some conditions caused by certain types of HPV. It is used in males or females aged 9 to 26 years to prevent vaginal cancer.

Vulvar Cancer

- **Blenoxane (Bleomycin).** Bleomycin is approved to be used alone or with other drugs as palliative treatment of:

  - Hodgkin lymphoma.

  - Non-Hodgkin lymphoma (NHL).

  - Penile cancer.

  - Squamous cell carcinoma of the cervix.

  - Squamous cell carcinoma of the head and neck (SCCHN).

  - Squamous cell carcinoma of the vulva.

  - Testicular cancer.

  Bleomycin is also approved to treat malignant pleural effusion and keep it from recurring.

Wilms Tumor and Other Childhood Kidney Cancers

- **Cosmegen (Dactinomycin).** Dactinomycin is approved to be used alone or with other drugs to treat:

  - Ewing sarcoma.

  - Gestational trophoblastic disease.

  - Rhabdomyosarcoma in children.

  - Solid tumors. It is used as palliative and/or adjuvant therapy for disease that has recurred (come back).

  - Testicular cancer. It is used for nonseminomas that have metastasized (spread to other parts of the body).

  - Wilms tumor.

- **Doxorubicin Hydrochloride**. Doxorubicin hydrochloride is approved to be used alone or with other drugs to treat:

  - Acute lymphoblastic leukemia (ALL).

  - Acute myeloid leukemia (AML).

  - Breast cancer. It is also used as adjuvant therapy for breast cancer that has spread to the lymph nodes after surgery.

  - Gastric (stomach) cancer.

  - Hodgkin lymphoma.

  - Neuroblastoma.

  - Non-Hodgkin lymphoma.

  - Ovarian cancer.

  - Small cell lung cancer.

  - Soft tissue and bone sarcomas.

  - Thyroid cancer.

  - Transitional cell bladder cancer.

  - Wilms tumor.

Doxorubicin hydrochloride is also available in a different form called doxorubicin hydrochloride liposome.

Section 10.2

Off-Label Drug Use in Cancer Treatment

This section includes text excerpted from "Off-Label Drug Use in Cancer Treatment," National Cancer Institute (NCI), January 1, 2014.

About Off-Label Drugs

Drugs can be legally sold in the U.S. only after the U.S. Food and Drug Administration (also known as the FDA) has approved them.

Drugs are approved after research shows they are safe and effective for a specific use.

Off-label drug use refers to the practice of prescribing a drug for a different purpose than what the FDA approved. This practice is called "off-label" because the drug is being used in a way not described on its package insert. This insert is known as its "label."

The label describes details of the drug, such as:

- What the drug is made of.

- How it works in the body.

- The research studies that led to its approval.

- Side effects it may cause.

The FDA must make sure that a drug is safe and effective for a specific use. However, it does not control the decision doctors make about which drugs to use for their patients. This means that once the FDA approves a drug, doctors can prescribe it for any purpose they think makes sense for the patient.

Off-label uses may include using an approved drug:

- For a different type of cancer than the one it is approved to treat

- At a different dose or frequency

- To treat a child when it is approved to treat adults

Off-label uses of a drug can become approved uses if the company that makes it obtains approval from the FDA. To gain the added approvals, the company must conduct research studies to show that the treatment is safe and effective for the new uses. However, a company may decide not to invest time and money in this research.

The Role of Off-Label Drug Use in Cancer Treatment

Research has shown that off-label use of drugs is very common in cancer treatment. Often, usual care for a specific type or stage of cancer includes the off-label use of one or more drugs.

Off-label drug use is common in cancer treatment because:

- Many cancer drugs are effective against more than one type of cancer.

- Cancer treatment often involves the use of combination chemotherapy.

Combination chemotherapy (which is treatment using more than one drug) is effective in treating many types of cancer. Examples of combination chemotherapy include:

- R-CVP to treat non-Hodgkin lymphoma

- CMF and TAC to treat breast cancer

- BEACOPP to treat Hodgkin lymphoma

- FOLFOX to treat colon cancer

These combinations might include one or more drugs not approved for the type of cancer they are being used to treat.

The FDA usually does not approve combinations of chemotherapy. There are so many of them that it would not be practical to approve each combination.

Research studies find new uses for drugs that are already approved. The results of research studies are published in medical journals and shared in the medical community. Doctors then adopt the new use and it may become an accepted and widely-used treatment for a different cancer, even if the FDA has not approved the drug for that use.

The Role of Off-Label Drug Use in Cancer Treatment

There are times when off-label drug use may cause harm, such as when:

- It has not been shown to be effective against certain cancer.

- There is no reason to believe the drug might be effective.

- The possible risks of giving the drug outweigh the possible benefits.

However, if your doctor prescribes a drug for an off-label use to treat your cancer, he or she is basing the decision on knowledge of and experience with the drug, as well as on research that shows it might be helpful for your stage and type of cancer.

Health Insurance Coverage of Off-Label Drugs in Cancer Treatment

Medicare and many insurance companies pay for off-label drugs for cancer treatment, as long as the off-label uses are listed in an approved compendium. A compendium is a collection of drug summaries put together by experts who have reviewed data about the drug's use in patients.

If your doctor prescribes an off-label drug for your treatment, check your plan to make sure the drug is covered. If coverage is denied, it may be helpful for the doctor to provide the insurance company with copies of documents that support the suggested off-label use.

Questions to Ask Your Doctor about Off-Label Drugs

Discussing these questions with your doctor can help you understand why your doctor might prescribe an off-label drug for you.

• Why do you think the off-label use of this drug will help the type of cancer that I have?

• Is the off-label drug likely to work better than an approved drug?

• What are the risks and benefits of treatment with this drug?

• Will my health insurance cover my treatment with this drug?

• If my treatment involves combination chemotherapy and one of the drugs is off-label, will my health insurance cover it?

Chapter 11

Complementary and Alternative Medicine (CAM) in Cancer Care

Complementary and alternative medicine (CAM) is the term for medical products and practices that are not part of standard medical care.

- **Standard medical care** is medicine that is practiced by health professionals who hold an M.D. (medical doctor) or D.O. (doctor of osteopathy) degree. It is also practiced by other health professionals, such as physical therapists, physician assistants, psychologists, and registered nurses. Standard medicine may also be called biomedicine or allopathic, Western, mainstream, orthodox, or regular medicine. Some standard medical care practitioners are also practitioners of CAM.

- **Complementary medicine** is treatments that are used along with standard medical treatments but are not considered to be standard treatments. One example is using acupuncture to help lessen some side effects of cancer treatment.

This chapter contains text excerpted from the following sources: Text in this chapter begins with excerpts from "Complementary and Alternative Medicine," National Cancer Institute (NCI), April 10, 2015; Text beginning with the heading "Acupuncture" is excerpted from "Topics in Integrative, Alternative, and Complementary Therapies (PDQ®)–Patient Version," National Cancer Institute (NCI), April 8, 2016.

- **Alternative medicine** is treatments that are used instead of standard medical treatments. One example is using a special diet to treat cancer instead of anticancer drugs that are prescribed by an oncologist.

- **Integrative medicine** is a total approach to medical care that combines standard medicine with the CAM practices that have shown to be safe and effective. They treat the patient's mind, body, and spirit.

Are CAM Approaches Safe?

Some CAM therapies have undergone careful evaluation and have found to be safe and effective. However there are others that have been found to be ineffective or possibly harmful. Less is known about many CAM therapies, and research has been slower for a number of reasons:

- Time and funding issues

- Problems finding institutions and cancer researchers to work with on the studies

- Regulatory issues

CAM therapies need to be evaluated with the same long and careful research process used to evaluate standard treatments. Standard cancer treatments have generally been studied for safety and effectiveness through an intense scientific process that includes clinical trials with large numbers of patients.

Natural Does Not Mean Safe

CAM therapies include a wide variety of botanicals and nutritional products, such as dietary supplements, herbal supplements, and vitamins. Many of these "natural" products are considered to be safe because they are present in, or produced by, nature. However, that is not true in all cases. In addition, some may affect how well other medicines work in your body. For example, the herb St. John's wort, which some people use for depression, may cause certain anticancer drugs not to work as well as they should.

Herbal supplements may be harmful when taken by themselves, with other substances, or in large doses. For example, some studies have shown that kava kava, an herb that has been used to help with stress and anxiety, may cause liver damage. Vitamins can also have unwanted effects in your body. For example, some studies show that high doses of vitamins, even vitamin C, may affect how chemotherapy and radiation work. Too much of any vitamin is not safe, even in a healthy person.

Tell your doctor if you're taking any dietary supplements, no matter how safe you think they are. This is very important. Even though there may be ads or claims that something has been used for years, they do not prove that it's safe or effective. Supplements do not have to be approved by the federal government before being sold to the public. Also, a prescription is not needed to buy them. Therefore, it's up to consumers to decide what is best for them.

National Cancer Institute (NCI) and the National Center for Complementary and Integrative Health (NCCIH) are currently sponsoring or cosponsoring various clinical trials that test CAM treatments and therapies in people. Some study the effects of complementary approaches used in addition to conventional treatments, and some compare alternative therapies with conventional treatments.

Things to Consider

Cancer patients who are using or considering using complementary or alternative therapy should talk with their doctor or nurse. Some therapies may interfere with standard treatment or even be harmful. It is also a good idea to learn whether the therapy has been proven to do what it claims to do.

To find a CAM practitioner, ask your doctor or nurse to suggest someone. Or ask if someone at your cancer center, such as a social worker or physical therapist can help you. Choosing a CAM practitioner should be done with as much care as choosing a primary care provider.

Patients, their families, and their healthcare providers can learn about CAM therapies and practitioners from the following government agencies:

- National Center for Complementary and Integrative Health (NCCIH)

- NCI Office of Cancer Complementary and Alternative Medicine (OCCAM)

- Office of Dietary Supplements (ODS)

Acupuncture

Acupuncture is a part of traditional Chinese medicine used in China and other Asian countries for thousands of years. In patients with cancer, acupuncture is usually used to relieve symptoms, treat side effects of therapy, and improve quality of life. It may help the immune system work better, control nausea and vomiting caused by chemotherapy, and relieve cancer pain. Acupuncture may treat weight loss, anxiety, depression, insomnia, poor appetite, and gastrointestinal symptoms (constipation and diarrhea).

Botanicals/Herbal Products

Black Cohosh

Black cohosh is a North American perennial herb. A substance found in the root of this plant has been used in some cultures to treat a number of medical conditions. Black cohosh has been studied to relieve hot flashes. However, randomized, placebo-controlled clinical trials using this herb have found that black cohosh is no better than a placebo in relieving hot flashes.

Cannabis and Cannabinoids (Also Known as Marijuana)

Cannabis is a plant from Central Asia that is grown in many parts of the world today. In the United States, it is a controlled substance and is classified as a Schedule I agent (a drug with increased potential for abuse and no known medical use). The Cannabis plant makes a resin that contains active chemicals called cannabinoids. Cannabinoids cause drug-like effects throughout the body, including the central nervous system and the immune system. Possible benefits of medicinal Cannabis for people living with cancer include control of nausea and vomiting, increasing appetite, relieving pain, and improving sleep.

Essiac/Flor Essence

Essiac and Flor Essence are herbal tea mixtures originally developed in Canada. They are marketed worldwide as dietary supplements. Supporters of Essiac and Flor Essence say that these products can help detoxify the body, make the immune system stronger, and fight cancer. There is no evidence in clinical trials that Essiac or Flor Essence can be effective in treating patients with cancer.

Flaxseed

Flaxseed comes from the flax plant. It is a rich source of omega-3 fatty acid, fiber, and a compound called lignin. It is being studied in the prevention of several types of cancer. Flaxseed has also been studied for its effect on hot flashes.

Ginger

Ginger is an herb that is used in cooking and in some cultures to treat medical conditions such as nausea. It can be used fresh, dried and powdered, or as a juice or oil. Ginger has been studied for the relief of nausea and vomiting in cancer patients.

Ginseng

Ginseng is an herb that is used to treat fatigue. It may be taken in capsules of ground ginseng root. Studies of ginseng have been done in patients either during or after their treatment for cancer. Patients who were given ginseng had less fatigue than patients who were given a placebo (inactive substance).

L-Carnitine

L-carnitine is a dietary supplement that is thought to be helpful in treating fatigue related to cancer. L-carnitine helps the body make energy and lowers inflammation that may be linked to fatigue.

Milk Thistle

Milk thistle is a plant whose fruit and seeds have been used for more than 2,000 years as a treatment for liver and bile duct disorders. The active substance in milk thistle is silymarin. Laboratory studies show that silymarin stimulates repair of liver tissue and acts as an antioxidant that protects against cell damage. It slows the growth of certain types of cancer cells and may make some types of chemotherapy less toxic and more effective.

Mistletoe Extracts

Mistletoe is a semiparasitic plant that has been used since ancient times to treat many ailments. It is used commonly in Europe, where a variety of different extracts are made and marketed as injectable prescription drugs. The FDA does not allow these injectable drugs to be sold in the United States and they are not approved as a treatment for patients with cancer.

PC-SPES

PC-SPES is a patented mixture of eight herbs. Each herb used in PC-SPES has been reported to have anti-inflammatory, antioxidant, or anticancer properties. PC-SPES was taken off the market because some batches were found to contain prescription medicines in addition to the herbs. The manufacturer is no longer in business and PC-SPES is no longer being made.

St. John's Wort

St. John's wort (*Hypericum perforatum*) is an herbal product sold as an over-the-counter treatment for depression. St. John's wort has not been proven to be better than standard antidepressant medicines. Many studies have been done to compare St. John's wort with antidepressants, placebo (inactive) medicines, or both, and have shown mixed results.

Be sure to talk with your doctor before taking St. John's wort. It may change the way some of your other medicines work, including anticancer medicines. Also, there are no standards for companies that make St. John's wort, so the amount of active ingredient may be different in each brand.

Selected Vegetables / Sun's Soup

"Selected Vegetables" and "Sun's Soup" are different mixtures of vegetables and herbs that have been studied as treatments for cancer. Dried and frozen forms of Selected Vegetables are sold in the United States as dietary supplements. The vegetables and herbs in Selected Vegetables/Sun's Soup are thought to have substances that block the growth of cancer cells and/or help the body's immune system kill cancer cells. There is limited evidence that Selected Vegetables/Sun's Soup is useful as a treatment for cancer and no randomized or controlled clinical trials have been done.

Mind-Body Therapies and Massage

Aromatherapy and Essential Oils

Aromatherapy is the use of essential oils from plants (flowers, herbs, or trees) as therapy to improve physical, emotional, and spiritual well-being. Patients with cancer use aromatherapy mainly as supportive care to improve their quality of life, such as lowering stress and anxiety.

Aromatherapy may be combined with other complementary treatments (e.g., massage and acupuncture) as well as with standard treatment.

Cognitive-Behavioral Therapy (CBT)

Cognitive-behavioral therapy (CBT) is a type of psychotherapy that helps patients change their behavior by changing the way they think and feel about certain things. CBT may be helpful in treating many side effects of cancer and cancer treatment.

Thinking and behavioral interventions focus on positive thoughts and images instead of negative thoughts and behaviors. Patients may gain a sense of control and develop coping skills to deal with the disease and its symptoms. These interventions also show promise for the treatment of insomnia in patients with cancer. Relaxation and imagery techniques may be used for short periods of pain or discomfort (e.g., during procedures). Quick, simple techniques are useful when the patient has trouble concentrating due to severe pain, anxiety, fatigue, or nausea.

CBT for may be helpful for depression in patients with cancer. Most counseling or talk therapy programs for depression are offered in both individual and small-group settings. CBT may also help decrease a cancer patient's fatigue by working on cancer-related factors that make fatigue worse. CBT may be used to treat posttraumatic stress disorder symptoms in patients with cancer. The treatment can focus on solving problems, teaching coping skills, and providing a supportive setting for the patient.

Hypnosis

Hypnosis is a trance-like state that allows a person to be more aware and focused and more open to suggestion. Under hypnosis, the person can concentrate more clearly on a specific thought, feeling, or sensation without becoming distracted.

Manual Lymphedema Therapy

Manual lymphedema therapy is a massage that helps move lymph fluid out of a swollen arm or leg into healthy lymph nodes where it can drain.

Qigong

Qigong is a form of traditional Chinese medicine that combines movement, meditation, and controlled breathing. Its purpose is to enhance the vital energy or life force that keeps a person's spiritual, emotional, mental, and physical health in balance. Some clinical trials, mostly in small numbers of patients with cancer, have shown that qigong may improve their quality of life and cancer-related fatigue.

Spirituality

Studies have shown that religious and spiritual values are important to most Americans. Many patients with cancer rely on spiritual or religious beliefs and practices to help them cope with their disease. For healthcare providers, spiritual or religious well-being are sometimes viewed as an aspect of complementary and alternative medicine.

Tai Chi

Tai chi is a form of traditional Chinese mind-body exercise and meditation that uses slow sets of body movements and controlled breathing. Tai chi is done to improve balance, flexibility, muscle strength, and overall health. Some clinical trials, mostly in small numbers of patients with cancer, have shown that tai chi may improve their quality of life and cancer-related fatigue.

Yoga

Yoga is an ancient system of practices used to balance the mind and body through exercise, meditation (focusing thoughts), and control of breathing and emotions. Yoga is being studied as a way to relieve stress and treat sleep problems in cancer patients.

Nutritional Therapies

Antioxidants and Cancer Prevention

Antioxidants are substances that may protect cells from the damage caused by unstable molecules known as free radicals. Free radical damage may lead to cancer. Examples of antioxidants include beta-carotene, lycopene, vitamins C, E, and A, and other substances. There has been some concern about whether antioxidants may make chemotherapy and radiation therapy less effective.

Coenzyme Q10

Coenzyme Q10 is made naturally by the human body. Coenzyme Q10 helps cells produce energy and acts as an antioxidant. Studies show that coenzyme Q10 may boost the immune system and protect the heart from damage caused by certain chemotherapy drugs. No report of a randomized clinical trial using coenzyme Q10 as a treatment for cancer has been published in a peer-reviewed scientific journal.

Dietary Supplements

Many studies suggest that the use of complementary and alternative medicine is common among prostate cancer patients, and the use of vitamins, supplements, and specific foods is frequently reported by these patients.

Gerson Therapy

The Gerson therapy is used by some practitioners as a treatment for cancer based on changes in diet and nutrient intake. An organic vegetarian diet plus nutritional and biological supplements, pancreatic enzymes, and coffee or other types of enemas are the main features of the Gerson therapy. Few clinical studies of the Gerson therapy have been published.

Gonzalez Regimen

The Gonzalez regimen is a cancer treatment that is tailored by the practitioner for each patient and is currently available only to the patients of its developer. It involves taking certain pancreatic enzymes thought to have anticancer activity. The regimen also includes specific diets, vitamin and mineral supplements, extracts of animal organs, and coffee enemas.

Lycopene

Lycopene is a carotenoid (a natural pigment made by plants). It is found in a number of fruits and vegetables, including apricots, guava, and watermelon. The main source of lycopene in the American diet is tomato-based products. Lycopene is thought to have antioxidant activity. Lycopene has been studied for its role in chronic diseases, including cardiovascular disease and cancer.

Melatonin

Melatonin is a hormone made by the pineal gland during the hours of darkness. It plays a major role in the sleep-wake cycle. Clinical studies in renal, breast, colon, lung, and brain cancer suggest that melatonin may make chemotherapy and radiation therapy more effective; however randomized, blinded trials are needed to study these results.

Modified Citrus Pectin

Citrus pectin is found in the peel and pulp of citrus fruits such as oranges, grapefruit, lemons, and limes. Citrus pectin can be modified with high pH and heat so that it can be digested and absorbed by the body. Modified citrus pectin (MCP) may have effects on cancer growth and metastasis. Some research suggests that MCP may be protective against various types of cancer, including colon, lung, and prostate cancer.

Pomegranate

The pomegranate (*Punica granatum L.*) is native to Asia and grown in many parts of the world. Different parts of the pomegranate fruit have bioactive compounds that may support good health, including antioxidants found in the peel. Certain pomegranate extracts have been shown in laboratory studies to slow the growth and spread of prostate cancer cells and to cause cell death.

Probiotics

Probiotics are live microorganisms used as a dietary supplement to help with digestion and normal bowel function. A bacterium found in yogurt called Lactobacillus acidophilus is the most common probiotic. The use of probiotics may be recommended in conditions related to diarrhea, gut-barrier dysfunction, and inflammatory response.

Selenium

Selenium is a trace mineral (a nutrient that is essential to humans in tiny amounts). Selenium is found in certain proteins that are active in many body functions, including reproduction and immunity. Selenium is being studied for its role in cancer.

Soy

Soy is from a plant native to Asia that grows beans used in many food products. Soy foods (e.g., soy milk, miso, tofu, and soy flour) contain phytochemicals that may have health benefits. Isoflavones are the most widely researched compounds in soy. Soy is being studied for the prevention of cancer, hot flashes during menopause, and osteoporosis (loss of bone density).

Tea

Tea has long been thought to have health benefits, and many believe it can help lower the risk of cancer. Tea contains polyphenol compounds including catechins, which are antioxidants that help protect cells from damage caused by free radicals.

Vitamin C, High-Dose

Vitamin C (ascorbic acid) is a nutrient that humans must get from food or supplements since it cannot be made in the body. Vitamin C is an antioxidant and helps prevent oxidative stress. It also works with enzymes to play a key role in making collagen. High-dose vitamin C has been studied as a treatment for cancer patients.

Vitamin D

Vitamin D is a nutrient involved in a number of functions that are essential for good health. Skin exposed to sunshine can make Vitamin D. It can also be consumed in the diet, but very few foods naturally contain vitamin D. These foods include fatty fish, fish liver oil, and eggs.

Vitamin E

Vitamin E is a nutrient that the body needs in small amounts to stay healthy and work the way it should. It is fat-soluble (can dissolve in fats and oils) and is found in seeds, nuts, leafy green vegetables, and vegetable oils. Vitamin E boosts the immune system and helps keep blood clots from forming. It also helps prevent cell damage caused by free radicals (unstable molecules in the body). Vitamin E is being studied in the prevention and treatment of some types of cancer. It is a type of antioxidant.

Pharmacologic Treatments

714-X

714-X is a chemical compound that contains camphor, a natural substance that comes from the wood and bark of the camphor tree.

Nitrogen, water, and salts are added to camphor to make 714-X. It is claimed that 714-X protects the immune system and helps the body fight cancer. No peer-reviewed studies of 714-X has been published to show that it is safe or effective in treating cancer.

Antineoplastons

Antineoplastons are drugs made of chemical compounds that are naturally present in the urine and blood. It has been claimed that antineoplaston therapy can be used to stop certain cancer cells from dividing, while healthy cells are not affected.

Cancell / Cantron / Protocel

Cancell/Cantron/Protocel is a liquid that has been made in different forms since the late 1930s. It is also known by the names Sheridan's Formula, Jim's Juice, JS-114, JS-101, 126-F, and the "Cancell-like" products Cantron and Protocel. The exact ingredients of Cancell/Cantron/Protocel are not known and it is not effective in treating any type of cancer.

Cartilage (Bovine and Shark)

Bovine (cow) cartilage and shark cartilage have been studied as treatments for people with cancer and other medical conditions for more than 30 years. Substances that prevent the body from making the new blood vessels that a tumor needs to grow have been found in bovine cartilage and shark cartilage. However, these substances have not shown an effect on the growth of normal cells or tumor cells.

Hydrazine Sulfate

Hydrazine sulfate is a chemical that has been studied as a treatment for cancer and as a treatment for body wasting (i.e., cachexia) that can develop with this disease. It has been claimed that hydrazine sulfate limits the ability of tumors to take in glucose, which is a type of sugar that tumor cells need to grow.

Laetrile / Amygdalin

Laetrile is another name for the chemical amygdalin, which is found in the pits of many fruits and in numerous plants. Cyanide is thought to be the active anticancer ingredient of laetrile. Laetrile has shown little anticancer activity in animal studies and no anticancer activity in human clinical trials.

Newcastle Disease Virus (NDV)

Newcastle Disease Virus (NDV) is usually thought to be an avian (bird) virus, but it also infects humans. It causes a potentially fatal, noncancerous disease (Newcastle disease) in birds, but causes only minor illness in humans. NDV appears to copy itself much better in human cancer cells than in most normal human cells and may have anticancer effects.

Chapter 12

Palliative Care

Dealing with the symptoms of any painful or serious illness is difficult. However, special care is available to make you more comfortable right now. It's called palliative care. You receive palliative care at the same time that you're receiving treatments for your illness. Its primary purpose is to relieve the pain and other symptoms you are experiencing and improve your quality of life.

Palliative care is a central part of treatment for serious or life-threatening illnesses. The information in this chapter will help you understand how you or someone close to you can benefit from this type of care.

What Is Palliative Care?

Palliative care is comprehensive treatment of the discomfort, symptoms and stress of serious illness. It does not replace your primary treatment; palliative care works together with the primary treatment you're receiving. The goal is to prevent and ease suffering and improve your quality of life.

This chapter includes text excerpted from "Palliative Care: The Relief You Need When You're Experiencing the Symptoms of Serious Illness," National Institute of Nursing Research (NINR), May 2011. Reviewed February 2017.

If You Need Palliative Care, Does That Mean You're Dying?

The purpose of palliative care is to address distressing symptoms such as pain, breathing difficulties or nausea, among others. Receiving palliative care does not necessarily mean you're dying.

Palliative care gives you a chance to live your life more comfortably. Palliative care provides relief from distressing symptoms including pain, shortness of breath, fatigue, constipation, nausea, loss of appetite, problems with sleep and many other symptoms. It can also help you deal with the side effects of the medical treatments you're receiving. Perhaps, most important, palliative care can help improve your quality of life.

Palliative care also provides support for you and your family and can improve communication between you and your healthcare providers.

Palliative care strives to provide you with:

- Expert treatment of pain and other symptoms so you can get the best relief possible.
- Open discussion about treatment choices, including treatment for your disease and management of your symptoms.
- Coordination of your care with all of your healthcare providers.
- Emotional support for you and your family.

Palliative Care Can Be Very Effective

Researchers have studied the positive effects palliative care has on patients. Recent studies show that patients who receive palliative care report improvement in:

- Pain and other distressing symptoms, such as nausea or shortness of breath.
- Communication with their healthcare providers and family members.

Emotional support. Other studies also show that palliative care:

- Ensures that care is more in line with patients' wishes.
- Meets the emotional and spiritual needs of patients.

Palliative Care Can Improve Quality of Life

Together with your primary healthcare provider, your palliative care team combines vigorous pain and symptom control into every part of your treatment. Team members spend as much time with you and your family as it takes to help you fully understand your condition, care options, and other needs. They also make sure you experience a smooth transition between the hospital and other services, such as home care or nursing facilities.

This results in well-planned, complete treatment for all of your symptoms throughout your illness—treatment that takes care of you in your present condition and anticipates your future needs.

Palliative Care versus Hospice Care

Palliative care is available to you at any time during your illness. Remember that you can receive palliative care at the same time you receive treatments that are meant to cure your illness. Its availability does not depend upon whether or not your condition can be cured. The goal is to make you as comfortable as possible and improve your quality of life.

You don't have to be in hospice or at the end of life to receive palliative care. People in hospice always receive palliative care, but hospice focuses on a person's final months of life. To qualify for some hospice programs, patients must no longer be receiving treatments to cure their illness.

Palliative Care Team

Palliative care is provided by a team of specialists that may include:

- palliative care doctors
- palliative care nurses
- social workers
- chaplains
- pharmacists
- nutritionists
- counselors and others

Palliative care supports you and those who love you by maximizing your comfort. It also helps you set goals for the future that lead to a meaningful, enjoyable life while you get treatment for your illness.

How Do You Know If You Need Palliative Care?

Many adults and children living with illnesses such as cancer, heart disease, lung disease, kidney failure, acquired immune deficiency syndrome (AIDS), and cystic fibrosis, among others, experience physical symptoms and emotional distress related to their diseases.

Sometimes these symptoms are related to the medical treatments they are receiving.

You may want to consider palliative care if you or your loved one:

- Suffers from pain or other symptoms due to any serious illness.

- Experiences physical or emotional pain that is not under control.

- Needs help understanding your situation and coordinating your care.

Start palliative care as soon as you need it. It's never too early to start palliative care. In fact, palliative care occurs at the same time as all other treatments for your illness and does not depend upon the course of your disease.

There is no reason to wait. Serious illnesses and their treatments can cause exhaustion, anxiety and depression. Palliative care teams understand that pain and other symptoms affect your quality of life and can leave you lacking the energy or motivation to pursue the things you enjoy. They also know that the stress of what you're going through can have a big impact on your family. And they can assist you and your loved ones as you cope with the difficult experience.

Working Together as a Team

Patients who are considering palliative care often wonder how it will affect their relationships with their current healthcare providers. Some of their questions include:

- Will I have to give up my primary healthcare provider?

- What do I say if there is resistance to referring me for palliative care services?

- Will I offend my healthcare provider if I ask questions?

Most important, you do not give up your own healthcare provider in order to get palliative care. The palliative care team and your healthcare provider work together.

Most clinicians appreciate the extra time and information the palliative care team provides to their patients. Occasionally a clinician may not refer a patient for palliative care services. If this happens to you, ask for an explanation. Let your healthcare provider know why you think palliative care could help you.

Getting palliative care is as easy as asking for it. In most cases, palliative care is provided in the hospital. The process begins when either your healthcare provider refers you to the palliative care team or you ask your healthcare provider for a referral. In the hospital, palliative care is provided by a team of professionals, including medical and nursing specialists, social workers, pharmacists, nutritionists, clergy and others.

Insurance Pays for Palliative Care

Most insurance plans cover all or part of the palliative care treatment you receive in the hospital, just as they would other services. Medicare and Medicaid also typically cover palliative care. If you have concerns about the cost of palliative care treatment, a social worker from the palliative care team can help you.

What Happens When You Leave the Hospital?

When you leave the hospital, your palliative care team will help you make a successful move to your home, hospice or other healthcare setting.

Ask for Palliative Care and Start Feeling Better Now

If you think you need palliative care, ask for it now. Tell your healthcare provider that you'd like to add palliative care specialists to your treatment team and request a consultation. If you want to find a hospital in your area that offers a palliative care program, you can go to the Palliative Care Provider Directory of Hospitals at www. getpalliativecare.org to search by state and city.

Chapter 13

Hospice Care

What Is Hospice Care?

Hospice is a special type of care in which medical, psychological, and spiritual support are provided to patients and their loved ones when cancer therapies are no longer controlling the disease. Hospice care focuses on controlling pain and other symptoms of illness so patients can remain as comfortable as possible near the end of life. Hospice focuses on caring, not curing. The goal is to neither hasten nor postpone death. If the patient's condition improves or the cancer goes into remission, hospice care can be discontinued and active treatment may resume. Choosing hospice care doesn't mean giving up. It just means that the goal of treatment has changed.

How Is Hospice Care Used in Cancer Care?

The hospice team usually includes doctors, nurses, home health aides, social workers, clergy or other counselors, and trained volunteers. The team may also include speech, physical, and occupational therapists, if needed. A hospice team member is on-call 24 hours a day, 7 days a week to provide support. The hospice team will work with the patient on the patient's goals for end-of-life care, not a predetermined plan or scenario. Hospice care is very individualized.

This chapter includes text excerpted from "Hospice Care," National Cancer Institute (NCI), October 25, 2012. Reviewed February 2017.

Hospice services may include doctor or nursing care, medical supplies and equipment, home health aide services, short-term respite (relief) services for caregivers, drugs to help manage cancer-related symptoms, spiritual support and counseling, and social work services. Patients' families are also an important focus of hospice care, and services are designed to give them assistance and support.

Hospice care most often takes place at home. However, hospice care can also be delivered in special in-patient facilities, hospitals, and nursing homes.

Who Is Eligible for Hospice Care?

Under most insurance plans in the United States, including Medicare, acceptance into hospice care requires a statement by a doctor and the hospice medical director that the patient has a life expectancy of 6 months or less if the disease runs its normal course. The patient also signs a statement saying that he or she is choosing hospice care. (Hospice care can be continued if the patient lives longer than 6 months, as long as the hospice medical director or other hospice doctor recertifies the patient's condition.)

The hospice team or insurance provider can answer questions about whether specific care decisions, such as getting a second opinion or participating in a clinical trial while in hospice care, would affect eligibility for hospice services.

How Can People Get Help Paying for Hospice Services?

Medicare and most Medicaid and private insurance plans cover hospice services.

Medicare is a government health insurance program for the elderly and disabled that is administered by the Centers for Medicare and Medicaid Services (CMS). The Medicare hotline can answer general questions about Medicare benefits and refer people to their regional home health intermediary for information about Medicare-certified hospice programs. The hotline number is 1–800–MEDICARE (1–800–633–4227); callers with TTY equipment can call 1–877–486–2048.

Medicaid, a federal-state partnership program that is part of CMS and is administered by each state, is designed for people who need financial assistance for medical expenses. Information about coverage is available from local state welfare offices, state public health departments, state social services agencies, or the state Medicaid office. Information about specific state locations can also be found online.

Information about the types of costs covered by a particular private policy is available from a hospital business office or hospice social worker, or directly from the insurance company.

Local civic, charitable, or religious organizations may also be able to help patients and their families with hospice expenses.

What Is the Difference between Hospice and Palliative Care?

Although hospice and palliative care share the same principles of providing comfort and support for patients, palliative care is available throughout a patient's experience with cancer, whereas hospice is offered only toward the end of life. A person's cancer treatment continues to be administered and assessed while he or she is receiving palliative care, but with hospice care the focus has shifted to just relieving symptoms and providing support.

Where Can People Learn More about Hospice?

The following organizations can provide more information about hospice.

National Hospice and Palliative Care Organization (NHPCO)
Helpline: 1–800–658–8898
Multilingual line1–877–658–8896
E-mail: caringinfo@nhpco.org
Website: www.caringinfo.org

The National Hospice and Palliative Care Organization's Caring-Info website (www.caringinfo.org) offers information and publications focused on improving end-of-life care for adults and children. The site includes a database of national hospice programs.

Chapter 14

Transitional Care Planning

"Transition of care" is a term that refers to the movement of cancer patients between environments, types of treatment, and healthcare professionals. Effective planning helps ensure that during these transitions appropriate care continues without interruption. Typically, this could mean shifting from the patient's primary care physician to a specialist and then from an office setting to a hospital, with a different team of physicians, nurses, and support staff. In many cases, there might then be another transition to a skilled nursing facility, with yet another new care team, and then either to the patient's home or a hospice, where care and support would likely come from another group of professionals, as well as family and friends.

Transitional Care Planning Assessments

Each time a patient is moved from one facility or team of healthcare professionals to another, or when treatment plans are altered, an assessment is conducted. Since each patient's condition, past treatment, family situation, and psychological state is different, assessments help the new team become familiar with all of these factors and effectively plan future care.

The team involved in the assessment may include physicians, nurses, dieticians, social workers, and therapists. And the basic assessment will typically consist of:

- a physical examination

- blood tests

- complete medical history

- psychological evaluation

- cognitive learning tests

- tests for physical abilities

In addition, the patient, and in many cases family members, will be interviewed to gather further information. Questions asked during an assessment may include:

- How well does the patient understand his or her condition?

- Was the patient independent prior to admission, and is he or she independent now?

- What kind of informal support people does the patient have, and what are their abilities?

- Is the patient capable of participating in his or her discharge planning? If not, who will be able to represent the patient?

- What are the patient's expectations for the transition?

- What healthcare professionals and services will be required to meet these expectations?

- Does the patient have preferences for care providers and facilities?

- Does he or she have full understanding of the risks and implications of these choices?

- Are the patient's resources adequate to manage the cost of the next level of care?

Transitional Care Options

Depending on the individual patient and his or her unique needs, there can be a wide variety of transition options available. In consultation with the transition team, the patient and family may need to consider some of the following options:

- **Facilities.** These can include hospitals, rehabilitation facilities, nursing homes, the patient's own home or the home of a caregiver, and hospice care, either in a dedicated facility or at home.

- **Caregivers.** The patient might be able to choose between professional caregivers, such as doctors, nurses, physical therapists, social workers, dieticians, mental-health counselors, trained home-care assistants, and members of the clergy.

- **Medications.** The options for medication can include chemotherapy, pain management, medications that address symptoms, antibiotics, wound care, blood transfusions, and drugs that improve lung or cell function.

- **Special programs.** There are likely to be programs available to help patients and families with the transition to the next phase. These can include palliative-care programs, community support groups, home healthcare assistance, employment counselors, legal-assistance specialists, hospice programs, and bereavement-counseling programs.

Implications for Caregivers

When family or friends are enlisted as caregivers, there are a number of questions that must be asked, both for the benefit of the patient and the caregiver him- or herself. Some of these include:

- Is the caregiver qualified to provide the level of care required? If not, the stress on the caregiver could rise to unacceptable levels, or the patient could actually be in danger.

- What training is available to ensure that the caregiver is adequately qualified?

- What professional support will be required to supplement the caregiver's responsibilities? This might include visiting nurses, social workers, physical therapists, or clergy.

- What decisions is the patient able to make, and which ones will be relegated to the caregiver?

- What special equipment will be needed for the patient's care? Will it fit into the home, and does the caregiver know how to operate it?

- What plans are in place to give the caregiver regular time away from the patient? This is a critical factor in maintaining the caregiver's mental and physical abilities.

End-of-Life Decisions

Patients with advanced cancer and their families are faced with a number of decisions that will affect the patient's quality of life as well as the mental well-being of his or her loved ones. Although many of these decisions are not pleasant to think about, it's important to discuss them, so family members are thoroughly familiar with the patient's wishes and are able to carry them out if he or she is unable to communicate them at a later point.

Some end-of-life decision includes:

- whether to begin, or continue, chemotherapy

- the choice of available symptom-control methods

- the choice of available pain-control medications

- whether or not cardiopulmonary resuscitation (CPR) is desired

- whether or not the patient wants to be put on a ventilator

- what religious or spiritual support the patient would like

Finally, a legal document known as an advance directive can be helpful in ensuring that the patient's decisions are known and that his or her wishes are carried out. There a two components to an advance directive, the living will and durable power of attorney. A living will covers medical decisions, such as whether the patient wants dialysis, breathing machines, or tube feeding to be employed, as well as issues like organ and tissue donation. A durable power of attorney is a legal document that names the person who will make healthcare decisions for the patient if he or she is unable to do so.

The best time to make end-of-life decisions is when the patient is still well enough to participate fully in the process. That way, the patient can be assured that his or her medical and legal wishes are clarified in writing, and family members are not burdened with the task of making these serious decisions for their loved one.

References

1. Naylor, Mary, PhD, RN, FAAN and Stacen A. Keating, PhD, RN. "Transitional Care: Moving Patients from One Care Setting to Another," *American Journal of Nursing*, September, 2008.

2. "Planning the Transition to End-of-Life Care in Advanced Cancer," National Cancer Institute (NCI), November 24, 2015.

3. "Transitional Care Planning," National Cancer Institute (NCI), April 27, 2014.

4. "Transitional Care Planning," The Regional Cancer Center, 2017.

5. "Transitions of Care: The Need for a More Effective Approach to Continuing Patient Care," JointCommission.org, June 27, 2012.

Part Three

Clinical Trials and Cancer Research Updates

Chapter 15

Should You Take Part in a Clinical Trial?

What Are Clinical Trials?

Clinical trials are research studies that involve people. Through clinical trials, doctors find new ways to improve treatments and the quality of life for people with disease.

Researchers design cancer clinical trials to test new ways to:

- Treat cancer

- Find and diagnose cancer

- Prevent cancer

- Manage symptoms of cancer and side effects from its treatment

Clinical trials are the final step in a long process that begins with research in a lab. Before any new treatment is used with people in clinical trials, researchers work for many years to understand its effects on cancer cells in the lab and in animals. They also try to figure out the side effects it may cause.

Any time you or a loved one needs treatment for cancer, clinical trials are an option to think about. Trials are available for all stages of cancer. It is a myth that they are only for people who have advanced cancer that is not responding to treatment.

This chapter includes text excerpted from "Clinical Trials Information," National Cancer Institute (NCI), June 22, 2016.

Every trial has a person in charge, usually a doctor, who is called the principal investigator. The principal investigator prepares a plan for the trial, called a protocol. The protocol explains what will be done during the trial. It also contains information that helps the doctor decide if this treatment is right for you. The protocol includes information about:

- The reason for doing the trial
- Who can join the trial (called "eligibility criteria")
- How many people are needed for the trial
- Any drugs or other treatments that will be given, how they will be given, the dose, and how often
- What medical tests will be done and how often
- What types of information will be collected about the people taking part

Why Are Clinical Trials Important?

People are living longer lives from successful cancer treatments that are the results of past clinical trials. Through clinical trials, doctors determine whether new treatments are safe and effective and work better than current treatments. Clinical trials also help find new ways to prevent and detect cancer. And they help improve the quality of life for people during and after treatment. When you take part in a clinical trial, you add to our knowledge about cancer and help improve cancer care for future patients. Clinical trials are the key to making progress against cancer.

Deciding to Take Part in a Clinical Trial

When you need treatment for cancer, you may want to think about joining a clinical trial. Like all treatment options, clinical trials have possible benefits and risks. By looking closely at all options, including clinical trials, you are taking an active role in a decision that affects your life. This section has information you can use when making your decision.

Possible Benefits

- You will have access to a new treatment that is not available to people outside the trial.
- The research team will watch you closely.

- If the treatment being studied is more effective than the standard treatment, you may be among the first to benefit.

- The trial may help scientists learn more about cancer and help people in the future.

Possible Risks

- The new treatment may not be better than, or even as good as, the standard treatment.

- New treatments may have side effects that doctors do not expect or that are worse than those of the standard treatment.

- You may be required to make more visits to the doctor than if you were receiving standard treatment. You may have extra expenses related to these extra visits, such as travel and child care costs.

- You may need extra tests. Some of the tests could be uncomfortable or time consuming.

- Even if a new treatment has benefits in some patients, it may not work for you.

- Health insurance may not cover all patient care costs in a trial.

Who Can Join

Every clinical trial has a protocol, or study plan, that describes what will be done during the trial, how the trial will be conducted, and why each part of the trial is necessary. The protocol also includes guidelines for who can and cannot take part in the trial. These guidelines are called eligibility criteria.

Common eligibility criteria include:

- Having a certain type or stage of cancer

- Having received (or not having received) a certain kind of therapy in the past

- Having specific genetic changes in your tumor

- Being in a certain age group

- Medical history

- Current health status

Criteria such as these help reduce the medical differences among people in the trial. When people taking part in a trial are alike in key ways, researchers can be more certain that the results are due to the treatment being tested and not to other factors.

Some people have health problems besides cancer that could be made worse by the treatments in a trial. If you are interested in joining a trial, you will receive medical tests to be sure that you fit for the trial.

Paying for Clinical Trials

As you think about taking part in a clinical trial, you will face the issue of how to cover the costs of care. There are two types of costs associated with a clinical trial: patient care costs and research costs.

Patient care costs. Patient care costs are those costs related to treating your cancer, whether you are in a trial or receiving standard therapy. These costs are often covered by health insurance. They include:

- Doctor visits

- Hospital stays

- Standard cancer treatments

- Treatments to reduce or eliminate symptoms of cancer or side effects from treatment

- Lab tests

- X-rays and other imaging tests

Research costs. Research costs are those related to taking part in the trial. Often these costs are not covered by health insurance, but they may be covered by the trial's sponsor. Examples include:

- The study drug

- Lab tests performed purely for research purposes

- Additional X-rays and imaging tests performed solely for the trial

When you take part in a trial, you may have extra doctor visits that you would not have with standard treatment. During these visits your doctor carefully watches for side effects and your safety in the study. These extra visits can add costs for transportation and child care.

Chapter 16

Joining a Cancer Clinical Trial

If you are thinking about joining a clinical trial as a treatment option, the best place to start is to talk with your doctor or another member of your healthcare team. Often, your doctor may know about a clinical trial that could be a good option for you. He or she may also be able to search for a trial for you, provide information, and answer questions to help you decide about joining a clinical trial.

Some doctors may not be aware of or recommend clinical trials that could be appropriate for you. If so, you may want to get a second opinion about your treatment options, including taking part in a clinical trial.

If you decide to look for trials on your own, the following steps can guide you in your search. This information should not be used in place of advice from your doctor or other members of your healthcare team. This chapter takes you through the following steps:

Step One: Gather Details about Your Cancer

If you decide to look for a clinical trial, you must know certain details about your cancer diagnosis. You will need to compare these details with the eligibility criteria of any trial that interests you. Eligibility criteria are the guidelines for who can and cannot take part in a certain clinical trial.

This chapter includes text excerpted from "How to Join a Cancer Clinical Trial," National Cancer Institute (NCI), June 23, 2016.

To help you gather details about your cancer, complete as much of the Cancer Details Checklist as possible. Refer to the form during your search for a clinical trial.

If you need help filling out the form, talk with your doctor, a nurse, or social worker at your doctor's office. The more information you can gather, the easier it will be to find a clinical trial to fit your situation.

Step Two: Find Clinical Trials

There are many lists of cancer clinical trials taking place in the United States. Some trials are funded by nonprofit organizations, including the U.S. government. Others are funded by for-profit groups, such as drug companies. Hospitals and academic medical centers also sponsor trials conducted by their own researchers. Because of the many types of sponsors, no single list contains every clinical trial.

Whichever website you use to search for clinical trials, be sure to bookmark or print a copy of the protocol summary for every trial that interests you. A protocol summary should explain the goal of the trial and describe which treatments will be tested. It should also list the locations where the trial is taking place. Keep in mind that protocol summaries are written for healthcare providers and use medical language to describe the trial that may be difficult to understand.

Step Three: Take a Closer Look at the Trials That Interest You

Once you have completed the Cancer Details Checklist and found some trials that interest you, you should now:

- Take a closer look at the protocol summary for each trial

- Use the questions below to narrow your list to include only those trials for which you would like to get more information

Don't worry if you can't answer all of the questions below just yet. The idea is to narrow your list of potential trials, if possible. However, don't give up on trials you're not sure about. You may want to talk with your doctor or another healthcare team member during this process, especially if you find the protocol summaries hard to understand.

Step Four: Contact the Team Running the Trial

There are a few ways to reach the clinical trial team.

- **Contact the trial team directly.** The protocol summary should include the phone number of a person or an office that you can contact for more information. You do not need to talk to the lead researcher (called the "protocol chair" or "principal investigator") at this time, even if his or her name is given along with the telephone number. Instead, call the number and ask to speak with the "trial coordinator." This person can answer questions from patients and their doctors. It is also the trial coordinator's job to decide whether you are likely to be eligible to join the trial. However, a final decision will probably not be made until you have met with a doctor who is part of the trial team.

- **Ask your doctor or another healthcare team member to contact the trial team for you.** The clinical trial coordinator will ask questions about your cancer diagnosis and your current general health that you may not be sure how to answer. So, you may want to ask your doctor or someone else on your healthcare team to contact the trial coordinator for you.

- **The trial team may contact you.** If you have registered to use the website of a clinical trial listing service and found a trial that interests you, the clinical trial team may contact you directly by using the phone number and email address you provide when you register.

Step Five: Ask Questions

Whether you or someone from your healthcare team speaks with the clinical trial team, this is the time to get answers to questions that will help you decide whether or not to take part in this particular clinical trial.

Step Six: Make an Appointment

If you decide to join a clinical trial for which you are eligible, schedule a visit with the team running the trial.

Chapter 17

Bioinformatics and Cancer

Big Data and Its Contribution to Biomedical Research

The volume of biological data collected during the course of biomedical research has exploded, thanks in large part to powerful new research technologies. The availability of these data, and the insights they may provide into the biology of disease, has many in the research community excited about the possibility of expediting progress toward precision medicine—that is, tailoring prevention, diagnosis, and treatment based on the molecular characteristics of a patient's disease.

Mining the sheer volume of "Big Data" to answer the complex biological questions that will bring precision medicine into the mainstream of clinical care, however, remains a challenge. Nowhere is this challenge more evident than in oncology. By some estimates, by the end of 2017, just the research performed using next-generation sequencing of patient genomes will produce one xabyte—one quintillion bytes, 10^{18} bytes, or a million times a million times a million bytes—of data annually. Much of these data will come from studies of patients with cancer.

Seeking Answers from Big Data in the Era of Precision Medicine

Establishing an infrastructure to store, analyze, integrate, and visualize large amounts of biological data and related information, as

This chapter includes text excerpted from "Bioinformatics and Cancer," National Cancer Institute (NCI), September 14, 2015.

well as providing access to it, is the focus of bioinformatics. Bioinformatics uses advanced computing, mathematics, and different technological platforms to physically store, manage, analyze, and understand the data.

Currently, researchers use many different tools and platforms to store and analyze the biological data they collect during the course of their research, including data from whole genome sequencing, advanced imaging studies, comprehensive analyses of the proteins in biological samples, and clinical annotations. It is often difficult to integrate and analyze data from these various platforms, however, and often researchers don't have access to the raw or primary data created by other studies or lack the computational tools and infrastructure necessary to integrate and analyze it.

In recent years, there has been a boom in the use of virtual repositories—"data clouds"—as a way to integrate and improve access to research data. Many of these efforts are still in their early stages, and questions remain about the optimal way to organize and coordinate clouds and their use.

National Cancer Institute's (NCI) Role in Bioinformatics

National Cancer Institute (NCI) has played a leading role in advancing the science of genomics, proteomics, imaging, and metabolomics, among other areas, to increase our understanding of the molecular basis of cancer.

The National Cancer Informatics Program (NCIP), part of NCI's Center for Biomedical Informatics and Information Technology (CBIIT), oversees the institute's bioinformatics-related initiatives. NCIP is involved in numerous research areas, including genomics and clinical and translational studies, and how to improve data sharing, analysis, and visualization. For instance, NCIP operates NCIP Hub, a centralized resource designed to create a community space to promote learning and the sharing of data and bioinformatics tools by cancer researchers. NCIP Hub itself is an experiment to see if the cancer research community finds the social and community aspects of the program useful for team science and multi-investigator research teams.

Under The Cancer Genome Atlas (TCGA), a research program that was supported by NCI and the National Human Genome Research Institute (NHGRI), researchers have conducted comprehensive molecular analyses of more than 11,000 patients using tumor and healthy tissue samples. More than 1,000 studies have been published based on TCGA-collected data.

Similarly, under NCI's TARGET (Therapeutically Applicable Research to Generate Effective Targets) program, researchers have identified genetic alterations in pediatric cancers, most of which are from children in clinical trials conducted by the Children's Oncology Group (COG). Data from these two initiatives and other NCI-supported studies have helped researchers better understand the biology of different cancers and identify potential new targets for therapies.

In some respects, however, these studies have only scratched the surface of what can be learned from the vast amount of data collected as part of this research. As a result, there has been a new push in the research community to find ways to make these data, and the tools to analyze them, more widely accessible.

Democratizing Big Data

As a federal agency, NCI is uniquely positioned to democratize access to cancer research data. The institute has launched several initiatives to provide researchers with easier access to data from TCGA, TARGET, and other NCI-funded research, and the resources to analyze the data.

Initiated in late 2014, the NCI Genomic Data Commons (GDC) will provide a single source for data from these initiatives and cancer research projects and the analytical tools needed to mine them. NCI is creating the GDC following a recommendation by the Institute of Medicine for a centralized "knowledge system" for cancer.

When it is publicly launched in mid-2016, the GDC will include data from TCGA and TARGET. However, it will be expanded over the next several years to include data from cancer research projects conducted by individual researchers or research teams. The GDC will provide the cancer genomics repository for projects falling under the NIH Genomic Data Sharing Policy. NCI is also funding several pilot programs that will use cloud technology to provide researchers with access to genomic and other data from NCI-funded studies. These NCI Cancer Genomics Cloud Pilots will be used to explore innovative methods for accessing, sharing, and analyzing molecular data.

Each pilot, implemented through commercial cloud providers, will operate under common standards but have distinct designs and means of sharing data and analytical tools, with the goal of identifying the most effective means for using cloud technology to advance cancer research.

Chapter 18

Cancer Vaccines

What Is the Immune System?

The immune system is a complex network of cells, tissues, organs, and the substances they make that helps the body fight infections and other diseases. The immune system's role in defending against disease-causing microbes has long been recognized. Scientists have also discovered that the immune system can protect the body against threats posed by certain damaged, diseased, or abnormal cells, including cancer cells.

White blood cells, or leukocytes, play the main role in immune responses. These cells carry out the many tasks required to protect the body against disease-causing microbes and abnormal cells.

Some types of leukocytes patrol the circulatory system, seeking foreign invaders and diseased, damaged, or dead cells. These white blood cells provide a general—or nonspecific—level of immune protection.

Other types of leukocytes, known as lymphocytes, provide targeted protection against specific threats, whether from a specific microbe or a diseased or abnormal cell. The most important groups of lymphocytes responsible for carrying out immune responses against such threats are B cells and T cells.

B cells make antibodies, which are large secreted proteins that bind to, inactivate, and help destroy foreign invaders or abnormal cells. Cytotoxic T cells, which are also known as killer T cells, kill infected

---

This chapter includes text excerpted from "Cancer Vaccines," National Cancer Institute (NCI), December 18, 2015.

or abnormal cells by releasing toxic chemicals or by prompting the cells to self-destruct (in a process known as apoptosis).

Other types of lymphocytes and leukocytes play supporting roles to ensure that B cells and killer T cells do their jobs effectively. These supporting cells include helper T cells and dendritic cells, which help activate both B cells and killer T cells and enable them to respond to specific threats.

Antigens are substances that have the potential to cause the body to mount an immune response against them. They help the immune system determine whether something is foreign, or "non-self." Normal cells in the body have antigens that identify them as "self." Self-antigens tell the immune system that normal cells are not a threat and should be ignored. In contrast, microbes are recognized by the immune system as a potential threat that should be destroyed because they carry foreign, or non-self, antigens.

Are Cancer Cells Recognized By the Immune System?

Cancer cells can carry both self-antigens as well as what are referred to as cancer-associated antigens. Cancer-associated antigens mark cancer cells as abnormal or foreign and can cause killer T cells to mount an attack against them. Cancer-associated antigens may be:

- Self-antigens that are made in much larger amounts by cancer cells than normal cells and, thus, are viewed as foreign by the immune system

- Self-antigens that are not normally made by the tissue in which the cancer developed (for example, antigens that are normally made only by embryonic tissue but are expressed in an adult cancer) and, thus, are viewed as foreign by the immune system

- Newly formed antigens, or neoantigens, that result from gene mutations in cancer cells and have not been seen previously by the immune system

However, several factors may make it difficult for the immune system to target growing cancers for destruction:

- Many cancer-associated antigens are only slightly altered versions of self-antigens and therefore may be hard for the immune system to recognize.

- Cancer cells may undergo genetic changes that may lead to the loss of cancer-associated antigens.

- Cancer cells can evade anticancer immune responses by killer T cells. As a result, even when the immune system recognizes a growing cancer as a threat, the cancer may still escape a strong attack by the immune system.

What Are Vaccines?

Vaccines are medicines that boost the immune system's natural ability to protect the body against "foreign invaders," mainly infectious agents that may cause disease.

When an infectious microbe invades the body, the immune system recognizes it as foreign, destroys it, and "remembers" it to prevent another infection should the microbe invade the body again in the future. Vaccines take advantage of this defensive memory response.

Most vaccines are made with harmless versions of microbes—killed or weakened microbes, or parts of microbes—that do not cause disease but are able to stimulate an immune response against the microbes. When the immune system encounters these substances through vaccination, it responds to them, eliminates them from the body, and develops a memory of them. This vaccine-induced memory enables the immune system to act quickly to protect the body if it becomes infected by the same microbes in the future.

What Are Cancer Vaccines?

Cancer vaccines belong to a class of substances known as biological response modifiers. Biological response modifiers work by stimulating or restoring the immune system's ability to fight infections and disease. There are two broad types of cancer vaccines:

- **Preventive (or prophylactic) vaccines,** which are intended to prevent cancer from developing in healthy people

- **Treatment (or therapeutic) vaccines,** which are intended to treat an existing cancer by strengthening the body's natural immune response against the cancer. Treatment vaccines are a form of immunotherapy.

Two types of cancer preventive vaccines (human papillomavirus vaccines and hepatitis B virus vaccines) are available in the United States, and one treatment vaccine (for metastatic prostate cancer) is available.

153

How Do Cancer Preventive Vaccines Work?

Cancer preventive vaccines target infectious agents that cause or contribute to the development of cancer. They are similar to traditional vaccines, which help prevent infectious diseases, such as measles or polio, by protecting the body against infection. Both cancer preventive vaccines and traditional vaccines are based on antigens that are carried by infectious agents and that are relatively easy for the immune system to recognize as foreign.

Most preventive vaccines, including those aimed at cancer-causing viruses (hepatitis B virus and human papillomavirus), stimulate the production of antibodies that bind to specific targeted microbes and block their ability to cause infection.

What Cancer Preventive Vaccines Are Approved in the United States?

- **Human papillomavirus (HPV) vaccines.** Persistent infections with high-risk HPV types can cause cervical cancer, anal cancer, oropharyngeal cancer, and vaginal, vulvar, and penile cancers. Three vaccines are approved by the U.S. Food and Drug Administration (FDA) to prevent HPV infection: Gardasil®, Gardasil 9®, and Cervarix®. Gardasil and Gardasil 9 are approved for use in females ages 9 through 26 for the prevention of HPV-caused cervical, vulvar, vaginal, and anal cancers; precancerous cervical, vulvar, vaginal, and anal lesions; and genital warts. Gardasil and Gardasil 9 are also approved for use in males for the prevention of HPV-caused anal cancer, precancerous anal lesions, and genital warts. Gardasil is approved for use in males ages 9 through 26, and Gardasil 9 is approved for use in males ages 9 through 15. Cervarix is approved for use in females ages 9 through 25 for the prevention of cervical cancer caused by HPV.

- **Hepatitis B virus (HBV) vaccines.** Chronic HBV infection can lead to liver cancer. The FDA has approved multiple vaccines that protect against HBV infection. Two vaccines, Engerix-B and Recombivax HB, protect against HBV infection only. Both vaccines are approved for use in individuals of all ages. Several other vaccines protect against infection with HBV as well as other viruses. Twinrix protects against HBV and hepatitis A virus, and Pediarix against HBV, poliovirus, and the bacteria that cause diphtheria, tetanus, and pertussis. Twinrix is approved for use in persons 18 years of age or older. Pediarix is approved for use in infants whose mothers are negative for the HBV surface antigen (HBsAg) and is given as early as 6 weeks of age through 6 years of age. The original HBV vaccine was approved by the FDA in 1981, making it the first cancer preventive vaccine to be successfully developed and marketed. Today, most children in the United States are vaccinated against HBV shortly after birth.

How Are Cancer Treatment Vaccines Designed to Work?

Cancer treatment vaccines are used to treat cancers that have already developed. They are intended to delay or stop cancer cell growth; to cause tumor shrinkage; to prevent cancer from coming back; or to eliminate cancer cells that have not been killed by other forms of treatment.

Cancer treatment vaccines are designed to work by activating cytotoxic T cells and directing them to recognize and act against specific types of cancer or by inducing the production of antibodies that bind to molecules on the surface of cancer cells. To do so, treatment vaccines introduce one or more antigens into the body, usually by injection, where they cause an immune response that results in T cell activation or antibody production. Antibodies recognize and bind to antigens on the surface of cancer cells, whereas T cells can also detect cancer antigens inside cancer cells.

Producing effective treatment vaccines has proven more difficult and challenging than developing cancer preventive vaccines. To be effective, cancer treatment vaccines must achieve two goals. First, like preventive vaccines, cancer treatment vaccines must stimulate specific immune responses against the correct target. Second, the immune responses must be powerful enough to overcome the barriers that cancer cells use to protect themselves from attack by killer T cells.

Has the FDA Approved Any Cancer Treatment Vaccines?

In April 2010, the FDA approved the first cancer treatment vaccine. This vaccine, sipuleucel-T (Provenge®), is approved for use in some men with metastatic prostate cancer. It is designed to stimulate an immune response to prostatic acid phosphatase (PAP), an antigen that is found on most prostate cancer cells. In clinical trials, sipuleucel-T increased the survival of men with a certain type of metastatic prostate cancer by about 4 months.

Unlike some other cancer treatment vaccines, sipuleucel-T is customized to each patient. The vaccine is created by isolating immune system cells called dendritic cells, which are a type of antigen-presenting cell (APC), from a patient's blood through a procedure called leukapheresis. These cells are sent to the vaccine manufacturer, where they are cultured together with a protein called PAP-GM-CSF. This protein consists of PAP linked to a protein called granulocyte-macrophage colony-stimulating factor (GM-CSF). The GM-CSF stimulates the immune system and enhances antigen presentation.

APC cells cultured with PAP-GM-CSF constitute the active component of sipuleucel-T. The cells are returned to the patient's treating physician and infused into the patient. Patients receive three treatments, usually 2 weeks apart, with each round of treatment requiring the same manufacturing process. Although the precise mechanism of action of sipuleucel-T is not known, it appears that the APCs that have taken up PAP-GM-CSF stimulate T cells of the immune system to kill tumor cells that express PAP.

In October 2015, the FDA approved the first oncolytic virus therapy, talimogene laherparepvec (T-VEC, or Imlygic®) for the treatment of some patients with metastatic melanoma that cannot be surgically removed. In addition to infecting and lysing cancer cells when injected directly into melanoma tumors, T-VEC induces responses in non-injected lesions, suggesting that it triggers an antitumor immune response similar to those of other anticancer vaccines.

How Are Cancer Vaccines Made?

All cancer preventive vaccines approved by the FDA to date have been made using antigens from microbes that cause or contribute to the development of cancer. These include antigens from HBV and specific types of HPV. These antigens are proteins that help make up the outer surface of the viruses. Because only part of these microbes is used, the resulting vaccines are not infectious and, therefore, cannot cause disease.

Researchers are also creating synthetic versions of antigens in the laboratory for use in cancer preventive vaccines. In doing this, they often modify the chemical structure of the antigens to stimulate immune responses that are stronger than those caused by the original antigens.

Similarly, cancer treatment vaccines are made using cancer-associated antigens or modified versions of them. Antigens that have been used thus far include proteins, carbohydrates (sugars), glycoproteins or glycopeptides (carbohydrate–protein combinations), and gangliosides (carbohydrate–lipid combinations).

Cancer treatment vaccines are also being developed using weakened or killed cancer cells that carry a specific cancer-associated antigen(s) or immune cells that are modified to present such an antigen(s) on their surface. These cells can come from a patient himself or herself (called an autologous vaccine, such as with sipuleucel-T) or from another patient (called an allogeneic vaccine).

Some cancer vaccines in late-stage development use viruses, yeast, or bacteria as vehicles (or vectors) to deliver one or more antigens into the body. The vectors themselves are naturally immunogenic (that is, they can stimulate an immune response) but are modified so that they cannot cause disease.

Other types of cancer treatment vaccines that are under development include those made using molecules of DNA or RNA that contain the genetic instructions for cancer-associated antigens. The DNA or RNA can be injected alone into a patient as a "naked nucleic acid" vaccine, or packaged into a harmless virus. After the naked nucleic acid or virus is injected into the body, the DNA or RNA is taken up by cells, which begin to manufacture the tumor-associated antigens. Researchers hope that the cells will make enough of the tumor-associated antigens to stimulate a strong immune response.

A number of different cancer-associated antigens are now being used to make experimental cancer treatment vaccines. Some of these antigens are found on or in many or most types of cancer cells. Others are unique to specific cancer types.

Are Adjuvants Used with Cancer Vaccines?

Substances known as adjuvants are often added to vaccines to boost their ability to induce potent anticancer immune responses.

Adjuvants used for cancer vaccines come from many different sources. Some microbes, such as the bacterium Bacillus Calmette-Guérin (BCG), can serve as adjuvants. Substances produced by bacteria, such as Detox B (an oil droplet emulsion of monophosphoryl lipid A and mycobacterial cell wall skeleton), are also frequently used as adjuvants. Biological products derived from nonmicrobial organisms can also be used as adjuvants. One example is keyhole limpet hemocyanin (KLH), which is a large protein produced by a marine mollusk. Attaching antigens to KLH has been shown to increase their ability to stimulate immune responses. Even some nonbiological substances, such as an emulsified oil known as montanide ISA–51, can be used as adjuvants.

Natural or synthetic cytokines can also be used as adjuvants. Cytokines are substances that are naturally produced by white blood cells to regulate and fine-tune immune responses. Some cytokines increase the activity of B cells and killer T cells, whereas other cytokines suppress the activities of these cells. Cytokines frequently used in cancer treatment vaccines or given together with them include interleukin 2 (IL2, also known as aldesleukin), interferon alpha, and granulocyte-macrophage colony-stimulating factor (GM–CSF, also known as sargramostim).

Do Cancer Vaccines Have Side Effects?

Before any vaccine is licensed, the FDA must conclude that it is both safe and effective. Vaccines intended to prevent or treat cancer appear to have safety profiles comparable to those of other vaccines. However, the side effects of cancer vaccines can vary among vaccine formulations and from one person to another.

The most commonly reported side effect of cancer vaccines is inflammation at the site of injection, including redness, pain, swelling, warming of the skin, itchiness, and occasionally a rash.

People sometimes experience flu-like symptoms after receiving a cancer vaccine, including fever, chills, weakness, dizziness, nausea or vomiting, muscle ache, fatigue, headache, and occasional breathing difficulties. Blood pressure may also be affected. These side effects, which usually last for only a short time, indicate that the body is responding to the vaccine and making an immune response, as it does when exposed to a virus.

Other, more serious health problems have been reported in smaller numbers of people after receiving a cancer vaccine. These problems may or may not have been caused by the vaccine. The reported problems have included asthma, appendicitis, pelvic inflammatory disease, and certain autoimmune diseases, including arthritis and systemic lupus erythematosus.

Vaccines that use cells or microbes might have additional side effects. For example, serious side effects of sipuleucel-T include infection near the site of injection and blood in the urine.

Vaccines, like any other medication affecting the immune system, can cause adverse effects that may prove life threatening. For example, severe hypersensitivity (allergic) reactions to specific vaccine ingredients have occurred following vaccination. However, such severe reactions are rare.

Can Cancer Treatment Vaccines Be Combined with Other Types of Cancer Therapy?

Yes. In many of the clinical trials of cancer treatment vaccines that are now under way, vaccines are being given with other forms of cancer therapy. Therapies that have been combined with cancer treatment vaccines include surgery, chemotherapy, radiation therapy, and some forms of targeted therapy, including therapies that are intended to boost immune system responses against cancer.

Several studies have suggested that cancer treatment vaccines may be most effective when given in combination with other forms of cancer therapy. For example, preclinical studies and early-phase clinical trials have demonstrated that radiation therapy can enhance the efficacy of cancer treatment vaccines. In addition, in some clinical trials, cancer treatment vaccines have appeared to increase the effectiveness of other cancer therapies.

Additional evidence suggests that surgical removal of large tumors may enhance the effectiveness of cancer treatment vaccines. In patients with extensive disease, the immune system may be overwhelmed by the cancer. Surgical removal of the tumor may make it easier for the body to develop an effective immune response.

Researchers are also designing clinical trials to answer questions such as whether cancer treatment vaccines work best when they are administered before, after, or at the same time as other therapies. Answers to such questions may not only provide information about how best to use a specific cancer treatment vaccine but also reveal additional basic principles to guide the future development of combination therapies involving vaccines.

Chapter 19

Drug May Reduce Treatment-Related Joint Pain for Some Breast Cancer Survivors

A drug most commonly used to treat depression may also reduce joint pain in some women being treated for early-stage breast cancer, according to the results of a randomized clinical trial.

After undergoing treatment for early-stage breast cancer, many postmenopausal women take drugs known as aromatase inhibitors to reduce the risk of the cancer returning. These drugs, however, can cause significant pain in women's joints and muscles.

The clinical trial showed that duloxetine (Cymbalta®), which is approved to treat depression and anxiety as well as fibromyalgia and nerve pain caused by diabetes, provided some relief from pain associated with aromatase inhibitors.

"Joint and muscle pain can lead some patients to discontinue treatment with these life-saving medications," said N. Lynn Henry, M.D., Ph.D., of the Huntsman Cancer Institute (HCI) at the University of Utah, who led the study. "Based on our results, duloxetine seems to be an effective drug for some patients who experience this pain."

Dr. Henry presented findings from the study, which was led by the National Cancer Institute (NCI)-supported clinical trials group SWOG,

This chapter includes text excerpted from "For Some Breast Cancer Survivors, Drug May Reduce Treatment-Related Joint Pain," National Cancer Institute (NCI), January 4, 2017.

formerly the Southwest Oncology Group, at the San Antonio Breast Cancer Symposium.

New Strategies Needed

The body uses an enzyme called aromatase to make estrogen. Drugs that block the activity of this enzyme, called aromatase inhibitors, have been found to reduce the risk of cancer returning in postmenopausal women whose breast tumors rely on estrogen to fuel their growth.

But many patients taking these drugs experience pain in the knees, hips, hands, and wrists, which can make everyday tasks difficult. About 20 percent of patients stop taking aromatase inhibitors due to side effects, according to Dr. Henry. She noted that patients are generally recommended to take aromatase inhibitors for 5 to 10 years, so new strategies for managing the side effects are needed.

For the duloxetine trial, the researchers enrolled 299 women at 43 NCI Community Oncology Research Program (NCORP) sites across the United States. The women had been treated with aromatase inhibitors for early-stage breast cancer and were experiencing joint pain caused by treatment. The women were randomly assigned to receive a 12-week course of duloxetine or a placebo.

Participants completed questionnaires about joint pain, depression, and quality of life at the beginning of the trial, and then again after 2, 6, 12, and 24 weeks. The pain questionnaire used a 0–10 scale; the researchers defined a clinically significant change in average pain as a decrease of 2 or more points from the time a patient entered the study.

Duloxetine and Placebo Reduced Pain

Over the first 12 weeks of the trial, the pain scores of women in the duloxetine group fell an average of 0.82 points more than those of the placebo group. Other measures, including worst pain, joint pain, and stiffness, underwent similar declines.

For the duloxetine group, the average pain score decreased from 5.44 at baseline to 2.91 at 12 weeks. But the average pain score also dropped in the placebo group during the same period, from 5.49 to 3.45. Both reductions were clinically significant, according to the standards of the trial.

The finding of a strong placebo effect in the control group was not entirely unexpected, noted Dr. Henry. Other studies of treatments for pain have reported similar effects, although the reasons are not clear.

"This trial demonstrates the need for more research" on responsiveness to placebo, she added.

By 12 weeks, 69 percent of patients in the duloxetine group and 60 percent of patients in the placebo group had a 2-point improvement in pain compared to before starting treatment. At 24 weeks, which was 12 weeks after the patients had stopped taking duloxetine or the placebo, the average pain scores were similar for the groups (3.37 in the duloxetine group and 3.42 for the placebo group).

The most common side effects of duloxetine were nausea, fatigue, and dry mouth, which is consistent with other studies involving the drug.

Exploring Multiple Approaches

"These results of the duloxetine study are very promising," said Ann O'Mara, Ph.D., of NCI's Division of Cancer Prevention, who was not involved in the study. "Duloxetine is the first drug to show a benefit for this population of patients in a large, randomized clinical trial."

Dr. O'Mara suggested that patients taking aromatase inhibitors might ultimately need to try multiple approaches to manage their pain. Exercise such as walking and acupuncture are among various strategies that are being studied as ways to reduce pain, she noted.

"Clinicians need to be clear with their patients about the potential side effects of duloxetine, but this drug may help patients decrease their pain and become functional again," she added.

Chapter 20

Better Care for Children with Cancer Linked to Longer Lifespans

Gradual refinements in the treatment of many childhood cancers over the last few decades have helped to extend the lifespans of many cancer survivors, a study suggests. An analysis of data on more than 34,000 childhood cancer survivors showed that the death rate among survivors at 15 years after their diagnoses fell from 12.4 percent to 6 percent between the early 1970s and early 1990s.

Gregory Armstrong, M.D., of the St. Jude Children's Research Hospital, presented the findings from the Childhood Cancer Survivor Study (CCSS) during a plenary session at the American Society of Clinical Oncology (ASCO) annual meeting in Chicago.

Although there have been tremendous advancements in the treatment of childhood cancers, some therapies can cause health problems that occur months or years after a disease is diagnosed or after treatment has ended. These so-called late effects may include a second primary cancer, heart or lung conditions, as well as other health issues such as cognitive declines and loss of fertility.

Compared with the general population, survivors of childhood cancer have a 15-fold increased risk of dying from a second cancer and a seven-fold increased risk of cardiac-related death, Dr. Armstrong noted.

This chapter includes text excerpted from "Better Care for Children with Cancer Linked to Longer Lifespans," National Cancer Institute (NCI), June 11, 2015.

165

The study found that, between the early 1970s and early 1990s, the cumulative incidence of death from "other health-related causes"—a category that primarily consists of mortality due to late effects of cancer therapy—decreased from 3.1 percent to 1.9 percent. And survivors diagnosed in the 1990s had a lower risk of dying from causes such as second cancers, heart disease, and lung disease than those diagnosed in the 1970s.

The reduction in mortality was most striking among survivors of Wilms tumor, Hodgkin lymphoma, and acute lymphoblastic leukemia (ALL).

The treatment changes that occurred during the study period included reductions in the doses of chemotherapy and radiation therapy that young patients received. These refinements were tested in clinical trials run through the National Cancer Institute (NCI)-funded Children's Oncology Group (COG), and the results showed that, in many cases, the intensity of a treatment could be reduced without compromising the therapy's effectiveness.

For example, in the 1970s, 85 percent of patients with ALL received cranial radiation, compared with only 19 percent in the 1990s. The dose of radiation used to treat patients with Hodgkin lymphoma and Wilms tumor has also been reduced substantially. The cumulative exposure to anthracyclines, a class of chemotherapy drugs that can have serious cardiac side effects, has also been reduced across these three diseases.

The results demonstrate the important role of risk-adapted therapy, said Malcolm A. Smith, M.D., Ph.D., of NCI's Division of Cancer Treatment and Diagnosis (DCTD). "Previously it had been shown that this strategy produced increased survival rates resulting from improved disease control, and now we know that mortality from late effects is also reduced by risk-adapted therapy," Dr. Smith said.

Improvements in the screening, detection, and treatment of late effects, as well as in supportive care, have also played an important role in extending the lifespan of these individuals, Dr. Armstrong noted.

Survivors of childhood cancer "have a lifetime to develop late effects," said Michael Link, M.D., of the Lucile Packard Children's Hospital Stanford (LPCH), in discussing these results during the American Society of Clinical Oncology (ASCO) plenary session. The reduction in mortality from treatment-related health effects confirms that when treating some children with cancer, "sometimes less is more," he said.

Even as treatment for childhood cancers begins to move toward the use of targeted therapies, Dr. Link continued, concerns about side effects and late effects will remain. He called for continued research to help clinicians learn about the factors, such as genetic variants, that can predict which patients are at the greatest risk of treatment toxicities and late effects.

Chapter 21

Advancements in Stem Cell Transplant

In a proof-of-concept study in mice, researchers from the Stanford University School of Medicine successfully performed hematopoietic (blood) stem cell (HSC) transplants (also called bone marrow transplants) without first using radiation or chemotherapy.

Instead of these toxic conditioning regimens, which are normally used to clear existing stem cells in the bone marrow before transplantation, the researchers used two biological agents that selectively eliminated HSCs in the host mice but left other tissues and organs undamaged.

If the technique can be translated to humans, "hematopoietic cell therapy could potentially be expanded to those who currently cannot safely tolerate the preparative therapy for bone marrow transplant," including frail, elderly patients, said Richard Little, M.D., of National Cancer Institute's (NCI) Cancer Therapy Evaluation Program (CTEP), who was not involved in the study.

Clearing the Way for New Stem Cells

Stem cell transplantation can be a lifesaving treatment for patients with some types of cancer, primarily blood cancers like leukemia and lymphoma.

This chapter includes text excerpted from "Approach May Allow for Stem Cell Transplant without Radiation, Chemotherapy," National Cancer Institute (NCI), September 7, 2016.

However, the procedure is sometimes grueling for patients and potentially dangerous. Prior to the transplant, patients are often treated with radiation and chemotherapy to kill existing stem cells in the bone marrow so the transplanted donor stem cells have a safe harbor in which to grow and repopulate the body with healthy blood cells (a process called engraftment). And, in the case of HSCs from a genetically similar but not identical donor (an allogeneic transplant), these conditioning treatments help to suppress an immune response against the transplanted cells.

But the conditioning regimen can damage a patient's healthy cells and tissues as well as their HSCs, resulting in side effects, including infections, respiratory problems, and organ damage that can be fatal in a small percentage of patients.

If the preparation for transplantation could be made less toxic to healthy cells, explained Judith Shizuru, M.D., Ph.D., the study's senior author, the procedure could potentially be used not just for cancer but for other indications. These include treating diseases caused by malfunctioning blood and immune cells, including autoimmune diseases and blood disorders marked by abnormal hemoglobin (such as sickle cell anemia or thalassemia), as well as improving gene therapy and organ transplantation.

Previous research, by the Stanford team and others, has shown that biological agents that target c-kit, a protein that HSCs use for many of their normal cellular functions, can deplete HSCs in mice lacking a functioning immune system. However, in earlier studies, targeting this single protein did not deplete the HSCs in mice with a functioning immune system.

So the Stanford researchers tested whether targeting a second protein, called CD47, in addition to c-kit could eliminate HSCs in mice with a healthy immune system. CD47 serves as a "marker of self" for HSCs and some other types of cells, telling the immune system not to attack them. By blocking CD47 with a specially designed molecule, the researchers hoped to make HSCs vulnerable to treatment with an agent targeting c-kit.

The combination worked. In mice with healthy immune systems that were treated with both agents, the researchers saw a 10,000-fold reduction in the targeted HSCs, to the point where "we could no longer measure them," said the study's lead author, Akanksha Chhabra, Ph.D.

In further experiments, mice with healthy immune systems were treated with both agents or with a c-kit-targeting agent alone and then underwent a modified form of an autologous stem cell transplant. The mice that received both agents showed 100 times more engraftment of the donor stem cells in their bone marrow than mice treated with the anti-c-kit agent alone, and healthy cells derived from the transplanted HSCs were found in the blood, spleen, bone marrow, and thymus.

The researchers also tested in mice whether the general approach would work in a type of allogeneic transplant. They treated mice with the two-agent conditioning regimen and with additional biological agents to deplete immune cells (T cells) to prevent the immune system from attacking the transplanted cells. The transplant was successful, with the donor cells successfully establishing themselves in the recipient's bone marrow and producing healthy blood and immune cells.

Toward Human Trials

Agents that target c-kit and CD47 have already been tested in human studies in healthy volunteers and cancer patients, respectively, explained Dr. Shizuru, and no major side effect have been observed. The team has also recently begun enrolling patients in a clinical trial using an agent that targets c-kit for children with severe combined immunodeficiency disease. In mice, added Dr. Chhabra, researchers have seen some graying of the fur and drops in sperm counts due to the c-kit antibody, but "when the treatment stopped, the sperm counts did go [back] up," she said. The study did not look at long-term effects on fertility.

The next step is to test the drug combination as a conditioning regimen for HSC transplantation in nonhuman primates, said Dr. Shizuru. Since the drugs have already begun human safety studies as single agents, she thinks early human trials of the combination for HSC transplantation could begin in the next 3 to 5 years.

"The goal of this study, and what we're hoping we've shown, is that we're going to change the way that blood and marrow transplants will be done in the near future," Dr. Shizuru said. "We foresee that transplants will be safer to perform and that many more patients can be treated with this potentially curative cellular therapy."

Chapter 22

Cancer Genomics

Why Genomics Research Is Critical to Progress against Cancer

The study of cancer genomes has revealed abnormalities in genes that drive the development and growth of many types of cancer. This knowledge has improved our understanding of the biology of cancer and led to new methods of diagnosing and treating the disease.

For example, the discovery of cancer-causing genetic and epigenetic changes in tumors has enabled the development of therapies that target these changes as well as diagnostic tests that identify patients who may benefit from these therapies. One such targeted drug is vemurafenib (ZELBORAF®), which was approved by the U.S. Food and Drug Administration (FDA) in 2011 for the treatment of some patients with melanoma who have a specific mutation in the *BRAF* gene as detected by an FDA-approved test.

Over the past decade, large-scale research projects have begun to survey and catalog the genomic changes associated with a number of types of cancer. These efforts have revealed unexpected genetic similarities across different types of tumors. Mutations in the *HER2* gene, for instance, have been found in a number of cancers, including breast, bladder, pancreatic, and ovarian.

Researchers have also shown that a given type of cancer, such as breast, lung, and stomach, may have several molecular subtypes. For

---

This chapter includes text excerpted from "Cancer Genomics," National Cancer Institute (NCI), March 13, 2015.

173

some types of cancer, the existence of certain subtypes had not been known until researchers began to profile the genomes of tumor cells.

The results of these projects illustrate the diverse landscape of genetic alterations in cancer and provide a foundation for understanding the molecular basis of this group of diseases.

Opportunities in Cancer Genomics Research

Although a large number of mutations that drive the development and progression of many types of cancer have been identified through large-scale research studies, some tumor types have not been deeply characterized. New technologies and the knowledge gained from previous genomic studies could be used to define the full set of driver mutations in many cancers. In some cancers, for example, the ability to compare tumor and normal DNA from the same patient allows researchers to discover potential driver mutations of those cancers.

Another opportunity is to expand the current use of genomic methods to investigate the molecular basis of clinical phenotypes. This approach could help researchers identify genetic changes that may distinguish aggressive cancers from indolent ones, for example. Similar approaches could be used to study the molecular basis of response to a given therapy, as well as mechanisms of resistance to treatment.

The wealth of data emerging from cancer genome studies increasingly will be integrated with patients' medical histories and clinical data. These integrated results could be used to develop more tailored approaches to cancer diagnosis and treatment, as well as to improve methods of predicting cancer risk, prognosis, and response to treatment.

Genomic tools will also be essential for analyzing results from precision medicine clinical trials, such as those being conducted by National Cancer Institute's (NCI) National Clinical Trials Network (NCTN).

Challenges in Cancer Genomics Research

Comprehensive analysis of cancer genomes has revealed a great deal of diversity in the genetic abnormalities found within cancers of a single type. Moreover, recurrent genetic alterations within these cancers are often involved in only a small percentage of cases. Discovering rare genetic alterations that drive cancers is therefore a challenge for the field.

Another challenge is acquiring high-quality biological samples needed for genomic studies, particularly for tumor types that are uncommon or rare, or those not treated primarily by surgery.

Developing cell lines and animal models that capture the diversity of human cancer is also an unmet need. Models of rare cancer subtypes may be nonexistent or underrepresented, and there are no models for many recurrent genetic lesions in human cancer.

Managing and analyzing the vast amounts of data involved in genomic studies are additional challenges for the field. This area of research requires an efficient bioinformatics infrastructure and increasingly involves contributions of data and expertise from cross-disciplinary teams.

Chapter 23

Missed Radiation Therapy Sessions Increase Risk of Cancer Recurrence

Risk of Cancer Recurrence

Patients who miss radiation therapy sessions during cancer treatment have an increased risk of their disease returning, even if they eventually complete their course of radiation treatment, according to a study.

The magnitude of the effect was higher than the researchers anticipated, which they believe suggests that noncompliance with radiation therapy may be an indicator for other risk factors that could negatively affect outcomes.

Worsening Outcomes

To conduct the study, Nitin Ohri, M.D., and Madhur Garg, M.D., of the Albert Einstein College of Medicine in New York, and their colleagues analyzed data from more than 1,200 patients at their hospital who had received external-beam radiation therapy as part of treatment

This chapter includes text excerpted from "Missed Radiation Therapy Sessions Increase Risk of Cancer Recurrence," National Cancer Institute (NCI), February 26, 2016.

with the intent to cure for cancer of the head and neck, breast, lung, cervix, uterus, or rectum between 2007 and 2012.

Patients who missed two or more scheduled radiation therapy appointments were categorized as noncompliant. On average, noncompliant patients (22 percent of the total) missed four radiation therapy appointments. Missing two or more appointments prolonged the course of radiation therapy by an average of 7.2 days. All of the patients in the study eventually completed their planned course of radiation therapy.

During the follow-up period, 9 percent of patients had their cancer recur and 19 percent died. After adjusting for demographic and clinical variables, including cancer type, patients who had been noncompliant with radiation therapy had an increased risk of disease recurrence and inferior rates of survival without disease recurrence.

"The conclusions are relatively intuitive: If you miss treatment, the outcome is not going to be as good," said Bhadrasain Vikram, M.D., chief of the Clinical Radiation Oncology Branch in NCI's Radiation Research Program. "But it's good to have objective scientific data to confirm that."

Some of the increased risk of recurrence, the authors believe, may be due to tumor repopulation—that is, cancer cells that remain after a halt in treatment dividing at an accelerated rate. But for many cancer types included in the study, previous studies have suggested that tumor repopulation does not have a significant impact on tumor recurrence and survival.

Instead, the authors suggested, noncompliance with radiation therapy may serve as a broader warning sign for additional risk factors that negatively affect outcomes, including unmet mental health needs, lack of social support, and noncompliance with other treatments, such as chemotherapy.

Mitigating Noncompliance

In their analyses, the researchers did not find independent effects of variables such as age, gender, race, and socioeconomic status on recurrence and survival, once noncompliance was taken into account.

Based on the results from this study, the radiation oncology unit at Einstein has instituted a new policy, Dr. Ohri explained.

"At every visit we look back and make sure that the patient has come to treatment every day that week, and [if not] ask the patient in real time: 'Why were you not here?'" he said.

The radiation oncologists can then provide immediate referrals to supportive care, mental health services, transportation assistance, or other resources.

Doing so, Dr. Ohri continued, allows them to more rapidly address these issues and help patients be compliant for the remainder of their treatment course.

"We're fighting cancer on two fronts," said Dr. Ohri. "On one front we're trying to enhance cancer care and come up with new treatments... that may be more effective than what we currently have available. But equally importantly...we also need to make sure that those advances are available to all of our patients. That's really what our goal is with this kind of research," he concluded.

Future research is needed to identify factors that reliably predict noncompliance before any treatment starts, said Dr. Vikram. "It would be very helpful to have something you could put your finger on, before you started treatment that says 'this person needs individual [help] in order to be compliant."

Chapter 24

Nanotechnology in Cancer Research

For more than 30 years cancers caused by oncogenic RAS mutants have resisted direct therapeutic attack. Using nanomedicines to target RAS-driven cancers at the genomic or RNA level while sparing normal tissues has engaged the imagination of researchers, yet these aspirations have not yet yielded any drugs used in human patients. As described below, the Nanotechnology Characterization Laboratory (NCL) of the National Cancer Institute (NCI) has helped universities, companies, and institutes evaluate hundreds of nanomedicine candidates. Rachael Crist and Scott McNeil of the NCL summarize the challenges that must be overcome on the path to successful nanomedicines, including those that may someday target mutant RAS.

Nanotechnology is often touted as one of the most promising drug delivery innovations in today's fight against cancer. Typically not drugs themselves, nanoparticles have the potential to deliver traditional cancer drugs to tumors with fewer side effects or to enable non-traditional drugs (e.g., proteins or nucleic acids) to be targeted to kill cancer cells. However, since the mid-nineties only two nanoparticle cancer treatments have been approved by the U.S. Food and Drug Administration (FDA). Doxil (Janssen Biotech), a liposomal formulation of doxorubicin, was the first nanomedicine approved (1995). In 2005 the albumin-bound paclitaxel formulation

This chapter includes text excerpted from "Nanotechnology for Treating Cancer: Pitfalls and Bridges on the Path to Nanomedicines," National Cancer Institute (NCI), June 8, 2015.

Abraxane (Celgene Corp.) was approved, largely by virtue of reduced side effects in the treatment of solid tumors. The question naturally arises, why aren't there more approved nanodrugs on the market? Why is their development taking so long? Based on experiences the lag between inception and delivery in the development of nanotechnology-based therapeutics can be ascribed to the complexity of the nanomaterials themselves. Nanomaterials are not pure entities. On the contrary, they are complex, polydisperse, and oftentimes multifunctional formulations—the term in the field is "non-biological complex drugs" (NBCDs). Many different physical and chemical traits must be fine-tuned for each application, including nanoparticle size, charge, surface chemistry, and hydrophobicity, and this tuning process requires a suite of skills and technologies that often must be developed iteratively. "One size does not fit all" is a truism in the field of nanomedicine.

For the past ten years the Nanotechnology Characterization Lab (NCL) of the National Cancer Institute has provided comprehensive nanomaterial characterization, testing and evaluation services to nanomedicine developers around the world. The NCL has analyzed over 300 different nanoformulations and worked with nearly 100 academic, government, and commercial organizations, affording a unique opportunity to study the advantages and disadvantages of various platforms, drugs, surface coatings, targeting ligands, etc.

With nanoparticle-enabled delivery of chemotherapeutics there is an opportunity to deliver more of the cytotoxic drug to the intended site, offering reduced off-target toxicities and/or enhanced efficacy (because the "maximum tolerated dose" can be higher). Formulation using nanotechnology can alter biodistribution, clearance, and pharmacokinetics compared to the legacy drug. Employing what is known as the enhanced permeability and retention (EPR) effect, nanoparticles can accumulate in tumor tissues because of their leaky vasculature and compromised lymphatic drainage. To take advantage of the EPR effect however, nanoparticles must be precisely engineered to evade the mononuclear phagocyte system (MPS). For example, nanomedicines should be small enough to avoid uptake by the liver and spleen (<250 nm), yet large enough to avoid clearance by the kidneys (>10 nm), and should remain in circulation long enough to allow for significant tumor accumulation (t1/2 > 3 hr). A nanomaterial's physicochemical properties are known to influence its biological performance. For example, a size difference as little as 2 nm has been shown to alter the route of clearance, and surface modification has been shown to alter biodistribution.

It goes without saying that the most critical step in nanomedicine evaluation is thorough and well-documented characterization of each batch of material. Without a comprehensive understanding of the formulation its biological analysis can be easily misinterpreted. Starting materials should be characterized; intermediate materials should be characterized and archived for side-by-side biological evaluation (e.g., non-targeted vs. targeted nanomaterials); and of course, the final material should be characterized. It is imperative to ascertain which parameters are the most important to measure, which ones affect biological activity, and what assay techniques are most appropriate.

A short list of essential parameters to investigate includes:

1. the level of polydispersity that is acceptable to maintain the desired efficacy;

2. whether or not the surface coatings/targeting ligands are covalently attached or simply physisorbed;

3. the level of surface coverage required for optimal biological performance; and

4. the stability (temperature, pH, shelf-life, in biological matrix, etc.) of the formulation.

There are a number of excellent articles that address the importance of these and other characterization aspects.

Additional challenges arise when delivering agents such as RNA, DNA, or proteins, especially avoiding undesired immune responses. Although many nanoparticles without these agents can also elicit immunological reactions, nanoparticles containing oligos or proteins are particularly susceptible. Some commonly observed toxicities include anemia, neutropenia, thrombosis, complement activation, cytokine induction, and allergic reactions. Screening for this variety of potential adverse conditions can be a challenge, and it is often difficult to predict which assays will be most relevant for a given formulation. The NCL has more than a dozen in vitro immunological assays tailored for nanomedicine evaluation.

Sterility and endotoxin contamination are other aspects many researchers fail to address in the developmental process. Almost one-third of the materials submitted to the NCL have endotoxin levels exceeding U.S. FDA limits. Even though materials submitted to the NCL are at the preclinical stage, high levels of endotoxin can interfere with the correct interpretation of many assays. Without a proper screen for endotoxin, toxicity may be mistakenly assigned to the nanomaterial, when in fact it stems from contamination during the synthesis and/or purification process. The NCL has studied endotoxin quantification in nanomaterials extensively and has several manuscripts offering more elaboration on the trials and tribulations of this topic.

Generic versions of nanomedicines, or nanosimilars, pose even more challenges. Recently the FDA approved the first "generic" nanomedicine. A generic version of Doxil (Sun Pharma) was approved for the treatment of ovarian cancer in 2013, nearly 20 years after approval of the innovator product. Researchers are now beginning to develop new and improved methods to verify the bioequivalence of these follow-on nanomedicines. However, there is an inherent challenge in defining similarity for a formulation that is naturally polydisperse, and determining whether or not these differences are meaningful. Because of the novelty of this area, the potential regulatory hurdles and additional characterization requirements for nanosimilars may not yet be fully realized.

Nanomedicine research is not unrealistic or unattainable. There are many who do this work superbly. But for the novice nano-researcher, here are a few key recommendations:

- Screen for endotoxin early.

- Ensure the biocompatibility of all formulation components.

- Monitor the complete removal of potentially toxic excipients and side products from the manufacturing and purification process.

- Certify batch-to-batch consistency and define acceptance criteria.

- Assess nanoparticle stability and drug release rates in vivo or in an appropriate biological matrix.

- Don't ignore immunological assessments.

- Don't skimp on proper controls and comparisons for in vivo studies. While this may save on costs in the short term, it usually doesn't in the long term.

- It is never too early to think about the big picture and how the research product should ultimately materialize. Researchers who focus on achieving a single optimal preclinical result often lose sight of clinical and regulatory requirements and end up facing unexpected (i.e., time consuming and costly) hurdles in their development path.

Chapter 25

Nanoparticle That Mimics Salmonella Counteracts Chemotherapy Resistance

Researchers at the University of Massachusetts Medical School have designed a nanoparticle that mimics the bacterium *Salmonella* and may help to counteract a major mechanism of chemotherapy resistance.

Working with mouse models of colon and breast cancer, Beth McCormick, Ph.D., and her colleagues demonstrated that when combined with chemotherapy, the nanoparticle reduced tumor growth substantially more than chemotherapy alone.

Chemotherapy Resistance

A membrane protein called P-glycoprotein (P-gp) acts like a garbage chute that pumps waste, foreign particles, and toxins out of cells. P-gp is a member of a large family of transporters, called ATP-binding cassette (ABC) transporters, that are active in normal cells but also have roles in cancer and other diseases. For instance, cancer cells can co-opt P-gp to rid themselves of chemotherapeutic agents, severely limiting the efficacy of these drugs.

This chapter includes text excerpted from "Nanoparticle That Mimics Salmonella Counteracts Chemotherapy Resistance," National Cancer Institute (NCI), August 22, 2016.

In previous work, Dr. McCormick and her colleagues serendipitously discovered that *Salmonella* enterica, a bacterium that causes food poisoning, decreases the amount of P-gp on the surface of intestinal cells. Because *Salmonella* has the capacity to grow selectively in cancer cells, the researchers wondered whether there was a way to use the bacterium to counteract chemotherapy resistance caused by P-gp.

"While trying to understand how *Salmonella* invades the human host, we made this other observation that may be relevant to cancer therapeutics and multidrug resistance," explained Dr. McCormick.

Salmonella and Cancer Cells

To determine the specific bacterial component responsible for reducing P-gp levels, the researchers engineered multiple *Salmonella* mutant strains and tested their effect on P-gp levels in colon cells. They found that a *Salmonella* strain lacking the bacterial protein SipA was unable to reduce P-gp levels in the colon of mice or in a human colon cancer cell line. *Salmonella* secretes SipA, along with other proteins, to help the bacterium invade human cells.

The researchers then showed that treatment with SipA protein alone decreased P-gp levels in cell lines of human colon cancer, breast cancer, bladder cancer, and lymphoma.

Because P-gp can pump drugs out of cells, the researchers next sought to determine whether SipA treatment would prevent cancer cells from expelling chemotherapy drugs.

When they treated human colon cancer cells with the chemotherapy agents doxorubicin or vinblastine, with or without SipA, they found that the addition of SipA increased drug retention inside the cells. SipA also increased the cancer cells' sensitivity to both drugs, suggesting that it could possibly be used to enhance chemotherapy.

"Through millions of years of co-evolution, *Salmonella* has figured out a way to remove this transporter from the surface of intestinal cells to facilitate host infection," said Dr. McCormick. "We capitalized on the organism's ability to perform that function."

A Nanoparticle Mimic

It would not be feasible to infect people with the bacterium, and SipA on its own will likely deteriorate quickly in the bloodstream, coauthor Gang Han, Ph.D., of the University of Massachusetts Medical School, explained in a press release. The researchers therefore fused SipA to gold nanoparticles, generating what they refer to as a nanoparticle mimic of *Salmonella*. They designed the nanoparticle to enhance the stability of SipA, while retaining its ability to interact with other proteins.

In an effort to target tumors without harming healthy tissues, the researchers used a nanoparticle of specific size that should only be able to access the tumor tissue due to its "leaky" architecture. "Because of this property, we are hoping to be able to avoid negative effects to healthy tissues," said Dr. McCormick. Another benefit of this technology is that the nanoparticle can be modified to enhance tumor targeting and minimize the potential for side effects, she added.

The researchers showed that this nanoparticle was 100 times more effective than SipA protein alone at reducing P-gp levels in a human colon cancer cell line. The enhanced function of the nanoparticle is likely due to stabilization of SipA, explained the researchers.

The team then tested the nanoparticle in a mouse model of colon cancer, because this cancer type is known to express high levels of P-gp. When they treated tumor-bearing mice with the nanoparticle plus doxorubicin, P-gp levels dropped and the tumors grew substantially less than in mice treated with the nanoparticle or doxorubicin alone. The researchers observed similar results in a mouse model of human breast cancer.

There are concerns about the potential effect of nanoparticles on normal tissues. "P-gp has evolved as a defense mechanism" to rid healthy cells of toxic molecules, said Suresh Ambudkar, Ph.D., deputy chief of the Laboratory of Cell Biology in NCI's Center for Cancer Research. It plays an important role in protecting cells of the blood-brain barrier, liver, testes, and kidney. "So when you try to interfere with that, you may create problems," he said.

The researchers, however, found no evidence of nanoparticle accumulation in the brain, heart, kidney, or lungs of mice, nor did it appear to cause toxicity. They did observe that the nanoparticles accumulated in the liver and spleen, though this was expected because these organs filter the blood, said Dr. McCormick.

Moving Forward

The research team is moving forward with preclinical studies of the SipA nanoparticle to test its safety and toxicity, and to establish appropriate dosage levels.

However, Dr. Ambudkar noted, "the development of drug resistance in cancer cells is a multifactorial process. In addition to the ABC transporters, other phenomena are involved, such as drug metabolism." And because there is a large family of ABC transporters, one transporter can compensate if another is blocked, he explained.

For the last 25 years, clinical trials with drugs that inhibit P-gp have failed to overcome chemotherapy resistance, Dr. Ambudkar said. Tackling the issue of multidrug resistance in cancer, he continued, "is not something that can be solved easily."

Dr. McCormick and her team are also pursuing research to better characterize and understand the biology of SipA. "We are not naïve about the complexity of the problem," she said. "However, if we know more about the biology, we believe we can ultimately make a better drug."

Chapter 26

Inherited Mutations in DNA-Repair Genes Found in Advanced Prostate Cancers

Nearly 12 percent of men with advanced prostate cancer have inherited mutations in genes that play a role in repairing damaged deoxyribonucleic acid (DNA), according to a study. Inherited mutations in DNA-repair genes—including *BRCA2*, *ATM*, and *CHEK2*—are associated with an increased risk of several other cancers, including breast, ovarian, and pancreatic cancer.

"This finding offers a new window into understanding how metastatic prostate cancers develop," said Peter Nelson, M.D., of the Fred Hutchinson Cancer Research Center, who co-led the study.

Reporting their results in the *New England Journal of Medicine* on July 6, the researchers noted that, in the future, men who have prostate cancer with these inherited mutations may be candidates for particular treatments, such as drugs that target molecular changes associated with defects in DNA repair.

Confirming an Unexpected Result

The study was sparked by an unexpected result of an earlier study. As the researchers were profiling genomic changes in metastatic

---

This chapter includes text excerpted from "Inherited Mutations in DNA-Repair Genes Found in Advanced Prostate Cancers," National Cancer Institute (NCI), July 25, 2016.

prostate cancers, they sequenced DNA from normal tissues in the same patients for comparison purposes. They found that 8 percent of men with metastatic prostate cancer in that study had inherited a mutation in a DNA-repair gene.

The proportion of inherited, or germline, mutations was so unexpectedly high that the researchers conducted the current study in part to see whether the high frequency of mutations was "reproducible when we were looking at a large population of men," explained coauthor Colin C. Pritchard, M.D., Ph.D., of the University of Washington.

The answer, he added, "was a resounding yes."

In fact, the frequency of germline mutations in 16 DNA-repair genes among 692 men with metastatic prostate cancer turned out to be even higher—11.8 percent. The researchers detected harmful germline mutations in a DNA repair gene among 82 of the 692 participants.

The frequency of inherited DNA-repair gene mutations in men in the study was higher than the prevalence of 4.6 percent among 499 men with localized prostate cancer who participated in The Cancer Genome Atlas project, the researchers noted.

"These findings raise the possibility that a high proportion of men with metastatic prostate cancer—1 in 8—may have germline mutations in DNA-repair genes," said James Gulley, M.D., Ph.D., chief of the Genitourinary Malignancy Branch in NCI's Center for Cancer Research, who was not involved in the research.

"DNA-repair genes may play a role in the progression to metastatic prostate cancer, and more research should be done to look at mutations in these genes in men with prostate cancer," Dr. Gulley added.

Potential Treatment Options

Given the high frequency of DNA-repair gene mutations in prostate cancer and the potential for information about these mutations to inform treatment decisions, Dr. Nelson recommends that all patients with metastatic prostate cancer discuss the possibility of germline testing for inherited mutations in DNA-repair genes with their physicians.

"The potential for new treatments for these patients is really exciting," said Dr. Pritchard.

For example, drugs known as PARP inhibitors, which block an enzyme that helps repair damaged DNA, have been approved for some patients with ovarian cancer and are being evaluated in men with prostate cancer. One of these agents, olaparib (Lynparza™), is approved for certain patients with ovarian cancer whose tumors have mutations in the *BRCA1* or *BRCA2* genes.

Although PARP inhibitors have not yet been approved for prostate cancer, the U.S. Food and Drug Administration (FDA) in January granted Breakthrough Therapy designation for olaparib for treating certain patients with prostate cancer. The decision was based on results from an early-stage clinical trial that showed a high response rate to olaparib among men with metastatic prostate cancer whose tumors did not respond to standard treatments and had defects in DNA-repair genes.

Another potential treatment is platinum-based chemotherapy, which has been tested in women with breast and ovarian cancers that have mutations in DNA-repair genes. A recent case report describes three patients with metastatic prostate cancer and *BRCA2* mutations who had exceptional responses to platinum-based chemotherapy, the study authors noted.

More research is needed to prospectively evaluate platinum-based chemotherapy in patients with metastatic prostate cancer, noted Dr. Nelson, who presented the study results in June at the annual meeting of the American Society of Clinical Oncology (ASCO). Nonetheless, he added, the findings have pointed "to potential treatments that we would not have thought of otherwise."

Additional Types of Cancer

Among all patients in the study (with and without germline DNA-repair gene mutations), 22 percent had a first-degree relative with prostate cancer. Some relatives had other types of cancer, including breast cancer, ovarian cancer, leukemia, lymphoma, pancreatic cancer, and other gastrointestinal cancers.

For instance, 51 of the 72 patients with an inherited DNA-repair gene mutation (71%) had a first-degree relative with a cancer other than prostate cancer, whereas 270 of the 537 patients without such a mutation (50%) did.

"The types of cancer in some of the family members of men with DNA-repair gene mutations were striking," said coauthor Michael Walsh, M.D., of Memorial Sloan Kettering Cancer Center. "We don't typically think of leukemia and lymphoma, for example, as being associated with mutations in DNA-repair genes."

The researchers have begun to investigate these cases to better understand the association between inherited DNA-repair gene mutations and various types of cancer.

"Based on our results," said Dr. Pritchard, "it looks as though asking men with metastatic prostate cancer about a family history of other cancers might be just as important as asking about their family history of prostate cancer."

"Sentinels" for Family Members

The findings may also have implications for family members who may have unknowingly inherited cancer-predisposing genetic mutations. Men with inherited DNA-repair gene mutations could serve as "sentinels" for family members who may carry the same genetic alterations, said Dr. Nelson.

For example, close female relatives of a patient with metastatic prostate cancer who carries an inherited harmful *BRCA1* mutation might want to be tested for the presence of the same mutation. If the relatives are found to have the mutation, they could consider taking steps to reduce their risk of developing breast or ovarian cancer.

Dr. Nelson noted that the investigators were conservative in their assessments of potential cancer-related mutations in DNA-repair genes, so the frequency of these mutations could be even higher. The patients in the study were nearly all white, however, and future studies need to include men of different racial and ethnic backgrounds, he added.

Guidelines on Genetic Screening

Tests for inherited mutations in DNA-repair genes are commercially available. But Dr. Walsh cautioned that, as with any type of genetic testing, "it is important for patients to go to centers that are familiar with the tests and how to interpret the results."

At the ASCO meeting, Judy Garber, M.D., M.P.H., of the Dana-Farber Cancer Institute discussed Dr. Nelson's presentation. She supported his recommendation to test all patients with metastatic prostate cancer for inherited mutations in DNA-repair genes.

A frequency of 11.8 percent is above the criteria for recommending genetic testing in nearly all European countries and "certainly for insurance coverage [of testing] in the United States," Dr. Garber said. There has been more interest in testing women for mutations in genes such as *BRCA2* than men, she continued, adding: "It's time we brought in the men."

By her calculation, only 4 of the 190 clinical trials involving PARP inhibitors include men with metastatic prostate cancer. Addressing the audience, she said, "You have a lot of opportunity, and now you have a real clue that you need to move forward."

In the meantime, some of the study authors have already begun to screen patients with metastatic prostate cancer for the mutations. "We are optimistic that this study and others will lead experts who create guidelines to takes a closer look at DNA-repair genes and metastatic prostate cancer," said Dr. Pritchard.

Chapter 27

Trials Produce Practice-Changing Results for Brain Cancer

The standard treatment that some patients with brain cancer receive is likely to change, based on findings from two large clinical trials presented at the American Society of Clinical Oncology (ASCO) annual meeting in Chicago this week.

Both trials showed that administering the chemotherapy drug temozolomide (Temodar®) in addition to radiation therapy increased how long patients lived overall and without their disease progressing. The trial investigators and other leading brain cancer researchers agreed that the results of the two trials will change the standard of care.

In addition to improving survival, both trials resolved important questions about whether specific groups of patients benefit from receiving temozolomide, said Mark Gilbert, M.D., chief of National Cancer Institute's (NCI) Neuro-Oncology Branch. "These are important studies in the brain cancer field," he said.

Improved Survival in Older Patients with Glioblastoma

One of the trials tested the regimen in patients with glioblastoma, one of the most aggressive types of brain cancer. The trial, led by the

This chapter includes text excerpted from "Trials Produce Practice-Changing Results for Brain Cancer," National Cancer Institute (NCI), June 9, 2016.

Canadian Cancer Trials Group (CCTG), focused on patients over the age of 65.

This is an important group of patients, said the trial's leader, James Perry, M.D., of Sunnybrook Research Institute in Toronto. The peak age for glioblastoma diagnoses is 64, Dr. Perry explained, and overall incidence of the disease has been creeping up in recent years. A pivotal 2005 trial showed that temozolomide can improve how long patients with glioblastoma live. The trial, however, was restricted to patients younger than 70, and very few patients over age 65 were included in the trial, he said.

Because of concerns about serious side effects of chemotherapy, radiation alone has been the standard of care for patients aged 70 and older, Dr. Gilbert explained.

"In fact, the radiation course is often truncated to 2, 3, or 4 weeks rather than the 6 weeks that is standardly used, along with chemotherapy, in the younger patient population," he said.

In the CCTG trial, more than 560 patients aged 65 and older with advanced glioblastoma were randomly assigned to receive either short-course radiation alone or radiation plus temozolomide, given both at the same time (concurrent) and for an additional 12 rounds after radiation (adjuvant).

Median overall survival in patients treated with both radiation and temozolomide was 9.3 months, compared with 7.6 months in patients who received radiation therapy alone. The radiation and temozolomide combination also modestly improved progression-free survival.

The 1-year and 2-year survival rates were 37.8 percent and 10.4 percent with radiation plus temozolomide, versus 22.2 percent and 2.8 percent with radiation therapy alone.

The researchers also identified a group of patients for whom the addition of temozolomide was especially beneficial: Patients whose tumors have an alteration of the *MGMT* gene, known as promoter methylation, had an overall survival of 13.5 months compared with 7.7 months in patients with the alteration who received only radiation therapy.

This was not necessarily a surprise, Dr. Perry noted. Earlier studies have shown that methylation of the *MGMT* promoter in glioblastoma is associated with better prognosis and improved response to chemotherapy. Approximately 46 percent of patients with glioblastoma have *MGMT* promoter methylation, Dr. Perry explained, a proportion that is consistent regardless of age at diagnosis.

Although there was "substantially more benefit" in patients whose tumors had *MGMT* promoter methylation, he said, "to our surprise, unmethylated patients also derived clinical benefit."

Adding temozolomide to radiation did not increase the toxicity of treatment, Dr. Perry said. In fact, he said, "most patients were able to easily complete the treatment plan."

Survival Improved for Rare Brain Cancer

The other trial, dubbed CATNON, included patients with a rare type of low-grade glioma called anaplastic glioma, of which only 1,200 to 1,500 cases are diagnosed each year in the United States. The trial enrolled only patients whose tumors lack the 1p/19q co-deletion, a molecular alteration in chromosomes 1 and 19 that is commonly seen in patients with some low-grade gliomas, named anaplastic oligodendroglioma.

Patients whose tumors have the 1p/19q co-deletion have a better prognosis and respond better to chemotherapy than patients whose tumors lack the alteration, explained the trial's lead investigator, Martin van den Bent, M.D., from the Erasmus MC Cancer Institute in the Netherlands.

So, given the need for new treatment options for patients whose tumors lack the 1p/19q co-deletion, Dr. van den Bent said, the CAT-NON trial was designed to determine whether these patients might benefit from adding temozolomide to standard radiation therapy.

The trial, which was led by the European Organization for Research and Treatment of Cancer (EORTC), involved nearly 120 institutions from around the world. Approximately 750 patients enrolled and were randomly assigned to one of four treatment arms: radiation therapy alone, concurrent radiation and temozolomide, radiation followed by adjuvant temozolomide, or radiation and concurrent temozolomide followed by adjuvant temozolomide.

At 5 years, 56 percent of patients who received adjuvant temozolomide (arms 3 and 4) were still alive compared with 44 percent of patients who did not (arms 1 and 2). Adjuvant temozolomide also more than doubled how long patients lived without their disease progressing: 42.8 months compared with 19 months.

Given the survival advantages seen when temozolomide is given to patients with glioblastoma, some oncologists already offer it to their patients with anaplastic glioma, explained Brian Alexander, M.D., of the Center for Neuro-Oncology at the Dana-Farber Cancer Institute.

From the perspective of potential side effects, it's not unexpected that temozolomide is given to such patients, Dr. Alexander continued. "Temozolomide has a degree of toxicity, but it is generally well tolerated," he said.

Of the two trials presented at ASCO, CATNON "will have the largest impact, because it has answered some fundamental questions about the role of adjuvant chemotherapy in patients with anaplastic glioma that does not have the 1p/19q chromosome loss," Dr. Gilbert said.

Dr. van den Bent and his colleagues are performing molecular analyses of tumor samples to determine whether patient treatment response correlates with the presence of other commonly seen genetic alterations in lower-grade gliomas, including mutations in the *IDH1* gene.

They are also continuing to follow the survival outcomes in patients treated with radiation alone and concurrent temozolomide, he said.

Chapter 28

Study Forecasts "Silver Tsunami" of Cancer Survivors

The aging of the U.S. population will result in a substantial increase in the number of older cancer survivors over the next quarter century, particularly those 85 and older, according to a study by National Cancer Institute (NCI) researchers.

Using statistical models to analyze population data, the researchers estimated that the overall number of cancer survivors in the United States will continue to grow substantially. But the proportion of survivors who are aged 65 or older will grow the most, with this group representing nearly three-quarters of cancer survivors by 2040, the researchers reported in a study published July 1 in *Cancer Epidemiology, Biomarkers & Prevention*.

"Current U.S. demographics will literally change the face of the survivor population in the decades to come," wrote Shirley Bluethmann, Ph.D., M.P.H., of NCI's Division of Cancer Control and Population Sciences (DCCPS), who led the study with her DCCPS colleagues.

A "Silver Tsunami" of Cancer Survivors

The number of long-term cancer survivors has continued to grow over the past several decades. With this growth has come the

This chapter includes text excerpted from "Study Forecasts "Silver Tsunami" of Cancer Survivors," National Cancer Institute (NCI), July 8, 2016.

recognition that many cancer survivors have unique healthcare needs as a consequence of their cancer or the treatments they received.

Concerns have been raised about whether the healthcare system has the capacity to satisfy the growing demand for cancer and survivorship care, with physician organizations forecasting shortages of oncologists and family physicians, both of which represent the primary medical providers for cancer survivors.

And the strain on the system is only expected to worsen as the U.S. population ages. Every day, thousands of "baby boomers" are turning 65 years old, and many of those with cancer will also have other medical conditions, from cardiac and respiratory diseases to diabetes and rheumatologic conditions.

These trends, the NCI researchers wrote, "foreshadow a 'silver tsunami' of cancer survivors whose health needs we are unprepared to meet."

To better understand the composition of the cancer survivor population and their other medical conditions, or comorbidities, the researchers made projections based on data from NCI's Surveillance, Epidemiology, and End Results (SEER) program, including the SEER-Medicare linked database, and the U.S. Census Bureau.

By 2040, the researchers estimated, the number of cancer survivors in the United States will increase by nearly 11 million: from 15.5 million in 2016 to 26.1 million in 2040. Moreover, they found, the makeup of the cancer survivor population will change substantially over that time period, with the proportion of survivors aged 65 or older increasing from 61 percent to 73 percent. By 2040, only 18 percent of cancer survivors will be between ages 50 and 64, and only 8 percent will be younger than 50.

A unique aspect of this study, Dr. Bluethmann explained in an interview, was that the researchers were able to assess specific cancer burden by age groups of older survivors.

"Many studies tend to group all older people together into a category of 'ages 65 and older,'" she said. "But, we know that the health and function of older adults is extremely diverse and thought it would be valuable to provide more discrete estimates of prevalence across the older population of survivors."

For example, they estimated that by 2040, a sizable portion of the older survivor population will be aged 85 or older. In fact, when they extended the starting point for their analysis back to 1975, they estimated that those aged 85 and older would have the sharpest increase in the number of cancer survivors by 2040.

The researchers also used SEER and Medicare data to assess the current extent of comorbidities in cancer survivors aged 65 and older compared with people in the same age range without a history of cancer. They tracked the prevalence of 16 common conditions that had been assessed in earlier population-based studies of older people, including a history of heart attack, liver disease, diabetes, and vascular conditions.

Overall, the comorbidity burden tracked more closely with age than with whether somebody had a prior cancer diagnosis. For example, the comorbidity burden among cancer survivors aged 66–74 was similar to the burden in the noncancer population of that age group.

But, not surprisingly, the extent of severe health problems in both cancer survivors and people without a history of cancer increased dramatically with age. For instance, 26 percent of survivors and 16 percent of those without a cancer history in their late 60s had severe comorbidities, compared with 47 percent and 42 percent, respectively, of those aged 85 years and older.

Cancer site also appears to be an important factor in comorbidity burden, the researchers found. In particular, most lung cancer survivors had a severe comorbidity burden compared with survivors of other cancer sites, even in the 65-69 age group.

The authors cautioned that their study may underestimate the extent of comorbidities among cancer survivors because it did not include other conditions—such as high blood pressure, arthritis, and atrial fibrillation—that are common in older populations and because medical records often don't capture all of a patient's health conditions.

Changes Needed to Address Older Survivors' Needs

The findings from this study and others make it clear that important changes are needed to meet the needs of older cancer survivors, noted study coauthor Julia Rowland, Ph.D., director of NCI's Office of Cancer Survivorship.

Those changes include enrolling more older and elderly patients in clinical trials, which will help researchers and clinicians better understand age-appropriate treatment plans and potentially reduce long-term treatment-related side effects. Greater participation by older adults in clinical trials may also provide much needed information about support resources and programs for cancer survivors in long-term recovery, Dr. Rowland said.

"Most older adults diagnosed with cancer present with two or more comorbid conditions," she continued. "Figuring out how to manage these in the context of cancer is an important goal."

And the expanding population of survivors clearly has repercussions for how their medical needs will be met, Dr. Rowland continued.

"Training diverse providers—including nurses, nurse practitioners, and physician assistants—to help with cancer-specific follow-up may be important to assist in the growing burden of caring for older survivors," she said.

Many informal caregivers of cancer survivors are poorly equipped to meet the demands of providing routine medical care to their loved ones. So Dr. Rowland said that researchers also need to continue to assess the impact of caregiving on these informal providers, including whether providing them with training "can improve their health as well as that of their loved one."

Part Four

Coping with Side Effects and Complications of Cancer Treatment

Chapter 29

Nausea and Vomiting

Nausea and vomiting are very distressing side effects of cancer therapy and affect most patients who have chemotherapy.

Nausea is an unpleasant wavelike feeling in the back of the throat and/or stomach that may lead to vomiting. Vomiting is throwing up the contents of the stomach through the mouth. Retching is the movement of the stomach and esophagus without vomiting and is also called dry heaves. Although treatments have improved, nausea and vomiting are still serious side effects of cancer therapy. Some patients are bothered more by nausea than by vomiting.

Prevention and Control

It is very important to prevent and control nausea and vomiting in patients with cancer so that they can continue treatment and perform activities of daily life. Nausea and vomiting that are not controlled can cause the following:

- Chemical changes in the body

- Mental changes

- Loss of appetite

- Malnutrition

- Dehydration

This chapter includes text excerpted from "Nausea and Vomiting (PDQ®)– Patient Version," National Cancer Institute (NCI), September 2, 2015.

- A torn esophagus

- Broken bones

- Reopening of surgical wounds

There are many types of nausea and vomiting that are caused by cancer therapy:

- Acute

- Delayed

- Anticipatory

- Breakthrough

- Refractory

- Chronic

Acute nausea and vomiting: Nausea and vomiting that happen within 24 hours after beginning chemotherapy.

Delayed nausea and vomiting: Nausea and vomiting that happen more than 24 hours after chemotherapy. Also called late nausea and vomiting.

Anticipatory nausea and vomiting: Nausea and vomiting that happen before a chemotherapy treatment begins. If a patient has had nausea and vomiting after an earlier chemotherapy treatment, he or she may have anticipatory nausea and vomiting before the next treatment. This usually begins after the third or fourth treatment. The smells, sights, and sounds of the treatment room may remind the patient of previous times and may trigger nausea and vomiting before chemotherapy has even begun.

Breakthrough nausea and vomiting: Nausea and vomiting that happen within five days after getting antinausea treatment. Different drugs or doses are needed to prevent more nausea and vomiting.

Refractory nausea and vomiting: Nausea and vomiting that does not respond to drugs taken to prevent it.

Chronic nausea and vomiting: In patients with advanced cancer, chronic nausea and vomiting may be caused by radiation therapy. Other causes of chronic nausea and vomiting include the following:

- Brain tumors or pressure on the brain

- Colon tumors

- Stomach ulcers

- Dehydration

- High or low levels of certain substances in the blood
- Medicines such as opioids or antidepressants

Causes

Chemotherapy is the most common cause of nausea and vomiting in patients being treated for cancer.

Nausea is controlled by a part of the central nervous system that controls involuntary body functions (like the heart beating). Vomiting is a reflex controlled by a vomiting center in the brain. Vomiting can be triggered by smell, taste, anxiety, pain, motion, poor blood flow, irritation, or changes in the body caused by inflammation.

Many Factors Increase the Risk for Nausea and Vomiting

Nausea and vomiting are more likely if the patient:

- Had severe or frequent periods of nausea and vomiting after past chemotherapy treatments
- Is female
- Is younger than 50 years
- Had motion sickness or vomiting with a past pregnancy
- Has a fluid and/or electrolyte imbalance (dehydration, too much calcium in the blood, or too much fluid in the body's tissues)
- Has a tumor in the gastrointestinal tract, liver, or brain
- Has constipation
- Is receiving certain drugs, such as opioids (pain medicine)
- Has an infection or blood poisoning
- Has kidney disease

Radiation Therapy

Radiation therapy may cause nausea and vomiting, especially in patients who are receiving radiation therapy to the gastrointestinal tract, liver, or brain. The risk for nausea and vomiting increases as the dose of radiation and the size of the area being treated increase. Nausea and vomiting caused by radiation therapy usually occur one-half hour to several hours after treatment. Patients may have fewer symptoms on days they do not have radiation therapy.

Anticipatory Nausea and Vomiting

Anticipatory nausea and vomiting occur in some patients after they have had several courses of treatment. This is caused by triggers, such as odors in the therapy room. For example, a person who begins chemotherapy and smells an alcohol swab at the same time may later have nausea and vomiting at the smell of alcohol alone. The more chemotherapy sessions a patient has, the more likely it is that anticipatory nausea and vomiting will occur. The following also may make anticipatory nausea and vomiting more likely:

- Being younger than 50 years

- Being female

- Having any of the following, after the last chemotherapy session:

- Nausea and vomiting

- Feeling warm or hot

- Feeling dizzy or lightheaded

- A history of motion sickness

- Having a high level of anxiety

- Certain types of chemotherapy (some are more likely to cause nausea and vomiting)

- A history of morning sickness during pregnancy

Treatment of anticipatory nausea and vomiting is more likely to work when symptoms are treated early. Antinausea drugs given for anticipatory nausea and vomiting do not seem to help. However, the following types of treatment may decrease symptoms:

- Muscle relaxation with guided imagery

- Hypnosis

- Behavior changing methods

- Biofeedback

- Distraction (such as playing video games)

Psychologists and other mental health professionals with special training in these treatments can often help patients with anticipatory nausea and vomiting.

Acute or Delayed Nausea and Vomiting

Acute and delayed nausea and vomiting are common in patients being treated for cancer. How often nausea and vomiting occur and how severe they are may be affected by the following:

- The specific drug

- The dose of the drug or if it is given with other drugs

- How often the drug is given

- The way the drug is given

- The individual patient

The following may make acute or delayed nausea and vomiting with chemotherapy more likely:

- Having nausea and vomiting after previous chemotherapy sessions

- Being female

- Being younger than 50 years

- Having chemotherapy in the past

- A history of motion sickness

- A history of morning sickness

- Dehydration

- Malnutrition

- Recent surgery

- Radiation therapy

Patients who have acute nausea and vomiting with chemotherapy are more likely to have delayed nausea and vomiting as well.

Acute and delayed nausea and vomiting are usually treated with antinausea drugs. Some types of chemotherapy are more likely to cause acute nausea and vomiting. Drugs may be given before each treatment to prevent nausea and vomiting. After chemotherapy, drugs may be given to prevent delayed vomiting. Some drugs last only a short time in the body and need to be given more often. Others last a long time and are given less often.

Drugs Used to Treat Nausea and Vomiting

The following table shows drugs that are commonly used to treat nausea and vomiting caused by cancer treatment:

Table 29.1. Drugs Used to Treat Nausea and Vomiting Caused by Cancer Treatment

Drug Name	Type of Drug
Prochlorperazine and other phenothiazines	Phenothiazines
Droperidol, haloperidol	Butyrophenones
Metoclopramide	Substituted benzamides
Dolasetron, granisetron, ondansetron, palonosetron	Serotonin receptor antagonists
Aprepitant, fosaprepitant, netupitant	Substance P/NK-1 antagonists
Dexamethasone, methylprednisolone	Corticosteroids
Alprazolam, lorazepam, midazolam	Benzodiazepines
Olanzapine	Antipsychotic /monoamine antagonists
Marijuana, nabilone	Cannabinoids

Treating Nausea and Vomiting Without Drugs

Non-drug treatments may help relieve nausea and vomiting, and may help antinausea drugs work better. These treatments include:

- Nutrition changes

- Acupuncture and acupressure

- Relaxation methods: Guided imagery and hypnosis are relaxation techniques that have been studied and shown to be helpful in anticipatory nausea and vomiting.

- Behavior therapy

Ginger is being studied in the treatment of nausea and vomiting.

Healthcare Costs for Treating Nausea and Vomiting

Healthcare costs for patients with severe nausea and vomiting caused by cancer therapy may be higher due to:

- Longer hospital stays

- Need for help with everyday activities

- Lost work hours

- Depression

When nausea and vomiting can be prevented or controlled, health-care costs are lower. However, even with preventive treatment for nausea and vomiting, many patients may still have uncontrolled symptoms that add to their medical costs and decrease their quality of life.

Chapter 30

Appetite Loss and Nutrition Therapy

Appetite Loss

Cancer treatments may lower your appetite or change the way food tastes or smells. Side effects such as mouth and throat problems, or nausea and vomiting can also make eating difficult. Cancer-related fatigue can also lower your appetite.

Talk with your healthcare team if you are not hungry or if your find it difficult to eat. Don't wait until you feel weak, have lost too much weight, or are dehydrated, to talk with your doctor or nurse. It's important to eat well, especially during treatment for cancer.

Ways to Manage

Take these steps to get the nutrition you need to stay strong during treatment:

- **Drink plenty of liquids.** Drinking plenty of liquids is important, especially if you have less of an appetite. Losing fluid can lead to dehydration, a dangerous condition. You may become

This chapter contains text excerpted from the following sources: Text under the heading "Appetite Loss" is excerpted from "Appetite Loss," National Cancer Institute (NCI), April 29, 2015; Text under the heading "Nutrition Therapy in Cancer Care" is excerpted from "Nutrition in Cancer Care (PDQ®)–Patient Version," National Cancer Institute (NCI), January 8, 2016.

weak or dizzy and have dark yellow urine if you are not drinking enough liquids.

- **Choose healthy and high-nutrient foods.** Eat a little, even if you are not hungry. It may help to have five or six small meals throughout the day instead of three large meals. Most people need to eat a variety of nutrient-dense foods that are high in protein and calories.

- **Be active.** Being active can actually increase your appetite. Your appetite may increase when you take a short walk each day.

Talking with Your Healthcare Team

Prepare for your visit by making a list of questions to ask. Consider adding these questions to your list:

- What symptoms or problems should I call you about?

- What steps can I take to feel better?

- What food and drink choices are best for me?

- Do you recommend supplemental nutrition drinks for me?

- Are there vitamins and supplements that I should avoid? Are there any I should take?

- Would you recommend a registered dietitian who could also help me?

Nutrition Therapy in Cancer Care

Screening and Assessment

Screening is used to look for nutrition risks in a patient who has no symptoms. This can help find out if the patient is likely to become malnourished, so that steps can be taken to prevent it. Assessment checks the nutritional health of the patient and helps to decide if nutrition therapy is needed to correct a problem.

Screening and assessment may include questions about the following:

- Weight changes over the past year.

- Changes in the amount and type of food eaten compared to what is usual for the patient.

- Problems that have affected eating, such as loss of appetite, nausea, vomiting, diarrhea, constipation, mouth sores, dry mouth, changes in taste and smell, or pain.

- Ability to walk and do other activities of daily living (dressing, getting into or out of a bed or chair, taking a bath or shower, and using the toilet).

A physical exam is also done to check the body for general health and signs of disease. The doctor will look for loss of weight, fat, and muscle, and for fluid buildup in the body.

Early Detection and Treatment of Nutrition Problems

Early nutrition screening and assessment help find problems that may affect how well the patient's body can deal with the effects of cancer treatment. Patients who are underweight or malnourished may not be able to get through treatment as well as a well-nourished patient. Finding and treating nutrition problems early can help the patient gain weight or prevent weight loss, decrease problems with the treatment, and help recovery.

Nutrition Support Team and Their Goal

A nutrition support team will check the patient's nutritional health often during cancer treatment and recovery. The team may include the following specialists:

- Physician

- Nurse

- Registered dietitian

- Social worker

- Psychologist

A patient whose religion doesn't allow eating certain foods may want to talk with a religious advisor about allowing those foods during cancer treatment and recovery.

Goals of Nutrition Therapy

The main goals of nutrition therapy for patients in active treatment and recovery are to provide nutrients that are missing, maintain nutritional health, and prevent problems. The healthcare team will use nutrition therapy to do the following:

- Prevent or treat nutrition problems, including preventing muscle and bone loss.
- Decrease side effects of cancer treatment and problems that affect nutrition.
- Keep up the patient's strength and energy.
- Help the immune system fight infection.
- Help the body recover and heal.
- Keep up or improve the patient's quality of life.

Good nutrition continues to be important for patients who are in remission or whose cancer has been cured.

The goals of nutrition therapy for patients who have advanced cancer include the following:

- Control side effects
- Lower the risk of infection
- Keep up strength and energy
- Improve or maintain quality of life

Methods of Nutrition Care*

Individuals diagnosed with cancer are at risk for malnutrition resulting from the disease itself; from anticancer therapy such as surgery, radiation, or pharmacologic therapy; and/or from anorexia due to emotional turmoil. The following sections highlight the benefits, contraindications, methods of administration, and home care issues for all forms of nutrition support—oral, enteral, and parenteral. The preferred method of nutrition support is via the oral route, with the use of dietary modifications to reduce the symptoms associated with cancer treatments. Enteral nutrition is indicated when the gastrointestinal (GI) tract is functional but oral intake is insufficient to meet nutritional requirements. Common situations in which enteral nutrition may be needed include malignancies of the head and neck regions, esophagus, and stomach. When the GI tract is dysfunctional, total parenteral nutrition (TPN) or enteral nutrition may be indicated; however, the widespread use of TPN is controversial because little evidence of improved survival has been demonstrated in patients with advanced cancer. Parenteral nutrition has been shown to be beneficial in only a small group of patients—specifically, postoperative patients who are being aggressively treated and who have demonstrated a positive response rate. One study reported that patients with GI cancer benefited from perioperative support with TPN, with one-third fewer complications and decreased mortality.

Oral Nourishment

Optimal nutrition can improve the clinical course, outcome, and quality of life of patients undergoing treatment for cancer. Virtually every cancer patient could benefit from consultation with a registered dietitian or physician to formulate a plan for nutrition and to begin meal planning. Oral nutrition, or eating by mouth, is the preferred method of feeding and should be used whenever possible. Appetite stimulants may be used to enhance the enjoyment of foods and to facilitate weight gain in the presence of significant anorexia. Recommendations during treatment may focus on eating foods that are high in energy, protein, and micronutrients to help maintain nutritional status. This may be especially true for individuals with early satiety, anorexia, and alteration in taste, xerostomia, mucositis, nausea, or diarrhea. Under most of these circumstances, eating frequently and including high-energy and high-protein snacks may help overall intake.

Enteral Nutrition

The benefits of enteral nutrition, or tube feeding, are that it continues to use the gut, has fewer complications such as infection and organ malfunction, is often easier to administer, and is cheaper than parenteral nutrition. In addition, nutrients are metabolized and utilized more efficiently by the body. Specific disease and condition-related indications for use consist of a diagnosis of a cancer of the alimentary canal (in particular, head and neck, esophageal, gastric, or pancreatic cancers) and severe complications/side effects from chemotherapy and/ or radiation that are seriously jeopardizing the treatment plan of an individual already suffering from malnutrition. Contraindications for enteral nutritional support include a malfunctioning gastrointestinal tract, malabsorptive conditions, mechanical obstructions, severe bleeding, severe diarrhea, intractable vomiting, gastrointestinal fistulas in locations difficult to bypass with an enteral tube, inflammatory bowel processes such as prolonged ileus and severe enterocolitis, and/ or an overall health prognosis not consistent with aggressive nutrition therapy. Thrombocytopenia and general pancytopenic conditions following anticancer treatments may also prevent placement of an enteral tube.

Parenteral Nutrition

Parenteral nutrition may be indicated in select individuals who are unable to use the oral or enteral route (i.e., those who have a nonfunctioning gut), such as those with obstruction, intractable nausea and/or vomiting, short-bowel syndrome, or ileus. Additional inclusive conditions common in the cancer population are severe diarrhea/malabsorption, severe mucositis or esophagitis, high-output gastrointestinal fistulas that cannot be bypassed by enteral intubation, and/or severe preoperative malnutrition. Contraindications for use of parenteral nutrition are a functioning gut, a need for nutritional support for a duration less than five days, an inability to obtain intravenous (IV) access, and poor prognosis not warranting aggressive nutritional support. Additional conditions that should cause hesitation are the following: patient or caregiver does not want parenteral nutrition, patient is hemodynamically unstable or has profound metabolic and/or electrolyte disturbances, and/or patient is anuric without dialysis.

Text under the heading "Methods of Nutrition" is excerpted from "Nutrition in Cancer Care (PDQ®)–Health Professional Version," National Cancer Institute (NCI), January 8, 2016.

Chapter 31

Gastrointestinal Complications of Cancer Treatment

The gastrointestinal (GI) tract is part of the digestive system, which processes nutrients (vitamins, minerals, carbohydrates, fats, proteins, and water) in foods that are eaten and helps pass waste material out of the body. The GI tract includes the stomach and intestines (bowels). The stomach is a J-shaped organ in the upper abdomen. Food moves from the throat to the stomach through a hollow, muscular tube called the esophagus. After leaving the stomach, partly-digested food passes into the small intestine and then into the large intestine. The colon (large bowel) is the first part of the large intestine and is about 5 feet long. Together, the rectum and anal canal make up the last part of the large intestine and are 6–8 inches long. The anal canal ends at the anus (the opening of the large intestine to the outside of the body).

GI complications are common in cancer patients. Complications are medical problems that occur during a disease, or after a procedure or treatment. They may be caused by the disease, procedure, or treatment, or may have other causes. This chapter describes the following GI complications and their causes and treatments:

- Constipation

This chapter includes text excerpted from "Gastrointestinal Complications (PDQ®)–Patient Version," National Cancer Institute (NCI), June 6, 2016.

- Fecal impaction
- Bowel obstruction
- Diarrhea
- Radiation enteritis

This chapter is about GI complications in adults with cancer. Treatment of GI complications in children is different than treatment for adults.

Constipation

Constipation is the slow movement of stool through the large intestine. The longer it takes for the stool to move through the large intestine, the more it loses fluid and the drier and harder it becomes. The patient may be unable to have a bowel movement, have to push harder to have a bowel movement, or have fewer than their usual number of bowel movements.

Causes

Constipation is a common problem for cancer patients. Cancer patients may become constipated by any of the usual factors that cause constipation in healthy people. These include older age, changes in diet and fluid intake, and not getting enough exercise. In addition to these common causes of constipation, there are other causes in cancer patients.

Other causes of constipation include:

- Medicines
- Diet
- Bowel movement habits
- Conditions that prevent activity and exercise
- Intestinal disorders
- Muscle and nerve disorders
- Changes in body metabolism
- Environment
- Narrow colon

Assessment

The assessment includes a physical exam and questions about the patient's usual bowel movements and how they have changed.

The following tests and procedures may be done to help find the cause of the constipation:

- Physical exam

- Digital rectal exam (DRE)

- Fecal occult blood test

- Proctoscopy

- Colonoscopy

- Abdominal X-ray

There is no "normal" number of bowel movements for a cancer patient. Each person is different. You will be asked about bowel routines, food, and medicines:

- How often do you have a bowel movement? When and how much?

- When was your last bowel movement? What was it like (how much, hard or soft, color)?

- Was there any blood in your stool?

- Has your stomach hurt or have you had any cramps, nausea, vomiting, gas, or feeling of fullness near the rectum?

- Do you use laxatives or enemas regularly?

- What do you usually do to relieve constipation? Does this usually work?

- What kind of food do you eat?

- How much and what type of fluids do you drink each day?

- What medicines are you taking? How much and how often?

- Is this constipation a recent change in your normal habits?

- How many times a day do you pass gas?

Treatment

It's easier to prevent constipation than to relieve it. The healthcare team will work with the patient to prevent constipation. Patients who take opioids may need to start taking laxatives right away to prevent constipation.

Constipation can be very uncomfortable and cause distress. If left untreated, constipation may lead to fecal impaction. This is a serious condition in which stool will not pass out of the colon or rectum. It's important to treat constipation to prevent fecal impaction.

Prevention and treatment are not the same for every patient. Do the following to prevent and treat constipation:

- Keep a record of all bowel movements.

- Drink eight 8-ounce glasses of fluid each day. Patients who have certain conditions, such as kidney or heart disease, may need to drink less.

- Get regular exercise. Patients who cannot walk may do abdominal exercises in bed or move from the bed to a chair.

- Increase the amount of fiber in the diet by eating more of the following:

  - Fruits, such as raisins, prunes, peaches, and apples.

  - Vegetables, such as squash, broccoli, carrots, and celery.

  - Whole grain cereals, whole grain breads, and bran.

- It's important to drink more fluids when eating more high-fiber foods, to avoid making constipation worse. Patients who have had a small or large intestinal obstruction or have had intestinal surgery (for example, a colostomy) should not eat a high-fiber diet.

- Drink a warm or hot drink about one half-hour before the usual time for a bowel movement.

- Find privacy and quiet when it is time for a bowel movement.

- Use the toilet or a bedside commode instead of a bedpan.

- Take only medicines that are prescribed by the doctor. Medicines for constipation may include bulking agents, laxatives, stool softeners, and drugs that cause the intestine to empty.

- Use suppositories or enemas only if ordered by the doctor. In some cancer patients, these treatments may lead to bleeding, infection, or other harmful side effects.

When constipation is caused by opioids, treatment may be drugs that stop the effects of the opioids or other medicines, stool softeners, enemas, and/or manual removal of stool.

Fecal Impaction

Fecal impaction is dry stool that cannot pass out of the body. Patients with fecal impaction may not have gastrointestinal (GI) symptoms. Instead, they may have problems with circulation, the heart, or breathing. If fecal impaction is not treated, it can get worse and cause death.

Causes

A common cause of fecal impaction is using laxatives too often. Repeated use of laxatives in higher and higher doses makes the colon less able to respond naturally to the need to have a bowel movement. This is a common reason for fecal impaction. Other causes include:

- Opioid pain medicines.

- Little or no activity over a long period.

- Diet changes.

- Constipation that is not treated. See the section above on causes of constipation.

Certain types of mental illness may lead to fecal impaction. Symptoms of fecal impaction include being unable to have a bowel movement and pain in the abdomen or back.

The following may be symptoms of fecal impaction:

- Being unable to have a bowel movement.

- Having to push harder to have a bowel movement of small amounts of hard, dry stool.

- Having fewer than the usual number of bowel movements.

- Having pain in the back or abdomen.

- Urinating more or less often than usual, or being unable to urinate.

- Breathing problems, rapid heartbeat, dizziness, low blood pressure, and swollen abdomen.

- Having sudden, explosive diarrhea (as stool moves around the impaction).

- Leaking stool when coughing.

- Nausea and vomiting

- Dehydration

Being confused and losing a sense of time and place, with rapid heartbeat, sweating, fever, and high or low blood pressure.

These symptoms should be reported to the healthcare provider.

Assessment

Assessment includes a physical exam and questions like those asked in the assessment of constipation.

The doctor will ask questions similar to those for the assessment of constipation:

- How often do you have a bowel movement? When and how much?

- When was your last bowel movement? What was it like (how much, hard or soft, color)?

- Was there any blood in your stool?

- Has your stomach hurt or have you had any cramps, nausea, vomiting, gas, or feeling of fullness near the rectum?

- Do you use laxatives or enemas regularly?

- What do you usually do to relieve constipation? Does this usually work?

- What kind of food do you eat?

- How much and what type of fluids do you drink each day?

- What medicines are you taking? How much and how often?

- Is this constipation a recent change in your normal habits?

- How many times a day do you pass gas?

The doctor will do a physical exam to find out if the patient has a fecal impaction. The following tests and procedures may be done:

- Physical exam

- X-rays

- Digital rectal exam (DRE)

- Sigmoidoscopy

- Blood tests

- Electrocardiogram (EKG)

Treatment

The main treatment for impaction is to moisten and soften the stool so it can be removed or passed out of the body. This is usually done with an enema. Enemas are given only as prescribed by the doctor since too many enemas can damage the intestine. Stool softeners or glycerin suppositories may be given to make the stool softer and easier to pass. Some patients may need to have stool manually removed from the rectum after it is softened.

Laxatives that cause the stool to move are not used because they can also damage the intestine.

Bowel Obstruction

A bowel obstruction is a blockage of the small or large intestine by something other than fecal impaction.

Bowel obstructions (blockages) keep the stool from moving through the small or large intestines. They may be caused by a physical change or by conditions that stop the intestinal muscles from moving normally. The intestine may be partly or completely blocked. Most obstructions occur in the small intestine.

Physical changes

- The intestine may become twisted or form a loop, closing it off and trapping stool.

- Inflammation, scar tissue from surgery, and hernias can make the intestine too narrow.

- Tumors growing inside or outside the intestine can cause it to be partly or completely blocked.

If the intestine is blocked by physical causes, it may decrease blood flow to blocked parts. Blood flow needs to be corrected or the affected tissue may die.

Conditions that affect the intestinal muscle:

- Paralysis (loss of ability to move).

- Blocked blood vessels going to the intestine.

- Too little potassium in the blood.

The most common cancers that cause bowel obstructions are cancers of the colon, stomach, and ovary. Other cancers, such as lung and breast cancers and melanoma, can spread to the abdomen and cause bowel obstruction. Patients who have had surgery on the abdomen or radiation therapy to the abdomen have a higher risk of a bowel obstruction. Bowel obstructions are most common during the advanced stages of cancer.

Assessment includes a physical exam and imaging tests.

The following tests and procedures may be done to diagnose a bowel obstruction:

- Physical exam

- Complete blood count (CBC)

- Electrolyte panel

- Urinalysis

- Abdominal X-ray

- Barium enema

Treatment for acute bowel obstruction. Acute bowel obstructions occur suddenly, may have not occurred before, and are not long-lasting. Treatment may include the following:

- **Fluid replacement therapy.** A treatment to get the fluids in the body back to normal amounts. Intravenous (IV) fluids may be given and medicines may be prescribed.

- **Electrolyte correction.** A treatment to get the right amounts of chemicals in the blood, such as sodium, potassium, and chloride. Fluids with electrolytes may be given by infusion.

- **Blood transfusion.** A procedure in which a person is given an infusion of whole blood or parts of blood.

- **Nasogastric or colorectal tube.** A nasogastric tube is inserted through the nose and esophagus into the stomach. A colorectal tube is inserted through the rectum into the colon. This is done to decrease swelling, remove fluid and gas buildup, and relieve pressure.

- **Surgery.** Surgery to relieve the obstruction may be done if it causes serious symptoms that are not relieved by other treatments.

Patients with symptoms that keep getting worse will have follow-up exams to check for signs and symptoms of shock and to make sure the obstruction isn't getting worse.

Chronic, Malignant Bowel Obstruction

Chronic bowel obstructions keep getting worse over time. Patients who have advanced cancer may have chronic bowel obstructions that cannot be removed with surgery. The intestine may be blocked or narrowed in more than one place or the tumor may be too large to remove completely. Treatments include the following:

- **Surgery.** The obstruction is removed to relieve pain and improve the patient's quality of life.

- **Stent.** A metal tube inserted into the intestine to open the area that is blocked.

- **Gastrostomy tube.** A tube inserted through the wall of the abdomen directly into the stomach. The gastrostomy tube can relieve fluid and air build-up in the stomach and allow medications and liquids to be given directly into the stomach by pouring them down the tube. A drainage bag with a valve may also be attached to the gastrostomy tube. When the valve is open, the patient may be able to eat or drink by mouth and the food drains directly into the bag. This gives the patient the experience of tasting the food and keeping the mouth moist. Solid food is avoided because it may block the tubing to the drainage bag.

- **Medicines.** Injections or infusions of medicines for pain, nausea and vomiting, and/or to make the intestines empty. This may be prescribed for patients who cannot be helped with a stent or gastrostomy tube.

Diarrhea

Diarrhea is frequent, loose, and watery bowel movements. Acute diarrhea lasts more than 4 days but less than 2 weeks. Symptoms of acute diarrhea may be loose stools and passing more than 3 unformed stools in one day. Diarrhea is chronic (long-term) when it goes on for longer than 2 months.

Diarrhea can occur at any time during cancer treatment. It can be physically and emotionally stressful for patients who have cancer.

Causes

Causes of diarrhea in cancer patients include the following:

- Cancer treatments, such as chemotherapy, radiation therapy, bone marrow transplant, and surgery.

- The cancer itself.

- Stress and anxiety from being diagnosed with cancer and having cancer treatment.

- Medical conditions and diseases other than cancer.

- Infections.

- Antibiotic therapy for certain infections. Antibiotic therapy can irritate the lining of the bowel and cause diarrhea that often does not get better with treatment.

- Laxatives.

- Fecal impaction in which the stool leaks around the blockage.

- Certain foods that are high in fiber or fat.

Assessment

Because diarrhea can be life-threatening, it is important to find out the cause so treatment can begin as soon as possible. The doctor may ask the following questions to help plan treatment:

- How often have you had bowel movements in the past 24 hours?

- When was your last bowel movement? What was it like (how much, how hard or soft, what color)? Was there any blood?

- Was there any blood in your stool or any rectal bleeding?

- Have you been dizzy, very drowsy, or had any cramps, pain, nausea, vomiting, or fever?

- What have you eaten? What and how much have you had to drink in the past 24 hours?

- Have you lost weight recently? How much?

- How often have you urinated in the past 24 hours?

- What medicines are you taking? How much and how often?

- Have you traveled recently?

Tests and procedures may include the following:

- Physical exam and history

- Digital rectal exam (DRE)

- Fecal occult blood test

- Stool tests

- Complete blood count (CBC)

- Electrolyte panel

- Urinalysis

- Abdominal X-ray

Treatment

Treatment depends on the cause of the diarrhea. The doctor may make changes in medicines, diet, and/or fluids.

- A change in the use of laxatives may be needed.

- Medicine to treat diarrhea may be prescribed to slow down the intestines, decrease fluid secreted by the intestines, and help nutrients be absorbed.

- Diarrhea caused by cancer treatment may be treated by changes in diet. Eat small frequent meals and avoid the following foods:

  - Milk and dairy products.

  - Spicy foods.

  - Alcohol.

  - Foods and drinks that have caffeine.

  - Certain fruit juices.

  - Foods and drinks that cause gas.

  - Foods high in fiber or fat.

- A diet of bananas, rice, apples, and toast (the BRAT diet) may help mild diarrhea.

- Drinking more clear liquids may help decrease diarrhea. It is best to drink up to 3 quarts of clear fluids a day. These include water, sports drinks, broth, weak decaffeinated tea, caffeine-free soft drinks, clear juices, and gelatin. For severe diarrhea, the patient may need intravenous (IV) fluids or other forms of IV nutrition.

- Diarrhea caused by graft-versus-host-disease (GVHD) is often treated with a special diet. Some patients may need long-term treatment and diet management.

- Probiotics may be recommended. Probiotics are live microorganisms used as a dietary supplement to help with digestion and normal bowel function. A bacterium found in yogurt called *Lactobacillus acidophilus*, is the most common probiotic.

- Patients who have diarrhea with other symptoms may need fluids and medicine given by IV.

Radiation Enteritis

Radiation enteritis is a condition in which the lining of the intestine becomes swollen and inflamed during or after radiation therapy to the abdomen, pelvis, or rectum. The small and large intestine are very sensitive to radiation. The larger the dose of radiation, the more damage may be done to normal tissue. Most tumors in the abdomen and pelvis need large doses of radiation. Almost all patients receiving radiation to the abdomen, pelvis, or rectum will have enteritis.

Radiation therapy to kill cancer cells in the abdomen and pelvis affects normal cells in the lining of the intestines. Radiation therapy stops the growth of cancer cells and other fast-growing cells. Since normal cells in the lining of the intestines grow quickly, radiation treatment to that area can stop those cells from growing. This makes it hard for tissue to repair itself. As cells die and are not replaced, gastrointestinal problems occur over the next few days and weeks.

Doctors are studying whether the order that radiation therapy, chemotherapy, and surgery are given affects how severe the enteritis will be.

Symptoms may begin during radiation therapy or months to years later.

Radiation enteritis may be *acute* or *chronic*:

- *Acute* radiation enteritis occurs during radiation therapy and may last up to 8 to 12 weeks after treatment stops.

- *Chronic* radiation enteritis may appear months to years after radiation therapy ends, or it may begin as acute enteritis and keep coming back.

Risks

Only 5 percent to 15 percent of patients treated with radiation to the abdomen will have chronic problems. The amount of time the enteritis lasts and how severe it is depend on the following:

- The total dose of radiation received.

- The amount of normal intestine treated.

- The tumor size and how much it has spread.

- If chemotherapy was given at the same time as the radiation therapy.

- If radiation implants were used.

- If the patient has high blood pressure, diabetes, pelvic inflammatory disease, or poor nutrition.

- If the patient has had surgery to the abdomen or pelvis.

Symptoms

Patients with acute enteritis may have the following symptoms:

- Nausea

- Vomiting

- Abdominal cramps

- Frequent urges to have a bowel movement

- Rectal pain, bleeding, or mucus in the stool

- Watery diarrhea

- Feeling very tired

Symptoms of acute enteritis usually go away 2 to 3 weeks after treatment ends.

Symptoms of chronic enteritis usually appear 6 to 18 months after radiation therapy ends. It can be hard to diagnose. The doctor will first check to see if the symptoms are being caused by a recurrent tumor in the small intestine. The doctor will also need to know the patient's full history of radiation treatments.

Patients with chronic enteritis may have the following signs and symptoms:

- Abdominal cramps

- Bloody diarrhea

- Frequent urges to have a bowel movement

- Greasy and fatty stools

- Weight loss

- Nausea

Assessment

Patients will be given a physical exam and be asked questions about the following:

- Usual pattern of bowel movements.
- Pattern of diarrhea:
  - When it started.
  - How long it has lasted.
  - How often it occurs.
  - Amount and type of stools.
  - Other symptoms with the diarrhea (such as gas, cramping, bloating, urgency, bleeding, and rectal soreness).
- Nutrition health:
  - Height and weight.
  - Usual eating habits.
  - Changes in eating habits.
  - Amount of fiber in the diet.
  - Signs of dehydration (such as poor skin tone, increased weakness, or feeling very tired).
- Stress levels and ability to cope.
- Changes in lifestyle caused by the enteritis.

Treatment

Treatment depends on whether the radiation enteritis is acute or chronic.

Acute radiation enteritis. Treatment of acute enteritis includes treating the symptoms. The symptoms usually get better with treatment, but if symptoms get worse, then cancer treatment may have to be stopped for a while.

Treatment of acute radiation enteritis may include the following:

- Medicines to stop diarrhea.
- Opioids to relieve pain.
- Steroid foams to relieve rectal inflammation.

- Pancreatic enzyme replacement for patients who have pancreatic cancer. A decrease in pancreatic enzymes can cause diarrhea.

- Diet changes. Intestines damaged by radiation therapy may not make enough of certain enzymes needed for digestion, especially lactase. Lactase is needed to digest lactose, which is found in milk and milk products. A lactose-free, low-fat, and low-fiber diet may help to control symptoms of acute enteritis.

- Foods to avoid:

  - Milk and milk products, except buttermilk, yogurt, and lactose-free milkshake supplements, such as Ensure.

  - Whole-bran bread and cereal.

  - Nuts, seeds, and coconut.

  - Fried, greasy, or fatty foods.

  - Fresh and dried fruit and some fruit juices (such as prune juice).

  - Raw vegetables.

  - Rich pastries.

  - Popcorn, potato chips, and pretzels.

  - Strong spices and herbs.

  - Chocolate, coffee, tea, and soft drinks with caffeine.

  - Alcohol and tobacco.

- Foods to choose:

  - Fish, poultry, and meat that are broiled or roasted.

  - Bananas.

  - Applesauce and peeled apples.

  - Apple and grape juices.

  - White bread and toast.

  - Macaroni and noodles.

  - Baked, boiled, or mashed potatoes.

  - Cooked vegetables that are mild, such as asparagus tips, green and waxed beans, carrots, spinach, and squash.

- Mild processed cheese. Processed cheese may not cause problems because the lactose is removed when it is made.

- Buttermilk, yogurt, and lactose-free milkshake supplements, such as Ensure.

- Eggs.

- Smooth peanut butter.

- Helpful hints:

  - Eat food at room temperature.

  - Drink about 12 eight-ounce glasses of fluid a day.

  - Let sodas lose their fizz before drinking them.

  - Add nutmeg to food. This helps slow down movement of digested food in the intestines.

  - Start a low-fiber diet on the first day of radiation therapy.

Chronic radiation enteritis. Treatment of chronic radiation enteritis may include the following:

- Same treatments as for acute radiation enteritis symptoms.

- **Surgery.** Few patients need surgery to control their symptoms. Two types of surgery may be used:

  - Intestinal bypass: A procedure in which the doctor creates a new pathway for the flow of intestinal contents around the damaged tissue.

  - Total intestinal resection: Surgery to completely remove the intestines.

Doctors look at the patient's general health and the amount of damaged tissue before deciding if surgery will be needed. Healing after surgery is often slow and long-term tube feeding may be needed. Even after surgery, many patients still have symptoms.

Chapter 32

Oral Complications of Cancer Treatment

Oral complications are common in cancer patients, especially those with head and neck cancer. Complications are new medical problems that occur during or after a disease, procedure, or treatment and that make recovery harder. The complications may be side effects of the disease or treatment, or they may have other causes. Oral complications affect the mouth.

Risks of Oral Complications

Cancer patients have a high risk of oral complications for a number of reasons:

- Chemotherapy and radiation therapy slow or stop the growth of new cells. These cancer treatments slow or stop the growth of fast growing cells, such as cancer cells. Normal cells in the lining of the mouth also grow quickly, so anticancer treatment can stop them from growing, too. This slows down the ability of oral tissue to repair itself by making new cells.

This chapter includes text excerpted from "Oral Complications of Chemotherapy and Head/Neck Radiation (PDQ®)–Patient Version," National Cancer Institute (NCI), December 16, 2016.

- Radiation therapy may directly damage and break down oral tissue, salivary glands, and bone.

- Chemotherapy and radiation therapy upset the healthy balance of bacteria in the mouth.

There are many different kinds of bacteria in the mouth. Some are helpful and some are harmful. Chemotherapy and radiation therapy may cause changes in the lining of the mouth and the salivary glands, which make saliva. This can upset the healthy balance of bacteria. These changes may lead to mouth sores, infections, and tooth decay.

This chapter is about oral complications caused by chemotherapy and radiation therapy.

Preventing and Controlling Oral Complications

Sometimes treatment doses need to be decreased or treatment stopped because of oral complications. Preventive care before cancer treatment begins and treating problems as soon as they appear may make oral complications less severe. When there are fewer complications, cancer treatment may work better and you may have a better quality of life.

Patients receiving treatments that affect the head and neck should have their care planned by a team of doctors and specialists. To manage oral complications, the oncologist will work closely with your dentist and may refer you to other health professionals with special training. These may include the following specialists:

- Oncology nurse

- Dental specialists

- Dietitian

- Speech therapist

- Social worker

The goals of oral and dental care are different before, during, and after cancer treatment:

- Before cancer treatment, the goal is to prepare for cancer treatment by treating existing oral problems.

- During cancer treatment, the goals are to prevent oral complications and manage problems that occur.

- After cancer treatment, the goals are to keep teeth and gums healthy and manage any long-term side effects of cancer and its treatment.

The most common oral complications from cancer treatment include the following:

- Oral mucositis (inflamed mucous membranes in the mouth).
- Infection.
- Salivary gland problems.
- Change in taste.
- Pain.

These complications can lead to other problems such as dehydration and malnutrition.

Causes

Cancer treatment can cause mouth and throat problems.

Complications of Chemotherapy

Oral complications caused by chemotherapy include the following:

- Inflammation and ulcers of the mucous membranes in the stomach or intestines.
- Easy bleeding in the mouth.
- Nerve damage.

Complications of Radiation Therapy

Oral complications caused by radiation therapy to the head and neck include the following:

- Fibrosis (growth of fibrous tissue) in the mucous membrane in the mouth.
- Tooth decay and gum disease.
- Breakdown of tissue in the area that receives radiation.
- Breakdown of bone in the area that receives radiation.
- Fibrosis of muscle in the area that receives radiation.

Complications Caused by Either Chemotherapy or Radiation Therapy

The most common oral complications may be caused by either chemotherapy or radiation therapy. These include the following:

- Inflamed mucous membranes in the mouth.

- Infections in the mouth or that travel through the bloodstream. These can reach and affect cells all over the body.

- Taste changes.

- Dry mouth.

- Pain.

- Changes in dental growth and development in children.

- Malnutrition (not getting enough of the nutrients the body needs to be healthy) caused by being unable to eat.

- Dehydration (not getting the amount of water the body needs to be healthy) caused by being unable to drink.

- Tooth decay and gum disease.

Oral complications may be caused by the treatment itself (directly) or by side effects of the treatment (indirectly).

Radiation therapy can directly damage oral tissue, salivary glands, and bone. Areas treated may scar or waste away. Total-body radiation can cause permanent damage to the salivary glands. This can change the way foods taste and cause dry mouth. Slow healing and infection are indirect complications of cancer treatment. Both chemotherapy and radiation therapy can stop cells from dividing and slow the healing process in the mouth. Chemotherapy may decrease the number of white blood cells and weaken the immune system (the organs and cells that fight infection and disease). This makes it easier to get an infection.

Complications May Be Acute or Chronic

Acute complications are ones that occur during treatment and then go away. Chemotherapy usually causes acute complications that heal after treatment ends.

Chronic complications are ones that continue or appear months to years after treatment ends. Radiation can cause acute complications but may also cause permanent tissue damage that puts you at a lifelong risk of oral complications. The following chronic complications may continue after radiation therapy to the head or neck has ended:

- Dry mouth

- Tooth decay

- Infections

- Taste changes

- Problems in the mouth and jaw caused by loss of tissue and bone

- Problems in the mouth and jaw caused by the growth of benign tumors in the skin and muscle

Oral surgery or other dental work can cause problems in patients who have had radiation therapy to the head or neck. Make sure that your dentist knows your health history and the cancer treatments you received.

Prevention Steps before Chemotherapy or Radiation Therapy

Finding and treating oral problems before cancer treatment begins can prevent oral complications or make them less severe.

Problems such as cavities, broken teeth, loose crowns or fillings, and gum disease can get worse or cause problems during cancer treatment. Bacteria live in the mouth and may cause an infection when the immune system is not working well or when white blood cell counts are low. If dental problems are treated before cancer treatments begin, there may be fewer or milder oral complications. Prevention of oral complications includes a healthy diet, good oral care, and dental checkups.

Ways to prevent oral complications include the following:

- Eat a well-balanced diet. Healthy eating can help the body stand the stress of cancer treatment, help keep up your energy, fight infection, and rebuild tissue.

- Keep your mouth and teeth clean. This helps prevent cavities, mouth sores, and infections.

- Have a complete oral health exam.

Your dentist should be part of your cancer care team. It is important to choose a dentist who has experience treating patients with oral complications of cancer treatment. A checkup of your oral health at least a month before cancer treatment begins usually allows enough time for the mouth to heal if any dental work is needed. The dentist will treat teeth that have a risk of infection or decay. This will help avoid the need for dental treatments during cancer treatment. Preventive care may help lessen dry mouth, which is a common complication of radiation therapy to the head or neck.

A preventive oral health exam will check for the following:

- Mouth sores or infections
- Tooth decay
- Gum disease
- Dentures that do not fit well
- Problems moving the jaw
- Problems with the salivary glands

Patients receiving high-dose chemotherapy, stem cell transplant, or radiation therapy should have an oral care plan in place before treatment begins. The goal of the oral care plan is to find and treat oral disease that may cause complications during treatment and to continue oral care during treatment and recovery. Different oral complications may occur during the different phases of a transplant. Steps can be taken ahead of time to prevent or lessen how severe these side effects will be.

Oral care during radiation therapy will depend on the following:

- Specific needs of the patient
- The radiation dose
- The part of the body treated
- How long the radiation treatment lasts
- Specific complications that occur

It is important that patients who have head or neck cancer stop smoking. Continuing to smoke tobacco may slow down recovery. It can also increase the risk that the head or neck cancer will recur or that a second cancer will form.

Managing Oral Complications during and after Chemotherapy or Radiation Therapy

Regular Oral Care

Good dental hygiene may help prevent or decrease complications. It is important to keep a close watch on oral health during cancer treatment. This helps prevent, find, and treat complications as soon as possible. Keeping the mouth, teeth, and gums clean during and after cancer treatment may help decrease complications such as cavities, mouth sores, and infections.

Everyday oral care for cancer patients includes keeping the mouth clean and being gentle with the tissue lining the mouth. Everyday oral care during chemotherapy and radiation therapy includes the following:

Brushing teeth

- Brush teeth and gums with a soft-bristle brush 2 to 3 times a day for 2 to 3 minutes. Be sure to brush the area where the teeth meet the gums and to rinse often.

- Rinse the toothbrush in hot water every 15 to 30 seconds to soften the bristles, if needed.

- Use a foam brush only if a soft-bristle brush cannot be used. Brush 2 to 3 times a day and use an antibacterial rinse. Rinse often.

- Let the toothbrush air-dry between brushings.

- Use a fluoride toothpaste with a mild taste. Flavoring may irritate the mouth, especially mint flavoring.

- If toothpaste irritates your mouth, brush with a mixture of 1/4 teaspoon of salt added to 1 cup of water.

Rinsing

- Use a rinse every 2 hours to decrease soreness in the mouth. Dissolve 1/4 teaspoon of salt and 1/4 teaspoon of baking soda in 1 quart of water.

- An antibacterial rinse may be used 2 to 4 times a day for gum disease. Rinse for 1 to 2 minutes.

- If dry mouth occurs, rinsing may not be enough to clean the teeth after a meal. Brushing and flossing may be needed.

Flossing

- Floss gently once a day.

Lip care

- Use lip care products, such as cream with lanolin, to prevent drying and cracking.

Denture care

- Brush and rinse dentures every day. Use a soft-bristle tooth-brush or one made for cleaning dentures.

- Clean with a denture cleaner recommended by your dentist.

- Keep dentures moist when not being worn. Place them in water or a denture soaking solution recommended by your dentist. Do not use hot water, which can cause the denture to lose its shape.

Oral Mucositis

Oral mucositis is an inflammation of mucous membranes in the mouth. The terms "oral mucositis" and "stomatitis" are often used in place of each other, but they are different.

- Oral mucositis is an inflammation of mucous membranes in the mouth. It usually appears as red, burn-like sores or as ulcer-like sores in the mouth.

- Stomatitis is an inflammation of mucous membranes and other tissues in the mouth. These include the gums, tongue, roof and floor of the mouth, and the inside of the lips and cheeks.

Mucositis may be caused by either radiation therapy or chemotherapy.

- Mucositis caused by chemotherapy will heal by itself, usually in 2 to 4 weeks if there is no infection.

- Mucositis caused by radiation therapy usually lasts 6 to 8 weeks, depending on how long the treatment was.

- In patients receiving high-dose chemotherapy or chemo-radiation for stem cell transplant: Mucositis usually begins 7 to 10 days after treatment begins, and lasts for about 2 weeks after treatment ends.

Swishing ice chips in the mouth for 30 minutes, beginning 5 minutes before patients receive fluorouracil, may help prevent mucositis. Patients who receive high-dose chemotherapy and stem cell transplant may be given medicine to help prevent mucositis or keep it from lasting as long.

Mucositis may cause the following problems:

- Pain

- Infection

- Bleeding, in patients receiving chemotherapy. Patients receiving radiation therapy usually do not have bleeding

- Trouble breathing and eating

Care of mucositis during chemotherapy and radiation therapy includes cleaning the mouth and relieving pain. Treatment of mucositis caused by either radiation therapy or chemotherapy is about the same. Treatment depends on your white blood cell count and how severe the mucositis is. The following are ways to treat mucositis during chemotherapy, stem cell transplant, or radiation therapy:

Cleaning the mouth

- Clean your teeth and mouth every 4 hours and at bedtime. Do this more often if the mucositis becomes worse.

- Use a soft-bristle toothbrush.

- Replace your toothbrush often.

- Use lubricating jelly that is water-soluble, to help keep your mouth moist.

- Use mild rinses or plain water. Frequent rinsing removes pieces of food and bacteria from the mouth, prevents crusting of sores, and moistens and soothes sore gums and the lining of the mouth.

- If mouth sores begin to crust over, the following rinse may be used:

- Three percent hydrogen peroxide mixed with an equal amount of water or saltwater. To make a saltwater mixture, put 1/4 teaspoon of salt in 1 cup of water.

This should not be used for more than 2 days because it will keep mucositis from healing.

243

Relieving mucositis pain

- Try topical medicines for pain. Rinse your mouth before putting the medicine on the gums or lining of the mouth. Wipe mouth and teeth gently with wet gauze dipped in saltwater to remove pieces of food.

- Painkillers may help when topical medicines do not. Nonsteroidal anti-inflammatory drugs (NSAIDS, aspirin-type painkillers) should not be used by patients receiving chemotherapy because they increase the risk of bleeding.

- Zinc supplements taken during radiation therapy may help treat pain caused by mucositis as well as dermatitis (inflammation of the skin).

- Povidone-iodine mouthwash that does not contain alcohol may help delay or decrease mucositis caused by radiation therapy.

Pain

There can be many causes of oral pain in cancer patients.

A cancer patient's pain may come from the following:

- The cancer
- Side effects of cancer treatments
- Other medical conditions not related to the cancer

Because there can be many causes of oral pain, a careful diagnosis is important. This may include:

- A medical history
- Physical and dental exams
- X-rays of the teeth

Oral pain in cancer patients may be caused by the cancer.

Cancer can cause pain in different ways:

- The tumor presses on nearby areas as it grows and affects nerves and causes inflammation.

- Leukemias and lymphomas, which spread through the body and may affect sensitive areas in the mouth. Multiple myeloma can affect the teeth.

- Brain tumors may cause headaches.

- Cancer may spread to the head and neck from other parts of the body and cause oral pain.

- With some cancers, pain may be felt in parts of the body not near the cancer. This is called referred pain. Tumors of the nose, throat, and lungs can cause referred pain in the mouth or jaw.

Oral pain may be a side effect of treatments. Oral mucositis is the most common side effect of radiation therapy and chemotherapy. Pain in the mucous membranes often continues for a while even after the mucositis is healed. Surgery may damage bone, nerves, or tissue and may cause pain. Bisphosphonates, drugs taken to treat bone pain, sometimes cause bone to break down. This is most common after a dental procedure such as having a tooth pulled. Patients who have transplants may develop graft-versus-host-disease (GVHD). This can cause inflammation of the mucous membranes and joint pain.

Certain anticancer drugs can cause oral pain. If an anticancer drug is causing pain, stopping the drug usually stops the pain. Because there may be many causes of oral pain during cancer treatment, a careful diagnosis is important. This may include a medical history, physical and dental exams, and X-rays of the teeth. Some patients may have sensitive teeth weeks or months after chemotherapy has ended. Fluoride treatments or toothpaste for sensitive teeth may relieve the discomfort.

Teeth grinding may cause pain in the teeth or jaw muscles. Pain in the teeth or jaw muscles may occur in patients who grind their teeth or clench their jaws, often because of stress or not being able to sleep. Treatment may include muscle relaxers, drugs to treat anxiety, physical therapy (moist heat, massage, and stretching), and mouth guards to wear while sleeping.

Pain control helps improve the patient's quality of life. Oral and facial pain can affect eating, talking, and many other activities that involve the head, neck, mouth, and throat. Most patients with head and neck cancers have pain. The doctor may ask the patient to rate the pain using a rating system. This may be on a scale from 0 to 10, with 10 being the worst. The level of pain felt is affected by many different things. It's important for patients to talk with their doctors about pain. Pain that is not controlled can affect all areas of the patient's life. Pain may cause feelings of anxiety and depression, and may prevent the patient from working or enjoying everyday life with friends and family. Pain may also slow the recovery from cancer or lead to new physical problems. Controlling cancer pain can help the patient enjoy normal routines and a better quality of life.

For oral mucositis pain, topical treatments are usually used. Other pain medicines may be also be used. Sometimes, more than one pain medicine is needed. Muscle relaxers and medicines for anxiety or depression or to prevent seizures may help some patients. For severe pain, opioids may be prescribed.

Non-drug treatments may also help, including the following:

- Physical therapy

- TENS (transcutaneous electrical nerve stimulation)

- Applying cold or heat

- Hypnosis

- Acupuncture

- Distraction

- Relaxation therapy or imagery

- Cognitive behavioral therapy

- Music or drama therapy

- Counseling

Infection

Damage to the lining of the mouth and a weakened immune system make it easier for infection to occur. Oral mucositis breaks down the lining of the mouth, which lets bacteria and viruses get into the blood. When the immune system is weakened by chemotherapy, even good bacteria in the mouth can cause infections. Germs picked up from the hospital or other places may also cause infections.

As the white blood cell count gets lower, infections may occur more often and become more serious. Patients who have low white blood cell counts for a long time have a higher risk of serious infections. Dry mouth, which is common during radiation therapy to the head and neck, may also raise the risk of infections in the mouth. Dental care given before chemotherapy and radiation therapy are started can lower the risk of infections in the mouth, teeth, or gums. Infections may be caused by bacteria, a fungus, or a virus.

Bacterial infections. Treatment of bacterial infections in patients who have gum disease and receive high-dose chemotherapy may include the following:

- Using medicated and peroxide mouth rinses
- Brushing and flossing
- Wearing dentures as little as possible

Fungal infections. The mouth normally contains fungi that can live on or in the oral cavity without causing any problems. However, an overgrowth (too much fungi) in the mouth can be serious and should be treated.

Antibiotics and steroid drugs are often used when a patient receiving chemotherapy has a low white blood cell count. These drugs change the balance of bacteria in the mouth, making it easier for a fungal overgrowth to occur. Also, fungal infections are common in patients treated with radiation therapy. Patients receiving cancer treatment may be given drugs to help prevent fungal infections from occurring.

Candidiasis is a type of fungal infection that is common in patients receiving both chemotherapy and radiation therapy. Symptoms may include a burning pain and taste changes. Treatment of fungal infections in the lining of the mouth only may include mouthwashes and lozenges that contain antifungal drugs. An antifungal rinse should be used to soak dentures and dental devices and to rinse the mouth. Drugs may be used to when rinses and lozenges do not get rid of the fungal infection. Drugs are sometimes used to prevent fungal infections.

Viral infections. Patients receiving chemotherapy, especially those with immune systems weakened by stem cell transplant, have an increased risk of viral infections. Herpesvirus infections and other viruses that are latent (present in the body but not active or causing symptoms) may flare up. Finding and treating the infections early is important. Giving antiviral drugs before treatment starts can lower the risk of viral infections.

Bleeding

Bleeding may occur when anticancer drugs make the blood less able to clot. High-dose chemotherapy and stem cell transplants can cause a lower-than-normal number of platelets in the blood. This can cause problems with the body's blood clotting process. Bleeding may be mild (small red spots on the lips, soft palate, or bottom of the mouth) or severe, especially at the gum line and from ulcers in the mouth. Areas of gum disease may bleed on their own or when irritated by eating, brushing, or flossing. When platelet counts are very low, blood may ooze from the gums.

Most patients can safely brush and floss while blood counts are low. Continuing regular oral care will help prevent infections that can make bleeding problems worse. Your dentist or medical doctor can explain how to treat bleeding and safely keep your mouth clean when platelet counts are low.

Treatment for bleeding during chemotherapy may include the following:

- Medicines to reduce blood flow and help clots form.

- Topical products that cover and seal bleeding areas.

- Rinsing with a mixture of saltwater and 3 percent hydrogen peroxide. (The mixture should have 2 or 3 times the amount of saltwater than hydrogen peroxide.) To make the saltwater mixture, put 1/4 teaspoon of salt in 1 cup of water. This helps clean wounds in the mouth. Rinse carefully so clots are not disturbed.

Dry Mouth

Dry mouth (xerostomia) occurs when the salivary glands don't make enough saliva. Saliva is made by salivary glands. Saliva is needed for taste, swallowing, and speech. It helps prevent infection and tooth decay by cleaning off the teeth and gums and preventing too much acid in the mouth.

Radiation therapy can damage salivary glands and cause them to make too little saliva. Some types of chemotherapy used for stem cell transplant may also damage salivary glands. When there is not enough saliva, the mouth gets dry and uncomfortable. This condition is called dry mouth (xerostomia). The risk of tooth decay, gum disease, and infection increases, and your quality of life suffers.

Symptoms of dry mouth include the following:

- Thick, stringy saliva

- Increased thirst

- Changes in taste, swallowing, or speech

- A sore or burning feeling (especially on the tongue)

- Cuts or cracks in the lips or at the corners of the mouth

- Changes in the surface of the tongue

- Problems wearing dentures

Salivary glands usually return to normal after chemotherapy ends. Dry mouth caused by chemotherapy for stem cell transplant is usually temporary. The salivary glands often recover 2 to 3 months after chemotherapy ends.

Salivary glands may not recover completely after radiation therapy ends. The amount of saliva made by the salivary glands usually starts to decrease within 1 week after starting radiation therapy to the head or neck. It continues to decrease as treatment goes on. How severe the dryness is depends on the dose of radiation and the number of salivary glands that receive radiation. Salivary glands may partly recover during the first year after radiation therapy. However, recovery is usually not complete, especially if the salivary glands received direct radiation. Salivary glands that did not receive radiation may start making more saliva to make up for the loss of saliva from the damaged glands.

Careful oral hygiene can help prevent mouth sores, gum disease, and tooth decay caused by dry mouth. Care of dry mouth may include the following:

- Clean the mouth and teeth at least 4 times a day.

- Floss once a day.

- Brush with a fluoride toothpaste.

- Apply fluoride gel once a day at bedtime, after cleaning the teeth.

- Rinse 4 to 6 times a day with a mixture of salt and baking soda (mix ½ teaspoon salt and ½ teaspoon baking soda in 1 cup of warm water).

- Avoid foods and liquids that have a lot of sugar in them.

- Sip water often to relieve mouth dryness.

A dentist may give the following treatments:

- Rinses to replace minerals in the teeth.

- Rinses to fight infection in the mouth.

- Saliva substitutes or medicines that help the salivary glands make more saliva.

- Fluoride treatments to prevent tooth decay.

Acupuncture may also help relieve dry mouth.

Tooth Decay

Dry mouth and changes in the balance of bacteria in the mouth increase the risk of tooth decay (cavities). Careful oral hygiene and regular care by a dentist can help prevent cavities.

Taste Changes

Changes in taste (dysguesia) are common during chemotherapy and radiation therapy. Changes in the sense of taste is a common side effect of both chemotherapy and head or neck radiation therapy. Taste changes can be caused by damage to the taste buds, dry mouth, infection, or dental problems. Foods may seem to have no taste or may not taste the way they did before cancer treatment. Radiation may cause a change in sweet, sour, bitter, and salty tastes. Chemotherapy drugs may cause an unpleasant taste.

In most patients receiving chemotherapy and in some patients receiving radiation therapy, taste returns to normal a few months after treatment ends. However, for many radiation therapy patients, the change is permanent. In others, the taste buds may recover 6 to 8 weeks or more after radiation therapy ends. Zinc sulfate supplements may help some patients recover their sense of taste.

Fatigue

Cancer patients who are receiving high-dose chemotherapy or radiation therapy often feel fatigue (a lack of energy). This can be caused by either the cancer or its treatment. Some patients may have problems sleeping. Patients may feel too tired for regular oral care, which may further increase the risk for mouth ulcers, infection, and pain.

Malnutrition

Loss of appetite can lead to malnutrition. Patients treated for head and neck cancers have a high risk of malnutrition. The cancer itself, poor diet before diagnosis, and complications from surgery, radiation therapy, and chemotherapy can lead to nutrition problems. Patients may lose the desire to eat because of nausea, vomiting, trouble swallowing, sores in the mouth, or dry mouth. When eating causes discomfort or pain, the patient's quality of life and nutritional well-being suffer. The following may help patients with cancer meet their nutrition needs:

- Serve food chopped, ground, or blended, to shorten the amount of time it needs to stay in the mouth before being swallowed.

- Eat between-meal snacks to add calories and nutrients.

- Eat foods high in calories and protein.

- Take supplements to get vitamins, minerals, and calories.

Meeting with a nutrition counselor may help during and after treatment.

Nutrition support may include liquid diets and tube feeding. Many patients treated for head and neck cancers who receive radiation therapy only are able to eat soft foods. As treatment continues, most patients will add or switch to high-calorie, high-protein liquids to meet their nutrition needs. Some patients may need to receive the liquids through a tube that is inserted into the stomach or small intestine. Almost all patients who receive chemotherapy and head or neck radiation therapy at the same time will need tube feedings within 3 to 4 weeks. Studies show that patients do better if they begin these feedings at the start of treatment, before weight loss occurs.

Normal eating by mouth can begin again when treatment is finished and the area that received radiation is healed. A team that includes a speech and swallowing therapist can help the patients with the return to normal eating. Tube feedings are decreased as eating by mouth increases, and are stopped when you are able to get enough nutrients by mouth. Although most patients will once again be able to eat solid foods, many will have lasting complications such as taste changes, dry mouth, and trouble swallowing.

Mouth and Jaw Stiffness

Treatment for head and neck cancers may affect the ability to move the jaws, mouth, neck, and tongue. There may be problems with swallowing. Stiffness may be caused by:

- Oral surgery.

- Late effects of radiation therapy. An overgrowth of fibrous tissue (fibrosis) in the skin, mucous membranes, muscle, and joints of the jaw may occur after radiation therapy has ended.

- Stress caused by the cancer and its treatment.

Jaw stiffness may lead to serious health problems, including:

- Malnutrition and weight loss from being unable to eat normally.
- Slower healing and recovery from poor nutrition.
- Dental problems from being unable to clean the teeth and gums well and have dental treatments.
- Weakened jaw muscles from not using them.
- Emotional problems from avoiding social contact with others because of trouble speaking and eating.

The risk of having jaw stiffness from radiation therapy increases with higher doses of radiation and with repeated radiation treatments. The stiffness usually begins around the time the radiation treatments end. It may get worse over time, stay the same, or get somewhat better on its own. Treatment should begin as soon as possible to keep the condition from getting worse or becoming permanent. Treatment may include the following:

- Medical devices for the mouth
- Pain treatments
- Medicine to relax muscles
- Jaw exercises
- Medicine to treat depression

Swallowing Problems

Pain during swallowing and being unable to swallow (dysphagia) are common in cancer patients before, during, and after treatment. Swallowing problems are common in patients who have head and neck cancers. Cancer treatment side effects, such as oral mucositis, dry mouth, skin damage from radiation, infections, and graft-versus-host-disease (GVHD), may all cause problems with swallowing.

Trouble swallowing increases the risk of other complications. Other complications can develop from being unable to swallow and these can further decrease the patient's quality of life:

- **Pneumonia and other respiratory problems:** Patients who have trouble swallowing may aspirate (inhale food or liquids into the lung) when trying to eat or drink. Aspiration can lead to serious conditions, including pneumonia and respiratory failure.

- **Poor nutrition:** Being unable to swallow normally makes it hard to eat well. Malnutrition occurs when the body doesn't get all the nutrients needed for health. Wounds heal slowly and the body is less able to fight off infections.

- **Need for tube feeding:** A patient who is not able to take in enough food by mouth may be fed through a tube. The health-care team and a registered dietitian can explain the benefits and risks of tube feeding for patients who have swallowing problems.

- **Side effects of pain medicine:** Opioids used to treat painful swallowing may cause dry mouth and constipation.

- **Emotional problems:** Being unable to eat, drink, and speak normally may cause depression and the desire to avoid other people.

Whether radiation therapy will affect swallowing depends on several factors. The following may affect the risk of swallowing problems after radiation therapy:

- Total dose and schedule of radiation therapy. Higher doses over a shorter time often have more side effects.

- The way the radiation is given. Some types of radiation cause less damage to healthy tissue.

- Whether chemotherapy is given at the same time. The risk of side effects is increased if both are given.

- The patient's genetic makeup.

- Whether the patient is taking any food by mouth or only by tube feeding.

- Whether the patient smokes.

- How well the patient copes with problems.

Swallowing problems sometimes go away after treatment. Some side effects go away within 3 months after the end of treatment, and patients are able to swallow normally again. However, some treatments can cause permanent damage or late effects. Late effects are health problems that occur long after treatment has ended. Conditions that may cause permanent swallowing problems or late effects include:

- Damaged blood vessels

- Wasting away of tissue in the treated areas

- Lymphedema (buildup of lymph in the body)

- Overgrowth of fibrous tissue in head or neck areas, which may lead to jaw stiffness

- Chronic dry mouth

- Infections

Swallowing problems are managed by a team of experts. The oncologist works with other healthcare experts who specialize in treating head and neck cancers and the oral complications of cancer treatment. These specialists may include the following:

- **Speech therapist:** A speech therapist can assess how well the patient is swallowing and give the patient swallowing therapy and information to better understand the problem.

- **Dietitian:** A dietitian can help plan a safe way for the patient to receive the nutrition needed for health while swallowing is a problem.

- **Dental specialist:** Replace missing teeth and damaged area of the mouth with artificial devices to help swallowing.

- **Psychologist:** For patients who are having a hard time adjusting to being unable to swallow and eat normally, psychological counseling may help.

Tissue and Bone Loss

Radiation therapy can destroy very small blood vessels within the bone. This can kill bone tissue and lead to bone fractures or infection. Radiation can also kill tissue in the mouth. Ulcers may form, grow, and cause pain, loss of feeling, or infection.

Preventive care can make tissue and bone loss less severe. The following may help prevent and treat tissue and bone loss:

- Eat a well-balanced diet.

- Wear removable dentures or devices as little as possible.

- Don't smoke.

- Don't drink alcohol.

- Use topical antibiotics.

- Use painkillers as prescribed.

- Surgery to remove dead bone or to rebuild bones of the mouth and jaw.

- Hyperbaric oxygen therapy (a method that uses oxygen under pressure to help wounds heal).

Oral Complications of Chemotherapy and Radiation Therapy in Children

Children who received high-dose chemotherapy or radiation therapy to the head and neck may not have normal dental growth and development. New teeth may appear late or not at all, and tooth size may be smaller than normal. The head and face may not develop fully. The changes are usually the same on both sides of the head and are not always noticeable.

Orthodontic treatment for patients with these dental growth and development side effects is being studied.

Chapter 33

Hair Loss (Alopecia)

Some types of chemotherapy cause the hair on your head and other parts of your body to fall out. Radiation therapy can also cause hair loss on the part of the body that is being treated. Hair loss is called alopecia. Talk with your healthcare team to learn if the cancer treatment you will be receiving causes hair loss. Your doctor or nurse will share strategies that have help others, including those listed below.

Ways to Manage

Talk with your healthcare team about ways to manage before and after hair loss:

- **Treat your hair gently.** You may want to use a hairbrush with soft bristles or a wide-tooth comb. Do not use hair dryers, irons, or products such as gels or clips that may hurt your scalp. Wash your hair with a mild shampoo. Wash it less often and be very gentle. Pat it dry with a soft towel.

- **You have choices.** Some people choose to cut their hair short to make it easier to deal with when it starts to fall out. Others choose to shave their head. If you choose to shave your head, use

---

This chapter contains text excerpted from the following sources: Text in this chapter begins with excerpts from "Hair Loss (Alopecia)," National Cancer Institute (NCI), April 29, 2015; Text beginning with the heading "Cooling Cap to Reduce Hair Loss during Chemotherapy" is excerpted from "FDA Allows Marketing of Cooling Cap to Reduce Hair Loss during Chemotherapy," U.S. Food and Drug Administration (FDA), December 8, 2015.

an electric shaver so you won't cut yourself. If you plan to buy a wig, get one while you still have hair so you can match it to the color of your hair. If you find wigs to be itchy and hot, try wearing a comfortable scarf or turban.

- **Protect and care for your scalp.** Use sunscreen or wear a hat when you are outside. Choose a comfortable scarf or hat that you enjoy and that keeps your head warm. If your scalp itches or feels tender, using lotions and conditioners can help it feel better.

- **Talk about your feelings.** Many people feel angry, depressed, or embarrassed about hair loss. It can help to share these feelings with someone who understands. Some people find it helpful to talk with other people who have lost their hair during cancer treatment. Talking openly and honestly with your children and close family members can also help you all. Tell them that you expect to lose your hair during treatment.

Ways to Care for Your Hair When It Grows Back

- **Be gentle.** When your hair starts to grow back, you will want to be gentle with it. Avoid too much brushing, curling, and blow-drying. You may not want to wash your hair as frequently.

- **After chemotherapy.** Hair often grows back in 2 to 3 months after treatment has ended. Your hair will be very fine when it starts to grow back. Sometimes your new hair can be curlier or straighter—or even a different color. In time, it may go back to how it was before treatment.

- **After radiation therapy.** Hair often grows back in 3 to 6 months after treatment has ended. If you received a very high dose of radiation your hair may grow back thinner or not at all on the part of your body that received radiation.

Talking with Your Healthcare Team

Prepare for your visit by making a list of questions to ask. Consider adding these questions to your list:

- Is treatment likely to cause my hair to fall out?

- How should I protect and care for my head? Are there products that you recommend? Ones I should avoid?

- Where can I get a wig or hairpiece?
- What support groups could I meet with that might help?
- When will my hair grow back?

Cooling Cap to Reduce Hair Loss during Chemotherapy

Hair loss is a common side effect of certain types of chemotherapy, commonly associated with the treatment of breast cancer. Hair may fall out entirely, gradually, in sections, or may become thin. Hair loss due to cancer treatment is usually temporary, but minimizing or relieving these kinds of side effects are considered important to overall treatment.

"We are pleased to see a product for breast cancer patients that can minimize chemotherapy-induced hair loss and contribute to the quality of life of these individuals," said William Maisel, M.D., M.P.H., acting director of the Office of Device Evaluation (ODE) in the U.S. Food and Drug Administration's (FDA) Center for Devices and Radiological Health (CDRH). "Managing the side effects of chemotherapy is a critical component to overall health and recovery."

The Dignitana DigniCap Cooling System is indicated to reduce the frequency and severity of alopecia during chemotherapy in breast cancer patients in which alopecia-inducing chemotherapeutic agents and doses are used. It is a computer-controlled system that circulates cooled liquid to a head-worn cooling cap during chemotherapy treatment. The cooling cap is covered by a second cap made from neoprene, which holds the cooling cap in place and acts as an insulation cover to prevent loss of cooling.

The cooling action is intended to constrict blood vessels in the scalp, which, in theory, reduces the amount of chemotherapy that reaches cells in the hair follicles (hair roots). The cold also decreases the activity of the hair follicles, which slows down cell division and makes them less affected by chemotherapy. The combined actions are thought to reduce the effect chemotherapy has on the cells, which may reduce hair loss. DigniCap may not work with some chemotherapy regimens. Interested patients should talk with their doctors.

The efficacy of the cooling system was studied in 122 Stage I and Stage II women with breast cancer who were undergoing chemotherapy, using recognized chemotherapy regimens that have been associated with hair loss. The data from this study may also be applied to some Stage III and IV breast cancer patients because they may have a benefit-risk profile comparable to the patients enrolled in this study.

The primary endpoint was a self-assessment of hair loss by the women using standardized photographs at one month (three-six weeks) after the last chemotherapy cycle. More than 66 percent of patients treated with the DigniCap reported losing less than half their hair.

Prevention of hair loss in these patients may be a significant benefit to their quality of life, and the risk of the chemotherapy drug missing an isolated grouping of the breast cancer cells in the scalp because of the cold cap is extremely rare.

The most common side effects of the cooling system include cold-induced headaches and neck and shoulder discomfort, chills, and pain associated with wearing the cooling cap for an extended period of time.

The FDA reviewed data for DigniCap cooling system through the de novo classification process, a regulatory pathway for some low- to moderate-risk devices that are novel and not substantially equivalent to any legally marketed device.

Chapter 34

Nervous System Disturbances

Some cancer treatments cause peripheral neuropathy, a result of damage to the peripheral nerves. These nerves carry information from the brain to other parts of the body. Side effects depend on which peripheral nerves (sensory, motor, or autonomic) are affected.

Damage to sensory nerves (nerves that help you feel pain, heat, cold, and pressure) can cause:

- tingling, numbness, or a pins-and-needles feeling in your feet and hands that may spread to your legs and arms

- inability to feel a hot or cold sensation, such as a hot stove

- inability to feel pain, such as from a cut or sore on your foot

Damage to motor nerves (nerves that help your muscles to move) can cause:

- Weak or achy muscles. You may lose your balance or trip easily. It may also be difficult to button shirts or open jars.

- Muscles that twitch and cramp or muscle wasting (if you don't use your muscles regularly).

- Swallowing or breathing difficulties (if your chest or throat muscles are affected).

This chapter includes text excerpted from "Nerve Problems (Peripheral Neuropathy)," National Cancer Institute (NCI), April 29, 2015.

Damage to autonomic nerves (nerves that control functions such as blood pressure, digestion, heart rate, temperature, and urination) can cause:

- digestive changes such as constipation or diarrhea

- dizzy or faint feeling, due to low blood pressure

- sexual problems; men may be unable to get an erection and women may not reach orgasm

- sweating problems (either too much or too little sweating)

- urination problems, such as leaking urine or difficulty emptying your bladder

If you start to notice any of the problems listed above, talk with your doctor or nurse. Getting these problems diagnosed and treated early is the best way to control them, prevent further damage, and to reduce pain and other complications.

Ways to Prevent or Manage Problems Related to Nerve Changes

You may be advised to take these steps:

- **Prevent falls.** Have someone help you prevent falls around the house. Move rugs out of your path so you will not trip on them. Put rails on the walls and in the bathroom, so you can hold on to them and balance yourself. Put bathmats in the shower or tub. Wear sturdy shoes with soft soles. Get up slowly after sitting or lying down, especially if you feel dizzy.

- **Take extra care in the kitchen and shower.** Use potholders in the kitchen to protect your hands from burns. Be careful when handling knives or sharp objects. Ask someone to check the water temperature, to make sure it's not too hot.

- **Protect your hands and feet.** Wear shoes, both inside and outside. Check your arms, legs, and feet for cuts or scratches every day. When it's cold, wear warm clothes to protect your hands and feet.

- **Ask for help and slow down.** Let people help you with difficult tasks. Slow down and give yourself more time to do things.

- **Ask about pain medicine and integrative medicine practices.** You may be prescribed pain medicine. Sometimes practices such as acupuncture, massage, physical therapy, yoga, and others may also be advised to lower pain. Talk with your healthcare team to learn what is advised for you.

Talking with Your Healthcare Team

Prepare for your visit by making a list of questions to ask. Consider adding these questions to your list:

- What symptoms or problems might I have? Which ones should I call you about?

- When will these problems start? How long might they last?

- What medicine, treatments, and integrative medicine practices could help me to feel better?

- What steps can I take to feel better? What precautions should I take to stay safe?

- Could you refer me to a specialist who could give me additional advice?

Chapter 35

Cancer-Related Fatigue

Cancer treatments such as chemotherapy, radiation therapy, and biologic therapy can cause fatigue in cancer patients. Fatigue is also a common symptom of some types of cancer. Patients describe fatigue as feeling tired, weak, worn-out, heavy, slow, or that they have no energy or get-up-and-go. Fatigue in cancer patients may be called cancer fatigue, cancer-related fatigue, and cancer treatment-related fatigue.

Fatigue Related to Cancer Is Different from Fatigue That Healthy People Feel

When a healthy person is tired by day-to-day activities, their fatigue can be relieved by sleep and rest. Cancer-related fatigue is different. Cancer patients get tired after less activity than people who do not have cancer. Also, cancer-related fatigue is not completely relieved by sleep and rest and may last for a long time. Fatigue usually decreases after cancer treatment ends, but patients may still feel some fatigue for months or years.

Fatigue Can Decrease a Patient's Quality of Life

Fatigue can affect all areas of life by making the patient too tired to take part in daily activities, relationships, social events, and community activities. Patients may miss work or school, spend less time with friends and family, or spend more time sleeping. In some cases,

This chapter includes text excerpted from "Fatigue (PDQ®)–Patient Version," National Cancer Institute (NCI), May 7, 2015.

physical fatigue leads to mental fatigue and mood changes. This can make it hard for the patient to pay attention, remember things, and think clearly. Money may become a problem if the patient needs to take leave from a job or stop working completely. Job loss can lead to the loss of health insurance. All these things can lessen the patient's quality of life and self-esteem.

Getting help with fatigue may prevent some of these problems and improve quality of life.

Causes of Fatigue in Cancer Patients

Doctors do not know all the reasons cancer patients have fatigue. Many conditions may cause fatigue at the same time.

Fatigue in cancer patients may be caused by the following:

- Cancer treatment with chemotherapy, radiation therapy, and some biologic therapies.

- Anemia (a lower than normal number of red blood cells).

- Hormone levels that are too low or too high.

- Trouble breathing or getting enough oxygen.

- Heart trouble.

- Infection.

- Pain.

- Stress.

- Loss of appetite or not getting enough calories and nutrients.

- Dehydration (loss of too much water from the body, such as from severe diarrhea or vomiting).

- Changes in how well the body uses food for energy.

- Loss of weight, muscle, and/or strength.

- Medicines that cause drowsiness.

- Problems getting enough sleep.

- Being less active.

- Other medical conditions.

Fatigue is common in people with advanced cancer who are not receiving cancer treatment.

Doctors are trying to better understand how cancer treatments such as surgery, chemotherapy, and radiation therapy cause fatigue. Some studies show that fatigue is caused by:

- The need for extra energy to repair and heal body tissue damaged by treatment.

- The build-up of toxic substances that are left in the body after cells are killed by cancer treatment.

- The effect of biologic therapy on the immune system.

- Changes in the body's sleep-wake cycle.

When they begin cancer treatment, many patients are already tired from medical tests, surgery, and the emotional stress of coping with the cancer diagnosis. After treatment begins, fatigue may get worse. Patients who are older, have advanced cancer, or receive more than one type of treatment (for example, both chemotherapy and radiation therapy) are more likely to have long-term fatigue.

Different cancer treatments have different effects on a patient's energy level. The type and schedule of treatments can affect the amount of fatigue caused by cancer therapy.

Fatigue Caused by Chemotherapy

Patients treated with chemotherapy usually feel the most fatigue in the days, right after each treatment. Then the fatigue decreases until the next treatment. Fatigue usually increases with each cycle. Some studies have shown that patients have the most severe fatigue about mid-way through all the cycles of chemotherapy. Fatigue decreases after chemotherapy is finished, but patients may not feel back to normal until a month or more after the last treatment. Many patients feel fatigued for months or years after treatment ends.

Fatigue during chemotherapy may be increased by the following:

- Pain.

- Depression.

- Anxiety.

- Anemia. Some types of chemotherapy stop the bone marrow from making enough new red blood cells, causing anemia (too few red blood cells to carry oxygen to the body).

- Lack of sleep caused by some anticancer drugs.

Fatigue Caused by Radiation Therapy

Many patients receiving radiation therapy have fatigue that keeps them from being as active as they want to be. After radiation therapy begins, fatigue usually increases until mid-way through the course of treatments and then stays about the same until treatment ends. For many patients, fatigue improves after radiation therapy stops. However, in some patients, fatigue will last months or years after treatment ends. Some patients never have the same amount of energy they had before treatment.

Cancer-related fatigue has been studied in patients with breast cancer and prostate cancer. The amount of fatigue they felt and the time of day the fatigue was worst was different in different patients.

In men with prostate cancer, fatigue was increased by having the following symptoms before radiation therapy started:

• Poor sleep

• Depression

In women with breast cancer, fatigue was increased by the following:

• Working while receiving radiation therapy.

• Having children at home.

• Depression.

• Anxiety.

• Trouble sleeping.

• Younger age.

• Being underweight.

• Having advanced cancer or other medical conditions.

Fatigue Caused by Biologic Therapy

Biologic therapy often causes flu-like symptoms. These symptoms include being tired physically and mentally, fever, chills, muscle pain, headache, and not feeling well in general. Some patients may also have problems thinking clearly. Fatigue symptoms depend on the type of biologic therapy used.

Fatigue Caused by Surgery

Fatigue is often a side effect of surgery, but patients usually feel better with time. However, fatigue caused by surgery can be worse when the surgery is combined with other cancer treatments.

Other Causes of Fatigue

Anemia. Anemia is a common cause of fatigue. Anemia affects the patient's energy level and quality of life. Anemia may be caused by the following:

- The cancer.
- Cancer treatments.
- A medical condition not related to the cancer.

The effects of anemia on a patient depend on the following:

- How quickly the anemia occurs.
- The patient's age.
- The amount of plasma (fluid part of the blood) in the patient's blood.
- Other medical conditions the patient has.

Nutrition. Side effects related to nutrition may cause or increase fatigue. The body's energy comes from food. Fatigue may occur if the body does not take in enough food to give the body the energy it needs. For many patients, the effects of cancer and cancer treatments make it hard to eat well. In people with cancer, three major factors may affect nutrition:

- A change in the way the body is able to use food. A patient may eat the same amount as before having cancer, but the body may not be able to absorb and use all the nutrients from the food. This is caused by the cancer or its treatment.
- A decrease in the amount of food eaten because of low appetite, nausea, vomiting, diarrhea, or a blocked bowel.
- An increase in the amount of energy needed by the body because of a growing tumor, infection, fever, or shortness of breath.

Anxiety and depression. Anxiety and depression are the most common psychological causes of fatigue in cancer patients. The emotional stress of cancer can cause physical problems, including fatigue. It's common for cancer patients to have changes in moods and attitudes. Patients may feel anxiety and fear before and after a cancer diagnosis. These feelings may cause fatigue. The effect of the disease on the patient's physical, mental, social, and financial well-being can increase emotional distress.

About 15 percent to 25 percent of patients who have cancer get depressed, which may increase fatigue caused by physical factors.

The following are signs of depression:

- Feeling tired mentally and physically

- Loss of interest in life

- Problems thinking

- Loss of sleep

- Feeling a loss of hope

Some patients have more fatigue after cancer treatments than others do.

Fatigue may be increased when it is hard for patients to learn and remember. During and after cancer treatment, patients may find they cannot pay attention for very long and have a hard time thinking, remembering, and understanding. This is called attention fatigue. Sleep helps to relieve attention fatigue, but sleep may not be enough when the fatigue is related to cancer. Taking part in restful activities and spending time outdoors may help relieve attention fatigue.

Poor Sleep. Not sleeping well may cause fatigue. Some people with cancer are not able to get enough sleep. The following problems related to sleep may cause fatigue:

- Waking up during the night.

- Not going to sleep at the same time every night.

- Sleeping during the day and less at night.

- Not being active during the day.

Poor sleep affects people in different ways. For example, the time of day that fatigue is worse may be different. Some patients who have trouble sleeping may feel more fatigue in the morning. Others may have severe fatigue in both the morning and the evening.

Even in patients who have poor sleep, fixing sleep problems does not always improve fatigue. A lack of sleep may not be the cause of the fatigue.

Medicines. Medicines other than chemotherapy may add to fatigue. Patients may take medicines for cancer symptoms, such as pain, or conditions other than the cancer. These medicines may cause the patient to feel sleepy. Opioids, antidepressants, and antihistamines have this side effect. If many of these medicines are taken at the same time, fatigue may be worse.

Taking opioids over time may lower the amount of sex hormones made in the testicles and ovaries. This can lead to fatigue as well as sexual problems and depression.

Assessment of Fatigue

An assessment is done to find out the level of fatigue and how it affects the patient's daily life. There is no test to diagnose fatigue, so it is important for the patient to tell family members and the healthcare team if fatigue is a problem. To assess fatigue, the patient is asked to describe how bad the fatigue is, how it affects daily activities, and what makes the fatigue better or worse. The doctor will look for causes of fatigue that can be treated.

An assessment of fatigue includes a physical exam and blood tests. The assessment process may include the following:

- Physical exam. This is an exam of the body to check general signs of health or anything that seems unusual. The doctor will check for problems such as trouble breathing or loss of muscle strength. The patient's walking, posture, and joint movements will be checked.

- Rating the level of fatigue. The patient is asked to rate the level of fatigue (how bad the fatigue is). There is no standard way to rate fatigue. The doctor may ask the patient to rate the fatigue on a scale from 0 to 10. Other ways to rate fatigue check for how much the fatigue affects the patient's quality of life.

- A series of questions about the following:

  - When the fatigue started, how long it lasts, and what makes it better or worse.

  - Symptoms or side effects, such as pain, the patient is having from the cancer or the treatments.

- Medicines being taken.

- Sleeping and resting habits.

- Eating habits and changes in appetite or weight.

- How the fatigue affects daily activities and lifestyle.

- How the fatigue affects being able to work.

- Whether the patient has depression, anxiety, or pain.

- Health habits and past illnesses and treatments.

- Blood tests to check for anemia: The most common blood tests to check if the number of red blood cells is normal are:

  - Complete blood count (CBC) with differential: A procedure in which a sample of blood is taken and checked for the following:

    - The number of red blood cells and platelets.

    - The number and type of white blood cells.

    - The amount of hemoglobin (the protein that carries oxygen) in the red blood cells.

    - The portion of the blood sample made up of red blood cells.

  - Peripheral blood smear: A procedure in which a sample of blood is checked for the number and kinds of white blood cells, the number of platelets, and changes in the shape of blood cells.

  - Other blood tests may be done to check for other conditions that affect red blood cells. These include a bone marrow aspiration and biopsy or a Coombs' test. Blood tests to check the levels of vitamin B12, iron, and erythropoietin may also be done.

- Checking for other causes of fatigue that can be treated.

A fatigue assessment is repeated at different times to see if there are patterns of fatigue. A fatigue assessment is repeated to see if there is a pattern for when fatigue starts or becomes worse. Fatigue may be worse right after a chemotherapy treatment, for example. The same method of measuring fatigue is used at each assessment. This helps show changes in fatigue over time.

Treatments for Fatigue

Fatigue in cancer patients is often treated by relieving related conditions such as anemia and depression. Treatment of fatigue depends on the symptoms and whether the cause of fatigue is known. When the cause of fatigue is not known, treatment is usually given to relieve symptoms and teach the patient ways to cope with fatigue.

Treatment of Anemia

Treating anemia may help decrease fatigue. When known, the cause of the anemia is treated. When the cause is not known, treatment for anemia is supportive care and may include the following:

- **Change in diet.** Eating more foods rich in iron and vitamins may be combined with other treatments for anemia.

- **Transfusions of red blood cells.** Transfusions work well to treat anemia. Possible side effects of transfusions include an allergic reaction, infection, graft-versus-host disease, immune system changes, and too much iron in the blood.

- **Medicine.** Drugs that cause the bone marrow to make more red blood cells may be used to treat anemia-related fatigue in patients receiving chemotherapy. Epoetin alfa and darbepoetin alfa are two of these drugs. This type of drug may shorten survival time, increase the risk of serious heart problems, and cause some tumors to grow faster or recur. The U.S. Food and Drug Administration (FDA) has not approved these drugs for the treatment of fatigue. Discuss the risks and benefits of these drugs with your doctor.

Treatment of Pain

If pain is making fatigue worse, the patient's pain medicine may be changed or the dose may be increased. If too much pain medicine is making fatigue worse, the patient's pain medicine may be changed or the dose may be decreased.

Treatment of Depression

Fatigue in patients who have depression may be treated with antidepressant drugs. Psychostimulant drugs may help some patients have more energy and a better mood, and help them think and concentrate. The use of psychostimulants for treating fatigue is still being studied. The FDA has not approved psychostimulants for the treatment of fatigue.

Psychostimulants have side effects, especially with long-term use. Different psychostimulants have different side effects. Patients who have heart problems or who take anticancer drugs that affect the heart may have serious side effects from psychostimulants. These drugs have warnings on the label about their risks. Talk to your doctor about the effects these drugs may have and use them only under a doctor's care. Some of the possible side effects include the following:

- Trouble sleeping

- Euphoria (feelings of extreme happiness)

- Headache

- Nausea

- Anxiety

- Mood changes

- Loss of appetite

- Nightmares

- Paranoia (feelings of fear and distrust of other people)

- Serious heart problems

The doctor may prescribe low doses of a psychostimulant to be used for a short time in patients with advanced cancer who have severe fatigue. Talk to your doctor about the risks and benefits of these drugs.

Certain drugs are being studied for fatigue related to cancer. The following drugs are being studied for fatigue related to cancer:

- Bupropion is an antidepressant that is being studied to treat fatigue in patients with or without depression.

- Dexamethasone is an anti-inflammatory drug being studied in patients with advanced cancer. In one clinical trial, patients who received dexamethasone reported less fatigue than the group that received a placebo. More trials are needed to study the link between inflammation and fatigue.

Certain dietary supplements are being studied for fatigue related to cancer. The following dietary supplements are being studied for fatigue related to cancer:

- L-carnitine is a supplement that helps the body make energy and lowers inflammation that may be linked to fatigue.

- Ginseng is an herb used to treat fatigue which may be taken in capsules of ground ginseng root. In a clinical trial, cancer patients who were either in treatment or had finished treatment, received either ginseng or placebo. The group receiving ginseng had less fatigue than the placebo group.

Treatment of fatigue may include teaching the patient ways to increase energy and cope with fatigue in daily life.

Exercise. Exercise (including walking) may help people with cancer feel better and have more energy. The effect of exercise on fatigue in cancer patients is being studied. One study reported that breast cancer survivors who took part in enjoyable physical activity had less fatigue and pain and were better able to take part in daily activities. In clinical trials, some patients reported the following benefits from exercise:

- More physical energy.
- Better appetite.
- More able to do the normal activities of daily living.
- Better quality of life.
- More satisfaction with life.
- A greater sense of well-being.
- More able to meet the demands of cancer and cancer treatment.

Moderate activity for 3 to 5 hours a week may help cancer-related fatigue. You are more likely to follow an exercise plan if you choose a type of exercise that you enjoy. The healthcare team can help you plan the best time and place for exercise and how often to exercise. Patients may need to start with light activity for short periods of time and build up to more exercise little by little. Studies have shown that exercise can be safely done during and after cancer treatment.

Mind and body exercises such as qigong, tai chi, and yoga may help relieve fatigue. These exercises combine activities like movement, stretching, balance, and controlled breathing with spiritual activity such as meditation.

A schedule of activity and rest. Changes in daily routine make the body use more energy. A regular routine can improve sleep and help the patient have more energy to be active during the day. A program of regular times for activity and rest help to make the most of a patient's energy. A healthcare professional can help patients plan an exercise program and decide which activities are the most important to them.

The following sleep habits may help decrease fatigue:

• Lie in bed for sleep only.

• Take naps for no longer than one hour.

• Avoid noise (like television and radio) during sleep.

Cancer patients should not try to do too much. Health professionals have information about support services to help with daily activities and responsibilities.

Talk therapy. Therapists use talk therapy (counseling) to treat certain emotional or behavioral disorders. This kind of therapy helps patients change how they think and feel about certain things. Talk therapy may help decrease a cancer patient's fatigue by working on problems related to cancer that make fatigue worse, such as:

• Stress from coping with cancer.

• Fear that the cancer may come back.

• Feeling hopeless about fatigue.

• Not enough social support.

• A pattern of sleep and activity that changes from day to day.

Self-care for fatigue. Fatigue is often a short-term side effect of treatment, but in some patients it becomes chronic (continues as a long-term condition). Managing chronic fatigue includes adjusting to life with fatigue. Learning the facts about cancer-related fatigue may help you cope with it better and improve quality of life. For example, some patients in treatment worry that having fatigue means the treatment is not working. Anxiety over this can make fatigue even worse. Some patients may feel that reporting fatigue is complaining. Knowing that fatigue is a normal side effect that should be reported and treated may make it easier to manage.

Working with the healthcare team to learn about the following may help patients cope with fatigue:

• How to cope with fatigue as a normal side effect of treatment.

• The possible medical causes of fatigue such as not enough fluids, electrolyte imbalance, breathing problems, or anemia.

- How patterns of rest and activity affect fatigue.

- How to schedule important daily activities during times of less fatigue, and give up less important activities.

- The kinds of activities that may help you feel more alert (walking, gardening, bird-watching).

- The difference between fatigue and depression.

- How to avoid or change situations that cause stress.

- How to avoid or change activities that cause fatigue.

- How to change your surroundings to help decrease fatigue.

- Exercise programs that are right for you and decrease fatigue.

- The importance of eating enough food and drinking enough fluids.

- Physical therapy for patients who have nerve problems or muscle weakness.

- Respiratory therapy for patients who have trouble breathing.

- How to tell if treatments for fatigue are working.

Fatigue after Cancer Treatment Ends

Fatigue continues to be a problem for many cancer survivors long after treatment ends and the cancer is gone. Studies show that some patients continue to have moderate-to-severe fatigue years after treatment. Long-term therapies such as tamoxifen can also cause fatigue. In children who were treated for brain tumors and cured, fatigue may continue after treatment.

The causes of fatigue after treatment ends are different than the causes of fatigue during treatment. Treating fatigue after treatment ends also may be different from treating it during cancer therapy.

Since fatigue may greatly affect the quality of life for cancer survivors, long-term follow-up care is important.

Chapter 36

Cancer Pain

Pain is one of the most common symptoms in cancer patients. Pain can be caused by cancer, treatment for cancer, or a combination of factors. Tumors, surgery, intravenous chemotherapy, radiation therapy, targeted therapy, supportive care therapies such as bisphosphonates, and diagnostic procedures, may cause you pain.

Younger patients are more likely to have cancer pain and pain flares than older patients. Patients with advanced cancer have more severe pain, and many cancer survivors have pain that continues after cancer treatment ends.

This chapter is about ways to control cancer pain.

Pain Control Can Improve Your Quality of Life

Pain can be controlled in most patients who have cancer. Although cancer pain cannot always be relieved completely, there are ways to lessen pain in most patients. Pain control can improve your quality of life all through your cancer treatment and after it ends.

Management of Cancer Pain

Many diagnostic and treatment procedures are painful. It helps to start pain control before the procedure begins. Some drugs may be used to help you feel calm or fall asleep. Treatments such as imagery or relaxation can also help control pain and anxiety related to treatment.

This chapter includes text excerpted from "Cancer Pain (PDQ®)–Patient Version," National Cancer Institute (NCI), September 23, 2016.

Knowing what will happen during the procedure and having a relative or friend stay with you may also help lower anxiety.

Different Cancer Treatments May Cause Specific Types of Pain

Patients may have different types of pain depending on the treatments they receive, including:

- Spasms, stinging, and itching caused by intravenous chemotherapy.

- Mucositis (sores or inflammation in the mouth or other parts of the digestive system) caused by chemotherapy or targeted therapy.

- Skin pain, rash, or hand-foot syndrome (redness, tingling, or burning in the palms of the hands and/or the soles of feet) caused by chemotherapy or targeted therapy.

- Pain in joints and muscles throughout the body caused by paclitaxel or aromatase inhibitor therapy.

- Osteonecrosis of the jaw caused by bisphosphonates given for cancer that has spread to the bone.

- Pain syndromes caused by radiation, including mucositis, pain flares, and dermatitis.

Cancer Pain and Quality of Life after Treatment

Pain that is severe or continues after cancer treatment ends increases the risk of anxiety and depression. Patients may be disabled by their pain, unable to work, or feel that they are losing support once their care moves from their oncology team back to their primary care team. Feelings of anxiety and depression can worsen cancer pain and make it harder to control.

Each Patient Needs a Personal Plan to Control Cancer Pain

Each person's diagnosis, cancer stage, response to pain, and personal likes and dislikes are different. For this reason, each patient needs a personal plan to control cancer pain. You, your family, and your healthcare team can work together to manage your pain. As part of your pain control plan, your healthcare provider can give you and your family members written instructions to control your pain at home. Find out who you should call if you have questions.

Assessment of Cancer Pain

It's important that the cause of the pain is found early and treated quickly. Your healthcare team will help you measure pain levels often, including at the following times:

- After starting cancer treatment.

- When there is new pain.

- After starting any type of pain treatment.

To learn about your pain, the healthcare team will ask you to describe the pain with the following questions:

- When did the pain start?

- How long does the pain last?

- Where is the pain? You will be asked to show exactly where the pain is on your body or on a drawing of a body.

- How strong is the pain?

- Have there been changes in where or when the pain occurs?

- What makes the pain better or worse?

- Is the pain worse during certain times of the day or night?

- Is there breakthrough pain (intense pain that flares up quickly even when pain control medicine is being used)?

- Do you have symptoms, such as trouble sleeping, fatigue, depression, or anxiety?

- Does pain get in the way of activities of daily life, such as eating, bathing, or moving around?

Your healthcare team will also take into account:

- Past and current pain treatments.

- Prognosis (chance of recovery).

- Other conditions you may have, such as kidney, liver, or heart disease.

- Past and current use of nicotine, alcohol, or sleeping pills.

- Personal or family history of substance abuse.

- Personal history of childhood sexual abuse.

• Your own choices.

This information will be used to decide how to help relieve your pain. This may include drugs or other treatments. In some cases, patients are referred to pain specialists or palliative care specialists. Your healthcare team will work with you to decide whether the benefits of treatment outweigh any risks and how much improvement you should expect. After pain control is started, the doctor will continue to assess how well it is working for you and make changes if needed.

A family member or caregiver may be asked to give answers for a patient who has a problem with speech, language, or understanding.

Physical and neurological exams will be done to help plan pain control. The following exams will be done:

• **Physical exam and history:** An exam of the body to check general signs of health, including checking for signs of disease, such as lumps or anything else that seems unusual. A history of your health habits and past illnesses and treatments will also be taken.

• **Neurological exam:** A series of questions and tests to check the brain, spinal cord, and nerve function. The exam checks your mental status, coordination, and ability to walk normally, and how well the muscles, senses, and reflexes work. This may also be called a neuro exam or a neurologic exam.

Your healthcare team will also assess your psychological, social, and spiritual needs.

Using Drugs to Control Cancer Pain

The doctor will prescribe drugs based on whether the pain is mild, moderate, or severe. Your doctor will prescribe drugs to help relieve your pain. These drugs need to be taken at scheduled times to keep a constant level of the drug in the body to help keep the pain from coming back. Drugs may be taken by mouth or given in other ways, such as by infusion or injection.

Your doctor may prescribe extra doses of a drug that can be taken as needed for pain that occurs between scheduled doses of the drug. The doctor will adjust the drug dose for your needs.

A scale from 0 to 10 is used to measure how severe the pain is and decide which pain medicine to use. On this scale:

• 0 means no pain.

- 1 to 3 means mild pain.

- 4 to 6 means moderate pain.

- 7 to 10 means severe pain.

Acetaminophen and nonsteroidal anti-inflammatory drugs (NSAIDs) may be used to relieve mild pain. They may be given with opioids for moderate to severe pain.

Pain relievers of this type include:

- Acetaminophen
- Ibuprofen
- Celecoxib
- Ketoprofen
- Diclofenac
- Ketorolac

Patients, especially older patients, who are taking acetaminophen or NSAIDs need to be closely watched for side effects.

Opioids are used to relieve moderate to severe pain. Opioids work very well to relieve moderate to severe pain. Some patients with cancer pain stop getting pain relief from opioids if they take them for a long time. This is called tolerance. Larger doses or a different opioid may be needed if your body stops responding to the same dose. Tolerance of an opioid is a physical dependence on it. This is not the same as addiction (psychological dependence).

Since 1999, there have been four times the number of prescriptions written for opioids and four times the number of deaths caused by drug overdose in the United States. Although most patients who are prescribed opioids for cancer pain use them safely, a small percentage of patients may become addicted to opioids. Your doctor will carefully prescribe and monitor your opioid doses so that you are treated for pain safely.

There are several types of opioids:

- Buprenorphine

- Codeine

- Diamorphine

- Fentanyl

- Hydrocodone

- Hydromorphone

- Methadone

- Morphine (the most commonly used opioid for cancer pain)

- Oxycodone

- Oxymorphone

- Tapentadol

- Tramadol

The doctor will prescribe drugs and the times they should be taken in order to best control your pain. Also, it is important that patients and family caregivers know how to safely use, store, and dispose of opioids.

Most patients with cancer pain will need to receive opioids on a regular schedule. Receiving opioids on a regular schedule helps relieve the pain and keeps it from getting worse. The amount of time between doses depends on which opioid you are using. The correct dose is the amount of opioid that controls your pain with the fewest side effects. The dose will be slowly adjusted until there is a good balance between pain relief and side effects. If opioid tolerance does occur, the dose may be increased or a different opioid may be needed.

Opioids may be given in different ways. Opioids may be given by the following ways:

- **Mouth:** If your stomach and intestines work normally, medicine is usually given by mouth. Opioids given orally are easy to use and usually low-cost. Oral opioids are sometimes placed under the tongue (sublingual route) or on the inside of the cheek (buccal route) to be absorbed.

- **Rectum:** If you cannot take opioids by mouth, they may be given as rectal suppositories.

- **Skin patches:** Opioid patches are placed on the skin (transdermal route).

- **Nose spray:** Opioids may be given in the form of a nasal spray.

- **Intravenous (IV) line:** Opioids are given into a vein only when simpler and less costly methods cannot be used, don't work, or are not wanted by the patient. Patient-controlled analgesia (PCA) pumps are one way to control pain through your IV line. A PCA pump allows you to control the amount of drug that is used. With a PCA pump, you can receive a preset opioid dose by pressing a button on a computerized pump that is connected to a small tube. Once the pain is controlled, the doctor may prescribe regular opioid doses based on the amount you used with the PCA pump.

- **Subcutaneous injection:** Opioids are given by injection into the fatty layer of tissue just under the skin.

- **Intraspinal injection:** Intraspinal opioids are injected into the fluid around the spinal cord. These may be combined with a local anesthetic to help some patients who have pain that is very hard to control.

There are common side effects caused by opioids. Your doctor will discuss the side effects with you before opioid treatment begins and will watch you for side effects. The following are the most common side effects:

- Constipation

- Nausea

- Drowsiness

- Dry mouth

Nausea and drowsiness most often occur when opioid treatment is first started and usually get better within a few days.

Opioids slow down the muscle contractions and movement in the stomach and intestines, which can cause hard stools. To keep the stool soft and prevent constipation, it's important to drink plenty of fluids. Unless there are problems such as a blocked bowel or diarrhea, you will be given a treatment plan to follow to prevent constipation and information on how to avoid problems with your intestines while taking opioids.

Other side effects of opioid treatment include the following:

- Vomiting
- Low blood pressure
- Dizziness
- Trouble sleeping
- Trouble thinking clearly
- Delirium or hallucinations
- Trouble urinating
- Problems with breathing
- Severe itching
- Problems with sexual function
- Hot flashes
- Depression
- Hypoglycemia

Talk with your doctor about side effects that bother you or become severe. Your doctor may decrease the dose of the opioid, change to a different opioid, or change the way the opioid is given to help decrease the side effects.

Other drugs may be added to help treat your pain. Other drugs may be given while you are taking opioids for pain relief. These are drugs that help the opioids work better, treat symptoms, and relieve certain types of pain. The following types of drugs may be used:

- Antidepressants

- Anticonvulsants

- Local anesthetics

- Corticosteroids

- Stimulants

- Bisphosphonates and denosumab

There are big differences in how patients respond to these drugs. Side effects are common and should be reported to your doctor.

Bisphosphonates (pamidronate and zoledronic acid) are drugs that are sometimes used when cancer has spread to the bones. They are given as an intravenous infusion and combined with other treatments to decrease pain and reduce risk of broken bones. However, bisphosphonates sometimes cause severe side effects. Talk to your doctor if you have severe muscle or bone pain. Bisphosphonate therapy may need to be stopped.

The use of bisphosphonates is also linked to the risk of bisphosphonate-associated osteonecrosis (BON).

Denosumab is another drug that may be used when cancer has spread to the bones. It is given as a subcutaneous injection and may help prevent and relieve pain. It is not used in certain patients, such as patients with myeloma.

Other Treatments for Cancer Pain

Most cancer pain can be controlled with drug treatments, but some patients have too many side effects from drugs or have pain in a certain part of the body that needs to be treated in a different way. You can talk to your doctor to help decide which methods work best to relieve your pain. These other treatments include:

Nerve blocks: A nerve block is the injection of either a local anesthetic or a drug into or around a nerve to block pain. Nerve blocks help control pain that can't be controlled in other ways. Nerve blocks may also be used to find where the pain is coming from, to predict how the pain will respond to long-term treatments, and to prevent pain after certain procedures.

Neurological treatments: Surgery can be done to insert a device that delivers drugs or stimulates the nerves with mild electric current. In rare cases, surgery may be done to destroy a nerve or nerves that are part of the pain pathway.

Cordotomy: Cordotomy is a less common surgical procedure that is used to relieve pain by cutting certain nerves in the spinal cord. This blocks pain and also hot/cold feelings. This procedure may be chosen for patients who are near the end of life and have severe pain that cannot be relieved in other ways.

Palliative care: Certain patients are helped by palliative care services. Palliative care providers may also be called supportive care providers. They work in teams that include doctors, nurses, mental health specialists, social workers, chaplains, pharmacists, and dietitians. Some of the goals of palliative care are to:

- Improve quality of life for patients and their families
- Manage pain and non-pain symptoms
- Support patients who need higher doses of opioids, have a history of substance abuse, or are coping with emotional and social problems

Radiation therapy: Radiation therapy is used to relieve pain in patients with skin lesions, tumors, or cancer that has spread to the bone. This is called palliative radiation therapy. It may be given as local therapy directly to the tumor or to larger areas of the body. Radiation therapy helps drugs and other treatments work better by shrinking tumors that are causing pain. Radiation therapy may help patients with bone pain move more freely and with less pain.

The following types of radiation therapy may be used:

External radiation therapy: External radiation therapy uses a machine outside the body to send high-energy X-rays or other types of radiation toward the cancer. External radiation therapy relieves pain from cancer that has spread to the bone. Radiation therapy may be given in a single dose or divided into several smaller doses given over a period of time. The decision whether to have a single or divided dose may depend on how easy it is to get the treatments and how much they cost.

Radiopharmaceuticals: Radiopharmaceuticals are drugs that have a radioactive substance that may be used to diagnose or treat disease, including cancer. Radiopharmaceuticals may also be used to relieve pain from cancer that has spread to the bone. A single dose of a radioactive agent injected into a vein may relieve pain when cancer has spread to several areas of bone and/or when there are too many areas to treat with external radiation therapy.

Physical medicine and rehabilitation: Patients with cancer and pain may lose their strength, freedom of movement, and ability to manage their daily activities. Physical therapy or occupational therapy may help these patients.

Physical medicine uses physical methods, such as exercise and machines to prevent and treat disease or injury.

Physical methods to treat weakness, muscle wasting, and muscle and bone pain include the following:

- Exercise to strengthen and stretch weak muscles, loosen stiff joints, help coordination and balance, and strengthen the heart.

- Changing position (for patients who are not able to move on their own).

- Limiting the movement of painful areas or broken bones.

Some patients may be referred to a physiatrist (a doctor who specializes in physical medicine) who can develop a personal plan for them. Some physiatrists are also trained in procedures to treat and manage pain.

Complementary therapies: Complementary and alternative therapies combined with standard treatment may be used to treat pain. They may also be called integrative therapies. Acupuncture, support groups, and hypnosis are a few integrative therapies that have been used to relieve pain.

Acupuncture: Acupuncture is an integrative therapy that applies needles, heat, pressure, and other treatments to one or more places on the skin called acupuncture points. Acupuncture may be used to control pain, including pain related to cancer.

Hypnosis: Hypnosis may help you relax and may be combined with other thinking and behavior methods. Hypnosis to relieve pain works best in people who are able to concentrate and use imagery and who are willing to practice the technique.

Treating Cancer Pain in Older Patients

Certain factors affect cancer pain treatment in older adults. Some problems are more likely in patients 65 years and older. For caregivers of these patients, the following should be kept in mind:

Lower Doses

Pain medicine should be started at lower doses in older patients and adjusted slowly to allow for differences in their pain threshold and the ways they respond and function.

Older patients may need lower doses of opioids since they are more sensitive to their effects. Side effects of opioids, such as drowsiness and constipation, are more likely in older patients.

Opioid doses may need to be lower in older patients for either acute or chronic pain. Lower doses may give older patients better pain relief that lasts longer than in younger patients.

Meperidine, and some drugs often used with opioids, are not given to certain older patients.

More than One Chronic Disease and Source of Pain

Older patients may have more than one chronic disease and take several drugs for different conditions. This can increase the risk of drug interactions. Drugs taken together can change how they work in the body and can affect the patient's chronic diseases.

Side Effects of Nonsteroidal Anti-Inflammatory Drugs (NSAIDs)

Side effects of NSAIDs, such as stomach and kidney damage, memory problems, constipation, and headaches, are more likely in older patients.

NSAIDs and tricyclic antidepressants are not given to certain older patients. When NSAIDs are used, older patients should be watched closely for side effects. Other drugs may be given with NSAIDs to help protect the stomach.

To avoid side effects from certain NSAIDs, some patients may be given the following:

- Acetaminophen
- Topical NSAIDs

- COX-2 -selective NSAIDs (NSAIDs that cause fewer problems with the stomach and intestines)

Risk of Under Treatment

In older patients there is a risk of under-treatment (not receiving enough treatment). This may be caused by the following:

- Patients do not report their pain.
- Patients are not able to talk about the pain they have.
- The doctor is concerned about side effects or changes in patient behavior that may be caused by pain medicine.

Poor pain control may cause other problems in older patients, including the following:

- Reduced physical or mental function.
- Slow recovery.
- Changes in appetite or sleep.
- Increased need for care of other health problems.
- Treating depression in patients can also help with pain treatment.

Chapter 37

Sexuality and Reproductive Concerns Related to Cancer Treatment

Chapter Contents

Section 37.1

Sexual and Fertility Concerns for Women

This section includes text excerpted from "Sexual and Fertility Problems (Women)," National Cancer Institute (NCI), April 29, 2015.

Many cancer treatments and some types of cancer can cause sexual and fertility-related side effects. Whether or not you have these problems depends on the type of treatment(s) you receive, your age at time of treatment, and the length of time since treatment.

It is important to get information about how the treatment recommended for you may affect your fertility before you start treatment. Many women also find it helpful to talk with their doctor or nurse about sexual problems they may have during treatment. Learning about these issues will help you make decisions that are best for you.

Treatments That May Cause Sexual and Fertility Problems

- Some types of chemotherapy may cause symptoms of early menopause (hot flashes, vaginal dryness, irregular or no periods, and feeling irritable) or lead to vaginal infections. It may also cause temporary or permanent infertility.

- Hormone therapy can stop or slow the growth of certain cancers, such as breast cancer. However, lower hormone levels can cause problems (hot flashes, vaginal discharge or pain, and trouble reaching orgasm). These problems are more likely in women over the age of 45.

- Radiation therapy to the pelvic area (vagina, uterus, or ovaries) can cause:

  - infertility

  - symptoms of menopause (hot flashes, vaginal dryness, and no periods)

- pain or discomfort during sex

- increased risk of birth defects; use a method of birth control to avoid pregnancy

- vaginal stenosis (less elastic, narrow, shorter vagina)

- vaginal itching, burning, or dryness

- vaginal atrophy (weak vaginal muscles and thin vaginal wall)

- Surgery for cancers of the uterus, bladder, vulvar, endometrium, cervix, or ovaries may cause sexual and infertility-related side effects, depending on the size and location of the tumor.

- Other side effects of cancer and its treatment, such as fatigue and anxiety, can also lower your interest in sexual activity.

What to Expect

Before starting treatment talk with your healthcare team to learn what to expect, based on the type of treatment you will be receiving. Get answers to questions about:

- **Infertility.** Ask if treatment could lower your fertility or make you infertile. If you would like to have children after treatment, talk with your doctor or nurse before you start treatment. Learn ahead of time about options such as embryo banking, ovarian tissue banking, ovarian transposition, and clinical trials for egg banking. Talk with your doctor or a fertility specialist to learn more about these procedures and others that may be available through a clinical trial.

- **Pregnancy.** It is important to prevent pregnancy during treatment and for some time after treatment. Ask your doctor or nurse about different methods of birth control, to choose one that may be best for you and your partner.

- **Sexual activity.** Ask your doctor or nurse if it is okay for you to be sexually active during your treatment period. Most women can be sexually active, but you will want to confirm this with your healthcare team.

Talking with Your Healthcare Team

Prepare for your visit by making a list of questions.

Consider adding these questions to your list:

Sexual and sexuality-related questions

- What problems or changes might I have during treatment?
- How long might these problems last? Will any be permanent?
- Is there treatment for these problems?
- Would you give me the name of a specialist that I could meet with?
- Is there a support group for women that you would recommend?

Fertility-related questions

- Will my fertility be affected by the treatment I receive?
- What are all of my options now if I would like to have children in the future?
- Could you give me the name of a fertility specialist who I can talk with to learn more?
- After treatment, how long should I use birth control?

Section 37.2

Sexual and Fertility Concerns for Men

This section includes text excerpted from "Sexual and Fertility Problems (Men)," National Cancer Institute (NCI), April 29, 2015.

Many cancer treatments and some types of cancer can cause sexual and fertility-related side effects. Whether you have these problems depends on the type of treatment(s) you receive, your age at time of treatment, and how long it has been since you had treatment.

It is important to learn how the treatment recommended for you may affect your fertility before you start treatment. Many men also find it helpful to talk with their doctor or nurse about sexual problems they may have during treatment. Learning about these issues will help you make decisions that are best for you.

Treatments That May Cause Sexual and Fertility Problems

- Radiation therapy to the pelvic area (such as to the anus, bladder, penis, or prostate) may make it difficult to get or keep an erection. It may also cause infertility, which may be temporary or permanent. Some men notice that changes in sexual function occur slowly over the period of about a year. Smoking, heart disease, high blood pressure, and diabetes can make some problems worse.

- Hormone therapy may cause mood changes, decreased sexual desire, erectile dysfunction, and trouble reaching orgasm.

- Some types of chemotherapy may cause low testosterone levels and lower your sexual desire. Chemotherapy may also cause infertility, which may be temporary or permanent.

- Surgery for penile, rectal, prostate, testicular, and other pelvic cancers may affect sexual function and fertility.

- Other side effects of cancer and its treatment, such as fatigue and anxiety, can also lower your interest in sexual activity.

Learn What to Expect

Before starting treatment talk with your healthcare team to learn what to expect based on the type of treatment you will be receiving. Get answers to questions about:

Sexual activity. Ask your doctor or nurse if it is okay for you to be sexually active during your treatment period. Most men can, but you will want to confirm this with your doctor or nurse.

Infertility. Ask if your treatment could affect your fertility or make you infertile. If you would like to have children after treatment, talk with your doctor or nurse before you start treatment. Learn ahead of time about your options, such as sperm banking. Procedures such as testicular sperm extraction, testicular tissue freezing and testicular tissue cryopreservation (for young boys) are available. Talk with your doctor or a fertility specialist to learn more about these procedures and other that may be available through a clinical trial.

Birth control. It is important to prevent pregnancy during treatment and for some time after treatment. Ask your doctor or nurse about different methods of birth control to choose one that may be best for you and your partner.

- **Condom use.** If you receive chemotherapy you will most likely be advised to use a condom during intercourse, even if your partner is on birth control or cannot have children. This is because your semen may have traces of the chemotherapy drugs.

Talking with Your Healthcare Team

Prepare for your visit by making a list of questions to ask. Consider adding these questions to your list:

Sexual and sexuality-related questions

- What problems or changes might I have during or after treatment?

- How long might these problems last? Will any of these problems be permanent?

- How can these problems be treated or managed?

- Could you give me the name of a specialist who I can talk with to learn more?

- What precautions do I need to take during treatment? For example, do I need to use a condom?

- Is there a support group for men that you would recommend for me?

Fertility-related questions

- Will the treatment I receive make me infertile (unable to have children in the future)?

- What are all of my options now if I would like to have children in the future?

- Could you give me the name of a fertility specialist who I can talk with to learn more?

- After treatment, how long should I use some method of birth control?

Chapter 38

Hot Flashes and Night Sweats

Sweating is the body's way of lowering body temperature by causing heat loss through the skin. In patients with cancer, sweating may be caused by fever, a tumor, or cancer treatment.

Hot flashes can also cause too much sweating. They may occur in natural menopause or in patients who have been treated for breast cancer or prostate cancer.

Hot flashes combined with sweats that happen while sleeping are often called night sweats or hot flushes.

Hot flashes and night sweats affect quality of life in many patients with cancer. A treatment plan to help manage hot flashes and night sweats is based on the patient's condition and goals of care. For some patients, relieving symptoms and improving quality of life is the most important goal.

This chapter describes the causes and treatment of hot flashes and night sweats in cancer patients.

Causes of Hot Flashes and Night Sweats

In patients with cancer, hot flashes and night sweats may be caused by the tumor, its treatment, or other conditions. Sweating happens with disease conditions such as fever and may occur without disease in warm climates, during exercise, and during hot flashes in menopause.

This chapter includes text excerpted from "Hot Flashes and Night Sweats (PDQ®)–Patient Version," National Cancer Institute (NCI), October 15, 2014.

Sweating helps balance body temperature by allowing heat to evaporate through the skin.

Hot flashes and night sweats are common in patients with cancer and in cancer survivors. They are more common in women but can also occur in men.

Many patients treated for breast cancer and prostate cancer have hot flashes. Menopause in women can have natural, surgical, or chemical causes. Chemical menopause in women with cancer is caused by certain types of chemotherapy, radiation, or hormone therapy with androgen (a male hormone).

"Male menopause" in men with cancer can be caused by orchiectomy (surgery to remove one or both testicles) or hormone therapy with gonadotropin-releasing hormone or estrogen.

Treatment for breast cancer and prostate cancer can cause menopause or menopause-like effects, including severe hot flashes.

Certain types of drugs can cause night sweats. Drugs that may cause night sweats include the following:

- Tamoxifen

- Aromatase inhibitors

- Opioids

- Tricyclic antidepressants

- Steroids

Drug Treatment for Hot Flashes and Night Sweats

Sweats are controlled by treating their cause. Sweats caused by fever are controlled by treating the cause of the fever. Sweats caused by a tumor are usually controlled by treatment of the tumor.

Hot flashes may be controlled with estrogen replacement therapy. Hot flashes during natural or treatment-related menopause can be controlled with estrogen replacement therapy. However, many women are not able to take estrogen replacement (for example, women who have or had breast cancer). Hormone replacement therapy that combines estrogen with progestin may increase the risk of breast cancer or breast cancer recurrence.

Treatment of hot flashes in men who have been treated for prostate cancer may include estrogens, progestin, antidepressants, and anticonvulsants. Certain hormones (such as estrogen) can make some cancers grow.

Other drugs may be useful in some patients. Studies of non-estrogen drugs to treat hot flashes in women with a history of breast cancer have reported that many of them do not work as well as estrogen replacement or have side effects. Megestrol (a drug like progesterone), certain antidepressants, anticonvulsants, and clonidine (a drug used to treat high blood pressure) are non-estrogen drugs used to control hot flashes. Some antidepressants may change how other drugs, such as tamoxifen, work in the body. Side effects of drug therapy may include the following:

- Antidepressants used to treat hot flashes over a short period of time may cause nausea, drowsiness, dry mouth, and changes in appetite.

- Anticonvulsants used to treat hot flashes may cause drowsiness, dizziness, and trouble concentrating.

- Clonidine may cause dry mouth, drowsiness, constipation, and insomnia.

Patients may respond in different ways to drug therapy. It is important that the patient's healthcare providers know about all medicines, dietary supplements, and herbs the patient is taking.

Drugs that may relieve nighttime hot flashes or night sweats and improve sleep at the same time are being studied in clinical trials.

If one medicine does not improve symptoms, switching to another medicine may help.

Non-Drug Treatment for Hot Flashes and Night Sweats

Treatments that help patients cope with stress and anxiety may help manage hot flashes. Treatments that change how patients deal with stress, anxiety, and negative emotions may help manage hot flashes. These are called psychological interventions. Psychological interventions help patients gain a sense of control and develop coping skills to manage symptoms. Staying calm and managing stress may lower levels of a hormone called serotonin that can trigger hot flashes.

Psychological interventions may help hot flashes and related problems when used together with drug treatment.

Hypnosis may help relieve hot flashes. Hypnosis is a trance-like state that allows a person to be more aware, focused, and open to suggestion. Under hypnosis, the person can concentrate more clearly on a specific thought, feeling, or sensation without becoming distracted.

Hypnosis is a newer treatment for hot flashes that has been shown to be helpful. In hypnosis, a therapist helps the patient to deeply relax and focus on cooling thoughts. This may lower stress levels, balance body temperature, and calm the heart rate and breathing rate.

Comfort measures may help relieve night sweats related to cancer. Comfort measures may be used to treat night sweats related to cancer. Since body temperature goes up before a hot flash, doing the following may control body temperature and help control symptoms:

- Wear loose-fitting clothes made of cotton.

- Use fans and open windows to keep air moving.

- Practice relaxation training and slow, deep breathing.

Herbs and dietary supplements should be used with caution. Studies of vitamin E for the relief of hot flashes show that it is only slightly better than a placebo (pill that has no effect). Most studies of soy and black cohosh show they are no better than a placebo in reducing hot flashes. Soy contains estrogen-like substances; the effect of soy on the risk of breast cancer growth or recurrence is not clear. Studies of ground flaxseed to treat hot flashes have shown mixed results.

Claims are made about several other plant-based and natural products as remedies for hot flashes. These include dong quai, milk thistle, red clover, licorice root extract, and chaste tree berry. Since little is known about how these products work or whether they affect the risk of breast cancer, women should be cautious about using them.

Acupuncture may be used to treat hot flashes. Pilot studies of acupuncture and randomized clinical trials that compare true acupuncture and sham (inactive) treatment have been done in patients with hot flashes. Results are not clear and more studies are needed.

Chapter 39

Pruritus (Itching)

Pruritus is an itchy feeling that makes you want to scratch your skin. It may occur without a rash or skin lesions. Pruritus sometimes feels like pain because the signals for itching and pain travel along the same nerve pathways. Scratching may cause breaks in the skin, bleeding, and infection. If your skin feels itchy, let your doctor know so it can be treated and relieved.

The way pruritus feels and how long it lasts is not the same in everyone.

The skin is the largest organ of the body. The most important job of skin is to protect against heat, sunlight, injury, and infection. The skin is also important to self-image and your ability to touch and be touched.

Causes of Pruritus

Certain conditions, cancers, and blood disorders may cause pruritus. Pruritus is a symptom of a certain condition, blood disorder, or a disease. These include:

- Cancer and conditions related to cancer

- Liver, kidney, or thyroid disorders

- Diabetes mellitus

- HIV or parasite infection

This chapter includes text excerpted from "Pruritus (PDQ®)–Patient Version," National Cancer Institute (NCI), June 15, 2016.

- Dry skin

- Drug reactions

- Conditions related to stress, anxiety, or depression

The cause of pruritus is not always known.

Certain cancer treatments may cause pruritus. Cancer treatments that may cause pruritus include chemotherapy, radiation therapy, and immunotherapy (biologic therapy).

- When chemotherapy causes pruritus, it may be a sign that you are sensitive to the drugs being used.

- Radiation therapy can kill skin cells and cause dryness, burning, and itching as the skin peels off.

- Drugs used in immunotherapy may also cause dryness and itching.

Skin can become thin and dry because many of these therapies make your skin less able to make new cells and heal. Long-term dry skin may occur when hair and sweat gland function does not return to normal right after cancer treatment.

Drugs may be used for supportive care. Some of the drugs used to prevent or treat cancer symptoms may cause pruritus, including the following:

- Pain medicine such as opioids

- Drugs for nausea and vomiting

- Hormones such as estrogens, testosterone, or progestins

Assessment of Pruritus

Finding the cause of the itching is the first step in relieving pruritus. Since pruritus is a symptom of a disease or condition, finding and treating the cause is the first step in bringing you relief. A physical exam, blood tests, and a chest X-ray are done to assess pruritus.

The following tests and procedures may be done to find the problem that is causing the itching:

- **Physical exam and history:** An exam of the body to check general signs of health, including checking for signs of disease, such as lumps or anything else that seems unusual.

The doctor will check your skin for the following:

- Signs of infection

- Signs of a drug reaction

- Redness, dryness, scratches, or lesions

- Abnormal color, texture, or temperature

A history of your health habits, past illnesses, and treatments will also be taken.

You may be asked about the following:

- When the pruritus started, how long it lasts, how bad it is, and what part of your body is itchy.

- How it affects your daily activities and sleep.

- What makes the itching better or worse.

- Whether other family members or pets are affected.

- Whether you have had pruritus before.

- Current cancer treatment or past history of cancer.

- Other diseases you have now or had in the past and their treatment.

- Pain medicines, antibiotics, or other drugs you are taking, including illegal drugs.

- Whether your diet is healthy and you drink enough fluids.

- Social history (hobbies, job, sexual history, and travel).

- How you care for your skin.

- Your emotional health.

- **Blood chemistry studies:** A procedure in which a blood sample is checked to measure the amounts of certain substances released into the blood by organs and tissues in the body. An unusual (higher or lower than normal) amount of a substance can be a sign of disease. These blood tests include:

  - Kidney function tests

  - Liver function tests

  - Lactate dehydrogenase test

- Thyroid function tests

- **Complete blood count (CBC) with differential:** A procedure in which a sample of blood is drawn and checked for the following:

  - The number of red blood cells and platelets

  - The number and type of white blood cells

  - The amount of hemoglobin (the protein that carries oxygen) in the red blood cells

  - The portion of the blood sample made up of red blood cells

- **Sedimentation rate:** A procedure in which a sample of blood is drawn and checked for the rate at which the red blood cells settle to the bottom of the test tube. The sedimentation rate is a measure of how much inflammation is in the body. A higher than normal sedimentation rate may be a sign of lymphoma or another condition. Also called erythrocyte sedimentation rate, sed rate, or ESR.

- **Chest X-ray:** An X-ray of the organs and bones inside the chest. An X-ray is a type of energy beam that can go through the body and onto film, making a picture of areas inside the body.

Depending on the results, further tests, such as a skin biopsy, may be done to diagnose the problem and decide on treatment.

Treatment of Pruritus

Treatment of pruritus in cancer patients involves learning what the triggers are and taking steps to avoid them. It is important for you and for caregivers to know what triggers itching, such as dry skin or hot baths, so you can take steps to prevent it. You may need more than one type of treatment to relieve or prevent pruritus, protect your skin, and keep you comfortable.

Good nutrition is very important for healthy skin. A good diet includes a balance of proteins, carbohydrates, fats, vitamins, minerals, and fluids. Eating a balanced diet and drinking plenty of fluids helps your skin stay healthy. It is best to drink at least 3 liters (about 100 ounces) of fluid each day, but this may not be possible for everyone.

Washing the skin every day or every two days is important to help remove dirt and keep the skin healthy.

Different types of treatment are used to help treat pruritus.

Self-Care

Self-care includes avoiding pruritus triggers and taking good care of your skin.

Pruritus triggers include:

- Dehydration caused by fever, diarrhea, nausea and vomiting, or low fluid intake.
- Hot baths or bathing more than once a day, or for longer than 30 minutes.
- Bubble baths or soaps with detergents.
- Reusable scrubbing sponges for the face or loofahs for the body.
- Scents, fragrances, and perfumes.
- Adding oil at the beginning of the bath.
- Dry indoor air.
- Laundry detergent with scents, dyes, or preservatives.
- Fabric softener sheets.
- Tight clothes or clothes made of wool, synthetics, or other harsh/ scratchy fabric.
- Underarm deodorants or antiperspirants.
- Skin care or cosmetics with scents, dyes, or preservatives.
- Emotional stress.

Ways to help lessen itching include:

- Using unscented, soothing creams or ointments.
- Bathing in slightly warm water no more than 30 minutes daily or every other day.
- Using mild skin cleansers (non-soap) or soaps made for sensitive skin (such as Cetaphil cleanser, Dove for Sensitive Skin, Oilatum, Basis).
- Adding oil and soap at the end of a bath or adding a colloidal oatmeal treatment early to the bath.
- Using soap only for dirty areas; otherwise water is good enough.
- Gently washing, if needed, with a clean, fresh, soft cotton washcloth.

- Rinsing all soap or other residue from bathing with fresh, slightly warm water.

- Drying off by patting skin instead of rubbing.

- Keeping home air cool and humid (including use of a humidifier).

- Washing sheets, clothes, and underwear in mild soap or baby soap that contains no scents, dyes, or preservatives (such as Dreft, All Free Clear, Tide Free and Gentle). Adding vinegar (one teaspoon per quart of water) to rinse water removes traces of detergent.

- Using liquid fabric softener that gets rinsed out in the wash (such as All Free Clear Fabric Softener) or avoiding fabric softener altogether.

- Using blankets that are soft, such as cotton flannel.

- Wearing loose-fitting clothes and clothes made of cotton or other soft fabrics.

- Using distraction, music therapy, relaxation, or positive imagery.

Over-the-Counter Treatments

Some over-the-counter (OTC) treatments (medicines that can be bought without a prescription) help prevent or relieve pruritus. However, you should read labels carefully to look for ingredients that may trigger skin reactions, including alcohol, topical antibiotics, and topical anesthetics.

Cornstarch and talc. Cornstarch can help prevent itching of dry skin caused by radiation therapy but should not be used where skin is moist. When cornstarch becomes moist, fungus may grow. Avoid using it on areas close to mucous membranes, such as the vagina or rectum, in skin folds, and on areas that have hair or sweat glands.

Some powders and antiperspirants, such as those that contain talc and aluminum, cause skin irritation during radiation therapy and should be avoided when you're receiving radiation treatment.

For itching not related to radiation therapy, talc-based treatments may be better than cornstarch-based treatments, especially where two skin surfaces touch or rub together (such as the underarm or between fingers or toes).

Creams and lotions. If pruritus is related to dry skin, emollient creams or lotions may be used. Emollients help soothe and soften the skin and increase moisture levels in the skin. It is important to know the ingredients in these creams and lotions because some may cause skin reactions. Such ingredients include:

- Petrolatum, which is not well absorbed in skin treated with radiation therapy and may build up too much or be hard to remove.

- Lanolin, which may cause allergic reactions in some people.

- Mineral oil, which may be combined with petrolatum and lanolin in creams and lotions and may be an ingredient in bath oils.

Other ingredients added to emollients, such as thickeners, preservatives, fragrances, and colorings, may also cause allergic skin reactions.

Emollient creams or lotions are applied at least two or three times a day and after bathing. Gels with a local anesthetic (0.5%–5% lidocaine) can be used on some small areas as often as every 2 hours if you aren't sensitive to alcohol ingredients.

To soothe or cool areas of severe pruritus, over-the-counter products containing menthol, camphor, pramoxine, or capsaicin can be used. These products soothe, cool, and decrease the urge to scratch. Capsaicin-based therapies may work best in pruritus related to nerve signals.

Prescription drugs applied to the skin. Your doctor may prescribe topical steroids (steroids applied to the skin) to reduce itching, but they cause thinning of the skin and make it more sensitive. They should be used only for pruritus related to inflammation. Topical steroids should not be used on skin being treated with radiation therapy, but may be used to relieve inflamed skin after radiation treatment ends.

For xerosis (abnormally dry skin) or keratoderma (a horn-like skin condition), moisturizer creams may be used to seal in moisture and peel off scaly layers of skin. Humectants with ingredients like salicylic acid, ammonium lactate, or urea may improve skin smoothness but can cause stinging if applied to broken skin.

Systemic therapies. Systemic therapies travel through the bloodstream and reach and affect cells all over the body. They may help treat the condition causing your pruritus or help control your symptoms.

Your doctor may prescribe an antibiotic if your pruritus is caused by an infection. You may also be given an oral antihistamine to relieve itching. A larger dose may sometimes be used at bedtime to help you sleep.

Other drug therapies. If other drug treatments do not work to control pruritus, sedatives and antidepressants are sometimes used.

Aspirin may relieve pruritus in some patients with polycythemia vera but may increase pruritus in others. Cimetidine alone or combined with aspirin may help control pruritus in patients with Hodgkin lymphoma and polycythemia vera.

Comfort measures. Other steps may be taken to help you keep from scratching and stop the itch-scratch-itch cycle. These may include:

- Applying emollients to help prevent skin breakdown.
- A cool washcloth or ice held over the itchy area.
- Firm pressure on the itchy area, on the same area on the opposite side of the body, and at acupressure points.
- Rubbing or vibration on the itchy area.
- Transcutaneous electrical nerve stimulation (TENS) or acupuncture.

Chapter 40

Lymphedema

Lymphedema is the build-up of fluid in soft body tissues when the lymph system is damaged or blocked. Lymphedema occurs when the lymph system is damaged or blocked. Fluid builds up in soft body tissues and causes swelling. It is a common problem that may be caused by cancer and cancer treatment. Lymphedema usually affects an arm or leg, but it can also affect other parts of the body. Lymphedema can cause long-term physical, psychological, and social problems for patients.

The lymph system is a network of lymph vessels, tissues, and organs that carry lymph throughout the body. The parts of the lymph system that play a direct part in lymphedema include the following:

- **Lymph:** A clear fluid that contains lymphocytes (white blood cells) that fight infection and the growth of tumors. Lymph also contains plasma, the watery part of the blood that carries the blood cells.

- **Lymph vessels:** A network of thin tubes that helps lymph flow through the body and returns it to the bloodstream.

- **Lymph nodes:** Small, bean-shaped structures that filter lymph and store white blood cells that help fight infection and disease. Lymph nodes are located along the network of lymph vessels found throughout the body. Clusters of lymph nodes are found in the underarm, pelvis, neck, abdomen, and groin.

This chapter includes text excerpted from "Lymphedema (PDQ®)–Patient Version," National Cancer Institute (NCI), May 29, 2015.

The spleen, thymus, tonsils, and bone marrow are also part of the lymph system but do not play a direct part in lymphedema.

Lymphedema occurs when lymph is not able to flow through the body the way that it should. When the lymph system is working as it should, lymph flows through the body and is returned to the bloodstream.

- Fluid and plasma leak out of the capillaries (smallest blood vessels) and flow around body tissues so the cells can take up nutrients and oxygen.

- Some of this fluid goes back into the bloodstream. The rest of the fluid enters the lymph system through tiny lymph vessels. These lymph vessels pick up the lymph and move it toward the heart. The lymph is slowly moved through larger and larger lymph vessels and passes through lymph nodes where waste is filtered from the lymph.

- The lymph keeps moving through the lymph system and collects near the neck, then flows into one of two large ducts:

  - The right lymph duct collects lymph from the right arm and the right side of the head and chest.

  - The left lymph duct collects lymph from both legs, the left arm, and the left side of the head and chest.

- These large ducts empty into veins under the collarbones, which carry the lymph to the heart, where it is returned to the bloodstream.

When part of the lymph system is damaged or blocked, fluid cannot drain from nearby body tissues. Fluid builds up in the tissues and causes swelling.

There are two types of lymphedema. Lymphedema may be either primary or secondary:

- Primary lymphedema is caused by the abnormal development of the lymph system. Symptoms may occur at birth or later in life.

- Secondary lymphedema is caused by damage to the lymph system. The lymph system may be damaged or blocked by infection, injury, cancer, removal of lymph nodes, radiation to the affected area, or scar tissue from radiation therapy or surgery.

This chapter is about secondary lymphedema in adults that is caused by cancer or cancer treatment.

Signs of Lymphedema

Possible signs of lymphedema include swelling of the arms or legs. Other conditions may cause the same symptoms. A doctor should be consulted if any of the following problems occur:

- Swelling of an arm or leg, which may include fingers and toes.
- A full or heavy feeling in an arm or leg.
- A tight feeling in the skin.
- Trouble moving a joint in the arm or leg.
- Thickening of the skin, with or without skin changes such as blisters or warts.
- A feeling of tightness when wearing clothing, shoes, bracelets, watches, or rings.
- Itching of the legs or toes.
- A burning feeling in the legs.
- Trouble sleeping.
- Loss of hair.

Daily activities and the ability to work or enjoy hobbies may be affected by lymphedema. These symptoms may occur very slowly over time or more quickly if there is an infection or injury to the arm or leg.

Risk Factors for Lymphedema

Cancer and its treatment are risk factors for lymphedema. Lymphedema can occur after any cancer or treatment that affects the flow of lymph through the lymph nodes, such as removal of lymph nodes. It may develop within days or many years after treatment. Most lymphedema develops within three years of surgery. Risk factors for lymphedema include the following:

- Removal and/or radiation of lymph nodes in the underarm, groin, pelvis, or neck. The risk of lymphedema increases with the number of lymph nodes affected. There is less risk with the removal of only the sentinel lymph node (the first lymph node to receive lymphatic drainage from a tumor).
- Being overweight or obese.
- Slow healing of the skin after surgery.

- A tumor that affects or blocks the left lymph duct or lymph nodes or vessels in the neck, chest, underarm, pelvis, or abdomen.

- Scar tissue in the lymph ducts under the collarbones, caused by surgery or radiation therapy.

Lymphedema often occurs in breast cancer patients who had all or part of their breast removed and axillary (underarm) lymph nodes removed. Lymphedema in the legs may occur after surgery for uterine cancer, prostate cancer, lymphoma, or melanoma. It may also occur with vulvar cancer or ovarian cancer.

Diagnosis of Lymphedema

Tests that examine the lymph system are used to diagnose lymphedema. It is important to make sure there are no other causes of swelling, such as infection or blood clots. The following tests and procedures may be used to diagnose lymphedema:

- **Physical exam and history:** An exam of the body to check general signs of health, including checking for signs of disease, such as lumps or anything else that seems unusual. A history of the patient's health habits and past illnesses and treatments will also be taken.

- **Lymphoscintigraphy:** A method used to check the lymph system for disease. A very small amount of a radioactive substance that flows through the lymph ducts and can be taken up by lymph nodes is injected into the body. A scanner or probe is used to follow the movement of this substance. Lymphoscintigraphy is used to find the sentinel lymph node (the first node to receive lymph from a tumor) or to diagnose certain diseases or conditions, such as lymphedema.

- **MRI (magnetic resonance imaging):** A procedure that uses a magnet, radio waves, and a computer to make a series of detailed pictures of areas inside the body. This procedure is also called nuclear magnetic resonance imaging (NMRI).

The swollen arm or leg is usually measured and compared to the other arm or leg. Measurements are taken over time to see how well treatment is working.

A grading system is also used to diagnose and describe lymphedema. Grades 1, 2, 3, and 4 are based on size of the affected limb and how severe the signs and symptoms are.

Stages may be used to describe lymphedema.

- Stage I: The limb (arm or leg) is swollen and feels heavy. Pressing on the swollen area leaves a pit (dent). This stage of lymphedema may go away without treatment.

- Stage II: The limb is swollen and feels spongy. A condition called tissue fibrosis may develop and cause the limb to feel hard. Pressing on the swollen area does not leave a pit.

- Stage III: This is the most advanced stage. The swollen limb may be very large. Stage III lymphedema rarely occurs in breast cancer patients. Stage III is also called lymphostatic elephantiasis.

Managing Lymphedema

Patients can take steps to prevent lymphedema or keep it from getting worse. Taking preventive steps may keep lymphedema from developing. Healthcare providers can teach patients how to prevent and take care of lymphedema at home. If lymphedema has developed, these steps may keep it from getting worse.

Preventive steps include the following:

- Tell your healthcare provider right away if you notice symptoms of lymphedema. Tell your doctor right away if you have any of these symptoms. The chance of improving the condition is better if treatment begins early. Untreated lymphedema can lead to problems that cannot be reversed.

- Keep skin and nails clean and cared for, to prevent infection. Bacteria can enter the body through a cut, scratch, insect bite, or other skin injury. Fluid that is trapped in body tissues by lymphedema makes it easy for bacteria to grow and cause infection. Look for signs of infection, such as redness, pain, swelling, heat, fever, or red streaks below the surface of the skin. Call your doctor right away if any of these signs appear. Careful skin and nail care helps prevent infection:

  - Use cream or lotion to keep the skin moist.

  - Treat small cuts or breaks in the skin with an antibacterial ointment.

  - Avoid needle sticks of any type into the limb (arm or leg) with lymphedema. This includes shots or blood tests.

- Use a thimble for sewing.

- Avoid testing bath or cooking water using the limb with lymph-edema. There may be less feeling (touch, temperature, pain) in the affected arm or leg, and skin might burn in water that is too hot.

- Wear gloves when gardening and cooking.

- Wear sunscreen and shoes when outdoors.

- Cut toenails straight across. See a podiatrist (foot doctor) as needed to prevent ingrown nails and infections.

- Keep feet clean and dry and wear cotton socks.

- Avoid blocking the flow of fluids through the body. It is import-ant to keep body fluids moving, especially through an affected limb or in areas where lymphedema may develop.

- Do not cross legs while sitting.

- Change sitting position at least every 30 minutes.

- Wear only loose jewelry and clothes without tight bands or elastic.

- Do not carry handbags on the arm with lymphedema.

- Do not use a blood pressure cuff on the arm with lymphedema.

- Do not use elastic bandages or stockings with tight bands.

- Keep blood from pooling in the affected limb.

- Keep the limb with lymphedema raised higher than the heart when possible.

- Do not swing the limb quickly in circles or let the limb hang down. This makes blood and fluid collect in the lower part of the arm or leg.

- Do not apply heat to the limb.

Studies have shown that carefully controlled exercise is safe for patients with lymphedema. Exercise does not increase the chance that lymphedema will develop in patients who are at risk for lymphedema. In the past, these patients were advised to avoid exercising the affected limb. Studies have now shown that slow, carefully controlled exercise is safe and may even help keep lymphedema from developing. Studies have also shown that, in breast-cancer survivors, upper-body exercise does not increase the risk that lymphedema will develop.

Treatment of Lymphedema

The goal of treatment is to control the swelling and other problems caused by lymphedema. Damage to the lymph system cannot be repaired. Treatment is given to control the swelling caused by lymphedema and keep other problems from developing or getting worse. Physical (non-drug) therapies are the standard treatment. Treatment may be a combination of several of the physical methods. The goal of these treatments is to help patients continue with activities of daily living, to decrease pain, and to improve the ability to move and use the limb (arm or leg) with lymphedema. Drugs are not usually used for long-term treatment of lymphedema.

Treatment of lymphedema may include the following:

Pressure garments. Pressure garments are made of fabric that puts a controlled amount of pressure on different parts of the arm or leg to help move fluid and keep it from building up. Some patients may need to have these garments custom-made for a correct fit. Wearing a pressure garment during exercise may help prevent more swelling in an affected limb. It is important to use pressure garments during air travel, because lymphedema can become worse at high altitudes. Pressure garments are also called compression sleeves and lymphedema sleeves or stockings.

Exercise. Both light exercise and aerobic exercise (physical activity that causes the heart and lungs to work harder) help the lymph vessels move lymph out of the affected limb and decrease swelling.

- **Talk with a certified lymphedema therapist before beginning exercise.** Patients who have lymphedema or who are at risk for lymphedema should talk with a certified lymphedema therapist before beginning an exercise routine.

- **Wear a pressure garment if lymphedema has developed.** Patients who have lymphedema should wear a well-fitting pressure garment during all exercise that uses the affected limb or body part.

When it is not known for sure if a woman has lymphedema, upper-body exercise without a garment may be more helpful than no exercise at all. Patients who do not have lymphedema do not need to wear a pressure garment during exercise.

- **Breast cancer survivors should begin with light upper-body exercise and increase it slowly.** Some studies with breast cancer survivors show that upper-body exercise is safe in women who have lymphedema or who are at risk for lymphedema. Weight-lifting that is slowly increased may keep lymphedema from getting worse. Exercise should start at a very low level, increase slowly over time, and be overseen by the lymphedema therapist. If exercise is stopped for a week or longer, it should be started again at a low level and increased slowly.

If symptoms (such as swelling or heaviness in the limb) change or increase for a week or longer, talk with the lymphedema therapist. It is likely that exercising at a low level and slowly increasing it again over time is better for the affected limb than stopping the exercise completely.

More studies are needed to find out if weight-lifting is safe for cancer survivors with lymphedema in the legs.

Bandages. Once the lymph fluid is moved out of a swollen limb, bandaging (wrapping) can help prevent the area from refilling with fluid. Bandages also increase the ability of the lymph vessels to move lymph along. Lymphedema that has not improved with other treatments is sometimes helped with bandaging.

Skin care. The goal of skin care is to prevent infection and to keep skin from drying and cracking.

Combined therapy. Combined physical therapy is a program of massage, bandaging, exercises, and skin care managed by a trained therapist. At the beginning of the program, the therapist gives many treatments over a short time to decrease most of the swelling in the limb with lymphedema. Then the patient continues the program at home to keep the swelling down. Combined therapy is also called complex decongestive therapy.

Compression device. Compression devices are pumps connected to a sleeve that wraps around the arm or leg and applies pressure on and off. The sleeve is inflated and deflated on a timed cycle. This pumping action may help move fluid through lymph vessels and veins and keep fluid from building up in the arm or leg. Compression devices may be helpful when added to combined therapy. The use of these devices should be supervised by a trained professional because too much pressure can damage lymph vessels near the surface of the skin.

Weight loss. In patients who are overweight, lymphedema related to breast cancer may improve with weight loss.

Laser therapy. Laser therapy may help decrease lymphedema swelling and skin hardness after a mastectomy. A hand-held, battery-powered device is used to aim low-level laser beams at the area with lymphedema.

Drug therapy. Lymphedema is not usually treated with drugs. Antibiotics may be used to treat and prevent infections. Other types of drugs, such as diuretics or anticoagulants (blood thinners), are usually not helpful and may make the lymphedema worse.

Surgery. Lymphedema caused by cancer is rarely treated with surgery.

Massage therapy. Massage therapy (manual therapy) for lymphedema should begin with someone specially trained in treating lymphedema. In this type of massage, the soft tissues of the body are lightly rubbed, tapped, and stroked. It is a very light touch, almost like a brushing. Massage may help move lymph out of the swollen area into an area with working lymph vessels. Patients can be taught to do this type of massage therapy themselves.

When done correctly, massage therapy does not cause medical problems. Massage should not be done on any of the following:

- Open wounds, bruises, or areas of broken skin.

- Tumors that can be seen on the skin surface.

- Areas with deep vein thrombosis (blood clot in a vein).

- Sensitive soft tissue where the skin was treated with radiation therapy.

When lymphedema is severe and does not get better with treatment, other problems may be the cause. Sometimes severe lymphedema does not get better with treatment or it develops several years after surgery. If there is no known reason, doctors will try to find out if the problem is something other than the original cancer or cancer treatment, such as another tumor.

Lymphangiosarcoma is a rare, fast-growing cancer of the lymph vessels. It is a problem that occurs in some breast cancer patients and appears an average of 10 years after a mastectomy. Lymphangiosarcoma begins as purple lesions on the skin, which may be flat or raised. A CT scan or MRI is used to check for lymphangiosarcoma. Lymphangiosarcoma usually cannot be cured.

Chapter 41

Infection and Neutropenia

Chapter Contents

Section 41.1

Infection during Cancer Treatment

This section includes text excerpted from "Infection and
Neutropenia," National Cancer Institute (NCI), April 29, 2015.

What Is an Infection?

An infection is the invasion and growth of germs in the body, such
as bacteria, viruses, yeast, or other fungi. An infection can begin anywhere in the body, may spread throughout the body, and can cause
one or more of these signs:

- fever of 100.5°F (38°C) or higher or chills

- cough or sore throat

- diarrhea

- ear pain, headache or sinus pain, or a stiff or sore neck

- skin rash

- sores or white coating in your mouth or on your tongue

- swelling or redness, especially where a catheter enters your body

- urine that is bloody or cloudy, or pain when you urinate

Call your healthcare team if you have signs of an infection. Infections
during cancer treatment can be life threatening and require urgent
medical attention. Be sure to talk with your doctor or nurse before
taking medicine—even aspirin, acetaminophen (such as Tylenol®), or
ibuprofen (such as Advil®) for a fever. These medicines can lower a
fever but may also mask or hide signs of a more serious problem.

Some types of cancer and treatments such as chemotherapy may
increase your risk of infection. This is because they lower the number of
white blood cells, the cells that help your body to fight infection. During
chemotherapy, there will be times in your treatment cycle when the
number of white blood cells (called neutrophils) is particularly low and

you are at increased risk of infection. Stress, poor nutrition, and not enough sleep can also weaken the immune system, making infection more likely.

You will have blood tests to check for neutropenia (a condition in which there is a low number of neutrophils). Medicine may sometimes be given to help prevent infection or to increase the number of white blood cells.

Ways to Prevent Infection

Your healthcare team will talk with you about these and other ways to prevent infection:

- **Wash your hands often and well.** Use soap and warm water to wash your hands well, especially before eating. Have people around you wash their hands well too.

- **Stay extra clean.** If you have a catheter, keep the area around it clean and dry. Clean your teeth well and check your mouth for sores or other signs of an infection each day. If you get a scrape or cut, clean it well. Let your doctor or nurse know if your bottom is sore or bleeds, as this could increase your risk of infection.

- **Avoid germs.** Stay away from people who are sick or have a cold. Avoid crowds and people who have just had a live vaccine, such as one for chicken pox, polio, or measles. Follow food safety guidelines; make sure the meat, fish, and eggs you eat are well cooked. Keep hot foods hot and cold foods cold. You may be advised to eat only fruits and vegetables that can be peeled, or to wash all raw fruits and vegetables very well.

Talking with Your Healthcare Team

Prepare for your visit by making a list of questions to ask. Consider adding these questions to your list:

- Am I at increased risk of infection during treatment? When am I at increased risk?

- What steps should I take to prevent infection?

- What signs of infection should I look for?

- Which signs signal that I need urgent medical care at the emergency room? Which should I call you about?

Section 41.2

Neutropenia after Receiving Chemotherapy

This section includes text excerpted from "What You Need to Know
Neutropenia and Risk for Infection," Centers for Disease Control and
Prevention (CDC), October 20, 2011. Reviewed February 2017.

What Is Neutropenia?

Neutropenia is a decrease in the number of white blood cells. These
cells are the body's main defense against infection. Neutropenia is common after receiving chemotherapy and increases your risk for infections.

Why Does Chemotherapy Cause Neutropenia?

These cancer-fighting drugs work by killing fast-growing cells in
the body—both good and bad. These drugs kill cancer cells as well as
healthy white blood cells.

How Do I Know If I Have Neutropenia?

Your doctor or nurse will tell you. Because neutropenia is common
after receiving chemotherapy, your doctor may draw some blood to
look for neutropenia.

When Will I Be Most Likely to Have Neutropenia?

Neutropenia often occurs between 7 and 12 days after you receive
chemotherapy. This period can be different depending upon the chemotherapy you get. Your doctor or nurse will let you know exactly when
your white blood cell count is likely to be at its lowest. You should
carefully watch for signs and symptoms of infection during this time.

How Can I Prevent Neutropenia?

There is not much you can do to prevent neutropenia from occurring, but you can decrease your risk for getting an infection while your
white blood cell count is low.

How Can I Prevent an Infection?

In addition to receiving treatment from your doctor, the following suggestions can help prevent infections:

- Clean your hands frequently.

- Try to avoid crowded places and contact with people who are sick.

- Do not share food, drink cups, utensils or other personal items, such as toothbrushes.

- Shower or bathe daily and use an unscented lotion to prevent your skin from becoming dry and cracked.

- Cook meat and eggs all the way through to kill any germs.

- Carefully wash raw fruits and vegetables.

- Protect your skin from direct contact with pet bodily waste (urine or feces) by wearing vinyl or household cleaning gloves when cleaning up after your pet. Wash your hands immediately afterwards.

- Use gloves for gardening.

- Clean your teeth and gums with a soft toothbrush, and if your doctor or nurse recommends one, use a mouthwash to prevent mouth sores.

- Try and keep all your household surfaces clean.

- Get the seasonal flu shot as soon as it is available.

What If I Have to Go to the Emergency Room?

Cancer patients receiving chemotherapy should not sit in a waiting room for a long time. While you are receiving chemotherapy, fever may be a sign of infection. Infections can become serious very quickly. When you check in, tell them right away that you are getting chemotherapy and have a fever. This may be an indication of an infection.

Chapter 42

Sleep Disorders

Certain Drugs or Treatments May Affect Sleep

Common cancer treatments and drugs can affect normal sleep patterns. How well a cancer patient sleeps may be affected by:

- Hormone therapy
- Corticosteroids
- Sedatives and tranquilizers
- Antidepressants
- Anticonvulsants

Long-term use of certain drugs may cause insomnia. Stopping or decreasing the use of certain drugs can also affect normal sleep. Other side effects of drugs and treatments that may affect the sleep-wake cycle include the following:

- Pain.
- Anxiety.
- Night sweats or hot flashes.
- Gastrointestinal problems such as nausea, constipation, diarrhea, and being unable to control the bowels.

This chapter includes text excerpted from "Sleep Disorders (PDQ®)–Patient Version," National Cancer Institute (NCI), January 27, 2016.

- Bladder problems, such as irritation or being unable to control urine.

- Breathing problems.

Being in the hospital may make it harder to sleep. Getting a normal night's sleep in the hospital is difficult. The following may affect how well a patient sleeps:

- **Hospital environment:** Patients may be bothered by an uncomfortable bed, pillow, or room temperature; noise; or sharing a room with a stranger.

- **Hospital routine:** Sleep may be interrupted when doctors and nurses come in to check on you or give you drugs, other treatments, or exams.

Getting sleep during a hospital stay may also be affected by anxiety and the patient's age.

Stress, anxiety, and depression are common reactions to learning you have cancer, receiving treatments, and being in the hospital. These are common causes of insomnia.

Cancer patients can have sleep disorders that are caused by other health problems. Conditions such as snoring, headaches, and daytime seizures increase the chance of having a sleep disorder.

Assessment of Sleep Disorders

An assessment is done to find problems that may be causing the sleep disorder and how it affects your life. Patients with mild sleep disorders may be irritable and unable to concentrate. Patients with moderate sleep disorders can be depressed and anxious. These sleep disorders may make it hard for you to stay alert and involved in activities during the day. You may not be able to remember treatment instructions and may have trouble making decisions. Being well-rested can improve energy and help you cope better with side effects of cancer and treatment.

Cancer patients should have assessments done from time to time because sleep disorders may become more or less severe over time.

A sleep disorder assessment includes a physical exam, health history, and sleep history. Your doctor will do a physical exam and take a medical history that includes:

- Side effects of your cancer and cancer treatments.

- Medicines, including vitamins, and other over-the-counter drugs.

- Emotional effects of the cancer and treatments.

- Diet.

- Exercise.

- Caregiver routines.

You and your family can tell your doctor about your sleep history and patterns of sleep.

A polysomnogram may be used to help diagnose the sleep disorder. A polysomnogram is a group of recordings taken during sleep that show:

- Brain wave changes

- Eye movements

- Breathing rate

- Blood pressure

- Heart rate and electrical activity of the heart and other muscles

This information helps the doctor find the cause of your sleeping problems.

Treatment of Sleep Disorders

Treating sleep disorders may include supportive care for side effects of cancer or cancer treatment. Sleep disorders that are caused by side effects of the cancer or cancer treatment may be helped by relieving the symptoms of those side effects. It's important to talk about your sleep problems with your family and the healthcare team so education and support can be given. Supportive care may improve your quality of life and ability to sleep.

Cognitive behavioral therapy (CBT) may reduce anxiety and help you relax. Cognitive behavioral therapy helps reduce anxiety about getting enough sleep. You learn to change negative thoughts and beliefs about sleep into positive thoughts and images, in order to fall asleep more easily. CBT helps replace the anxiety of "I need to sleep" with the idea of "just relax." You learn how to change sleep habits that keep you from sleeping well. If in-person CBT sessions with a health professional are not available, video CBT sessions have been shown to be helpful. CBT may include the following:

- **Stimulus control:** When you have sleep problems for a long time, just getting ready for bed or getting into bed to sleep may cause you to start worrying that you will have another sleepless night. That worry then makes it very hard to fall asleep. Stimulus control can help you learn to connect getting ready for bed and being in bed only with being asleep. By using the bed and bedroom only when you're sleepy, the bed and sleep are linked in your mind. Stimulus control may include the following changes in your sleeping habits:

  - Go to bed only when sleepy and get out of bed if you do not fall asleep after a short time. Return to bed only when you feel sleepy.

  - Use the bed and bedroom only for sleeping, not for other activities.

- **Sleep restriction:** Sleep restriction decreases the time you spend in bed sleeping. This makes you more likely to feel sleepy the next night. The time you can set aside for sleeping is increased when your sleep improves.

- **Relaxation therapy:** Relaxation therapy is used to relieve muscle tension and stress, lower blood pressure, and control pain. It may involve tensing and relaxing muscles throughout the body. It is often used with guided imagery (focusing the mind on positive images) and meditation (focusing thoughts). Self-hypnosis at bedtime can also help you feel relaxed and sleepy. Relaxation therapy exercises can make it easier for stimulus control and sleep restriction to work for you.

Learning good sleep habits is important. Good sleep habits help you fall asleep more easily and stay asleep. Habits and routines that may help improve sleep include the following:

A comfortable bed and bedroom. Making your bed and bedroom more comfortable may help you sleep. Some ways to increase bedroom comfort include:

- Keep the room quiet.

- Dim or turn off lights.

- Keep the room at a comfortable temperature.

- Keep skin clean and dry.

- Dress in loose, soft clothing.

- Keep bedding and pillows clean, dry, and smooth, without wrinkles.

- Use blankets to keep warm.

- Use pillows to get into a comfortable position.

Regular bowel and bladder habits. Regular bowel and bladder habits reduce the number of times you have to get up during the night. Waking during the night to go to the bathroom may be reduced by doing the following:

- Drink more fluids during the day.

- Eat more high-fiber foods during the day.

- Avoid drinking a lot before bedtime.

- Empty your bowel and bladder before going to bed.

Diet and exercise. The following diet and exercise habits may improve sleep:

- Stay active during the day.

- Get regular exercise but don't exercise within 3 hours of bedtime.

- Eat a high-protein snack (such as milk or turkey) 2 hours before bedtime.

- Avoid heavy, spicy, or sugary foods before bedtime.

- Avoid drinking alcohol or smoking before bedtime.

- Avoid foods and drinks that have caffeine, including dietary supplements to control appetite.

Other habits that may improve sleep include:

- Avoid naps.

- Avoid watching TV or working in the bedroom.

- Relax before bedtime.

- Go to sleep and wake up at the same hours every day, no matter how little you slept.

Hospital routines. Getting a good night's sleep in a hospital or other care facility can be hard to do. The good sleep habits listed above may help you. As a hospital patient, you may also:

- Ask caregivers to plan care so they wake you up the least number of times during the night.

- Ask for a back rub or massage to relieve pain or help you relax.

If treatment without drugs does not help, sleep medicines may be used for a short time. Treatment without drugs does not always work. Sometimes cognitive behavioral therapies are not available or they do not help. Also, some sleep disorders are caused by conditions that need to be treated with drugs, such as hot flashes, pain, anxiety, depression, or mood disorders. The drug used will depend on your type of sleep problem (such as trouble falling asleep or trouble staying asleep) and other medicines you're taking. All of your other medicines and health conditions will affect which sleeping medicines are safe and will work well for you.

Some drugs that help you sleep should not be stopped suddenly. Suddenly stopping them may cause nervousness, seizures, and a change in the rapid eye movement (REM) phase of sleep that increases dreaming, including nightmares. This change in REM sleep may be dangerous for patients with peptic ulcers or heart conditions.

Chapter 43

Urinary and
Bladder Problems

Some cancer treatments, such as those listed below, may cause urinary and bladder problems:

- Radiation therapy to the pelvis (including reproductive organs, the bladder, colon, and rectum) can irritate the bladder and urinary tract. These problems often start several weeks after radiation therapy begins and go away several weeks after treatment has been completed.

- Some types of chemotherapy and biological therapy can also affect or damage cells in the bladder and kidneys.

- Surgery to remove the prostate (prostatectomy), bladder cancer surgery, and surgery to remove a woman's uterus, the tissue on the sides of the uterus, the cervix, and the top part of the vagina (radical hysterectomy) can also cause urinary problems. These types of surgery may also increase the risk of a urinary tract infection.

Symptoms of a Urinary Problem

Talk with your doctor or nurse to learn what symptoms you may experience and ask which ones to call about. Some urinary or bladder

This chapter includes text excerpted from "Urinary and Bladder Problems," National Cancer Institute (NCI), April 29, 2015.

changes may be normal, such as changes to the color or smell of your urine caused by some types of chemotherapy. Your healthcare team will determine what is causing your symptoms and will advise on steps to take to feel better.

Irritation of the bladder lining (radiation cystitis):

• pain or a burning feeling when you urinate

• blood in your urine

• trouble starting to urinate

• trouble emptying your bladder completely

• feeling that you need to urinate urgently or frequently

• leaking a little urine when you sneeze or cough

• bladder spasms, cramps, or discomfort in the pelvic area

Urinary tract infection (UTI):

• pain or a burning feeling when you urinate

• urine that is cloudy or red

• a fever of 100.5°F (38°C) or higher, chills, and fatigue

• pain in your back or abdomen

• difficulty urinating or not being able to urinate

In people being treated for cancer, a UTI can turn into a serious condition that needs immediate medical care. Antibiotics will be prescribed if you have a bacterial infection.

Symptoms that may occur after surgery:

• leaking urine (incontinence)

• trouble emptying your bladder completely

Ways to Prevent or Manage

Here are some steps you may be advised to take to feel better and to prevent problems:

Drink plenty of liquids. Most people need to drink at least 8 cups of fluid each day, so that urine is light yellow or clear. You'll want to stay away from things that can make bladder problems worse. These include caffeine, drinks with alcohol, spicy foods, and tobacco products.

- **Prevent urinary tract infections.** Your doctor or nurse will talk with you about ways to lower your chances of getting a urinary tract infection. These may include going to the bathroom often, wearing cotton underwear and loose fitting pants, learning about safe and sanitary practices for catheterization, taking showers instead of baths, and checking with your nurse before using products such as creams or lotions near your genital area.

Talking with Your Healthcare Team

Prepare for your visit by making a list of questions to ask. Consider adding these questions to your list:

- What symptoms or problems should I call you about?

- What steps can I take to feel better?

- How much should I drink each day? What liquids are best for me?

- Are there certain drinks or foods that I should avoid?

Chapter 44

Late Effects of Treatment for Childhood Cancer

Late effects are health problems that occur months or years after treatment has ended. The treatment of cancer may cause health problems for childhood cancer survivors months or years after successful treatment has ended. Cancer treatments may harm the body's organs, tissues, or bones and cause health problems later in life. These health problems are called late effects.

Treatments that may cause late effects include the following:

- Surgery

- Chemotherapy

- Radiation therapy

- Stem cell transplant

Doctors are studying the late effects caused by cancer treatment. They are working to improve cancer treatments and stop or lessen late effects. While most late effects are not life-threatening, they may cause serious problems that affect health and quality of life.

Late effects in childhood cancer survivors affect the body and mind. Late effects in childhood cancer survivors may affect the following:

- Organs, tissues, and body function

This chapter includes text excerpted from "Late Effects of Treatment for Childhood Cancer (PDQ®)–Patient Version," National Cancer Institute (NCI), August 11, 2016.

- Growth and development

- Mood, feelings, and actions

- Thinking, learning, and memory

- Social and psychological adjustment

- Risk of second cancers

Second Cancers

Childhood cancer survivors have an increased risk of a second cancer later in life. A different primary cancer that occurs at least two months after cancer treatment ends is called a second cancer. A second cancer may occur months or years after treatment is completed. The type of second cancer that occurs depends in part on the original type of cancer and the cancer treatment. Benign tumors (not cancer) may also occur.

Second cancers that occur after cancer treatment include the following:

- Solid tumors.

- Myelodysplastic syndrome and acute myeloid leukemia.

Cardiovascular System

Heart and blood vessel late effects are more likely to occur after treatment for certain childhood cancers. Treatment for these and other childhood cancers may cause heart and blood vessel late effects:

- Acute lymphoblastic leukemia (ALL)

- Acute myelogenous leukemia (AML)

- Brain and spinal cord tumors

- Head and neck cancer

- Hodgkin lymphoma

- Non-Hodgkin lymphoma

- Wilms tumor

- Cancers treated with a stem cell transplant

Radiation to the chest and certain types of chemotherapy increase the risk of heart and blood vessel late effects. The risk of health problems involving the heart and blood vessels increases after treatment with the following:

- Radiation to the chest, spine, brain, neck, kidneys, or total-body irradiation (TBI) as part of a stem cell transplant. The risk of problems depends on the area of the body that was exposed to radiation, the amount of radiation given, and whether the radiation was given in small or large doses.

- Certain types of chemotherapy and the total dose of anthracycline given. Chemotherapy with anthracyclines such as doxorubicin, daunorubicin, idarubicin, and epirubicin, and with anthraquinones such as mitoxantrone increase the risk of heart and blood vessel problems. The risk of problems depends on the total dose of chemotherapy given and the type of drug used. It also depends on whether a drug called dexrazoxane was given during treatment with anthracyclines. Dexrazoxane may lessen heart and blood vessel damage. Ifosfamide, methotrexate, and chemotherapy with platinum, such as carboplatin and cisplatin, may also cause heart and blood vessel late effects.

- Stem cell transplant.

- Nephrectomy (surgery to remove all or part of a kidney).

Childhood cancer survivors who were treated with radiation to the heart or blood vessels and certain types of chemotherapy are at greatest risk.

The following may also increase the risk of heart and blood vessel late effects:

- Longer time since treatment.

- Having high blood pressure or other risk factors for heart disease, such as a family history of heart disease, being overweight, smoking, high cholesterol, or diabetes. When these risk factors are combined, the risk of late effects is even higher.

- Having lower than normal amounts of thyroid, growth, or sex hormones.

Late effects that affect the heart and blood vessels may cause certain health problems. Childhood cancer survivors who received radiation or certain types of chemotherapy have an increased risk of late

337

effects to the heart and blood vessels and related health problems. These include the following:

- Abnormal heartbeat
- Weakened heart muscle
- Inflamed heart or sac around the heart
- Damage to the heart valves
- Coronary artery disease (hardening of the heart arteries)
- Congestive heart failure
- Chest pain or heart attack
- Blood clots or one or more strokes
- Carotid artery disease

Central Nervous System

Brain and spinal cord late effects are more likely to occur after treatment for certain childhood cancers. Treatment for these and other childhood cancers may cause brain and spinal cord late effects:

- Acute lymphoblastic leukemia (ALL)
- Brain and spinal cord tumors
- Head and neck cancers

Radiation to the brain increases the risk of brain and spinal cord late effects. The risk of health problems that affect the brain or spinal cord increases after treatment with the following:

- Radiation to the brain or spinal cord, especially high doses of radiation. This includes total-body irradiation given as part of a stem cell transplant.
- Intrathecal or intraventricular chemotherapy.
- Chemotherapy with high-dose methotrexate or cytarabine that can cross the blood-brain barrier (protective lining around the brain). This includes high-dose chemotherapy given as part of a stem cell transplant.
- Surgery to remove a tumor on the brain or spinal cord.

When radiation to the brain and intrathecal chemotherapy are given at the same time, the risk of late effects is higher.

The following may also increase the risk of brain and spinal cord late effects:

- Being about 5 years old or younger at the time of treatment.

- Being female.

- Having hydrocephalus and a shunt placed to remove the extra fluid from the ventricles.

- Having hearing loss.

- Having cerebellar mutism following surgery to remove the brain tumor. Cerebellar mutism includes not being able to speak, loss of coordination and balance, mood swings, being irritable, and having a high-pitched cry.

- Having a personal history of stroke.

Central nervous system late effects are also affected by where the tumor has formed in the brain and spinal cord.

Late effects that affect the brain and spinal cord may cause certain health problems. Childhood cancer survivors who received radiation, certain types of chemotherapy, or surgery to the brain or spinal cord have an increased risk of late effects to the brain and spinal cord and related health problems. These include the following:

- Headaches.

- Loss of coordination and balance.

- Seizures.

- Loss of the myelin sheath that covers nerve fibers in the brain.

- Movement disorders that affect the legs and eyes or the ability to speak and swallow.

- Nerve damage in the hands or feet.

- Stroke. A second stroke may be more likely in survivors who received radiation to the brain, have a history of high blood pressure, or were older than 40 years when they had their first stroke.

- Hydrocephalus.

- Loss of bladder and/or bowel control.

- Cavernomas (clusters of abnormal blood vessels).

- Back pain.

Survivors may also have late effects that affect thinking, learning, memory, emotions, and behavior.

New ways of using more targeted and lower doses of radiation to the brain may lessen the risk of brain and spinal cord late effects.

Some childhood cancer survivors have posttraumatic stress disorder (PTSD). Being diagnosed and treated for a life-threatening disease may be traumatic. This trauma may cause posttraumatic stress disorder. PTSD is defined as having certain behaviors following a stressful event that involved death or the threat of death, serious injury, or a threat to oneself or others.

PTSD can affect cancer survivors in the following ways:

- Reliving the time they were diagnosed and treated for cancer, in nightmares or flashbacks, and thinking about it all the time.

- Avoiding places, events, and people that remind them of the cancer experience.

In general, childhood cancer survivors show low levels of PTSD, depending in part on the coping style of patients and their parents. Survivors who received radiation therapy to the head when younger than 4 years or survivors who received intensive treatment may be at higher risk of PTSD. Family problems, little or no social support from family or friends, and stress not related to the cancer may increase the chances of having PTSD.

Because avoiding places and persons connected to the cancer may be part of PTSD, survivors with PTSD may not get the medical treatment they need.

Digestive System

Teeth and Jaws

Problems with the teeth and jaws are late effects that are more likely to occur after treatment for certain childhood cancers. Treatment for these and other childhood cancers may cause the late effect of problems with teeth and jaws:

- Head and neck cancers

- Hodgkin lymphoma

- Leukemia that spread to the brain and spinal cord

- Nasopharyngeal cancer

- Neuroblastoma

- Cancers treated with a stem cell transplant

Radiation to the head and neck and certain types of chemotherapy increase the risk of late effects to the teeth and jaws. The risk of health problems that affect the teeth and jaws increases after treatment with the following:

- Radiation therapy to the head and neck

- Total-body irradiation (TBI) as part of a stem cell transplant

- Chemotherapy, especially with higher doses of alkylating agents such as cyclophosphamide

- Surgery in the head and neck area

Risk is also increased in survivors who were younger than 5 years at the time of treatment because their permanent teeth had not fully formed.

Late effects that affect the teeth and jaws may cause certain health problems. Teeth and jaw late effects and related health problems include the following:

- Teeth that are not normal

- Tooth decay (including cavities) and gum disease

- Salivary glands do not make enough saliva

- Death of the bone cells in the jaw

- Changes in the way the face, jaw, or skull form

Digestive Tract

Digestive tract late effects are more likely to occur after treatment for certain childhood cancers. Treatment for these and other childhood cancers may cause late effects of the digestive tract (esophagus, stomach, small and large intestines, rectum, and anus):

- Rhabdomyosarcoma of the bladder or prostate, or near the testicles

- Non-Hodgkin lymphoma

- Germ cell tumors

- Neuroblastoma

- Wilms tumor

341

Radiation to the bladder, prostate, or testicles and certain types of chemotherapy increase the risk of digestive tract late effects. The risk of health problems that affect the digestive tract increases after treatment with the following:

- Radiation therapy to the abdomen or areas near the abdomen, such as the esophagus, bladder, prostate, or testicles, may cause digestive tract problems that begin quickly and last for a short time. In some patients, however, digestive tract problems are delayed and long-lasting. These late effects are caused by radiation therapy that damages the blood vessels. Receiving higher doses of radiation therapy or receiving chemotherapy such as dactinomycin or anthracyclines together with radiation therapy may increase this risk.

- Abdominal surgery or pelvic surgery to remove the bladder.

- Chemotherapy with alkylating agents such as cyclophosphamide, procarbazine, and ifosfamide, or with platinum agents such as cisplatin or carboplatin, or with anthracyclines such as doxorubicin, daunorubicin, idarubicin, and epirubicin.

- Stem cell transplant.

The following may also increase the risk of digestive tract late effects:

- Older age at diagnosis or when treatment begins

- Treatment with both radiation therapy and chemotherapy

- A history of chronic graft-versus-host disease

Late effects that affect the digestive tract may cause certain health problems. Digestive tract late effects and related health problems include the following:

- A narrowing of the esophagus or intestine.

- Diarrhea, constipation, or blocked bowel.

- Bowel perforation (a hole in the intestine).

- Inflammation of the intestines.

- Death of part of the intestine.

- Intestine is not able to absorb nutrients from food.

Liver and Bile Ducts

Liver and bile duct late effects are more likely to occur after treatment for certain childhood cancers. Treatment for these and other childhood cancers may cause liver or bile duct late effects:

- Liver cancer

- Wilms tumor

- Acute lymphoblastic leukemia (ALL)

- Cancers treated with a stem cell transplant

Certain types of chemotherapy and radiation to the liver or bile ducts increase the risk of late effects. The risk of liver or bile duct late effects may be increased in childhood cancer survivors treated with one of the following:

- Surgery to remove part of the liver or a liver transplant.

- Chemotherapy that includes high-dose cyclophosphamide as part of a stem cell transplant.

- Chemotherapy such as 6-mercaptopurine, 6-thioguanine, and methotrexate.

- Radiation therapy to the liver and bile ducts. The risk depends on the following:

  - The dose of radiation and how much of the liver is treated.

  - Age when treated (the younger the age, the higher the risk).

  - Whether there was surgery to remove part of the liver.

  - Whether chemotherapy, such as doxorubicin or dactinomycin, was given together with radiation therapy.

  - Stem cell transplant (and a history of chronic graft-versus-host disease).

Late effects that affect the liver and bile ducts may cause certain health problems. Liver and bile duct late effects and related health problems include the following:

- Liver doesn't work the way it should or stops working.

- Gallstones.

- Benign liver lesions.

343

- Hepatitis B or C infection.

- Liver damage caused by veno-occlusive disease/sinusoidal obstruction syndrome (VOD/SOS).

- Liver fibrosis (an overgrowth of connective tissue in the liver) or cirrhosis.

- Fatty liver with insulin resistance (a condition in which the body makes insulin but cannot use it well).

- Tissue and organ damage from the buildup of extra iron after having many blood transfusions.

Pancreas

Radiation therapy increases the risk of pancreatic late effects. The risk of pancreatic late effects may be increased in childhood cancer survivors after treatment with one of the following:

- Radiation therapy to the abdomen.

- Total-body irradiation (TBI) as part of a stem cell transplant.

Late effects that affect the pancreas may cause certain health problems. Pancreatic late effects and related health problems include the following:

- **Insulin resistance:** A condition in which the body does not use insulin the way it should. Insulin is needed to help control the amount of glucose (a type of sugar) in the body. Because the insulin does not work the way it should, glucose and fat levels rise.

- **Diabetes mellitus:** A disease in which the body does not make enough insulin or does not use it the way it should. When there is not enough insulin, the amount of glucose in the blood increases and the kidneys make a large amount of urine.

Endocrine System

Thyroid Gland

Thyroid late effects are more likely to occur after treatment for certain childhood cancers. Treatment for these and other childhood cancers may cause thyroid late effects:

- Acute lymphoblastic leukemia (ALL)

- Brain tumors

- Head and neck cancers

- Hodgkin lymphoma

- Neuroblastoma

- Cancers treated with a stem cell transplant

Radiation therapy to the head and neck increases the risk of thyroid late effects. The risk of thyroid late effects may be increased in childhood cancer survivors after treatment with any of the following:

- Radiation therapy to the thyroid as part of radiation therapy to the head and neck or to the pituitary gland in the brain.

- Total-body irradiation (TBI) as part of a stem cell transplant.

- Chemotherapy.

- mIBG (radioactive iodine) therapy for neuroblastoma.

The risk also is increased in females, in survivors who were a young age at the time of treatment, in survivors who had a higher radiation dose, and as the time since diagnosis and treatment gets longer.

Pituitary Gland

Neuroendocrine late effects may be caused after treatment for certain childhood cancers. The neuroendocrine system is the nervous system and the endocrine system working together.

Childhood cancer survivors who have neuro endocrine late effects may have low levels of any of the following hormones made in the pituitary gland and released into the blood:

- Growth hormone (GH; helps promote growth and control metabolism).

- Adrenocorticotropic hormone (ACTH; controls the making of glucocorticoids).

- Prolactin (controls the making of breast milk).

- Thyroid-stimulating hormone (TSH; controls the making of thyroid hormones).

- Luteinizing hormone (LH; controls reproduction).

- Follicle-stimulating hormone (FSH; controls reproduction).

Metabolic Syndrome

Metabolic syndrome may cause heart and blood vessel disease and diabetes. Metabolic syndrome is linked to an increased risk of heart and blood vessel disease and diabetes. Health habits that decrease these risks include:

- Having a healthy weight
- Eating a heart-healthy diet
- Having regular exercise
- Not smoking

Weight

Being underweight, overweight, or obese is a late effect that is more likely to occur after treatment for certain childhood cancers. The risk of obesity increases after treatment with the following:

- Radiation therapy to the brain
- Surgery that damages the hypothalamus or pituitary gland

The following may also increase the risk of obesity:

- Being diagnosed with cancer when aged 5 to 9 years.
- Being female.
- Having growth hormone deficiency or low levels of the hormone leptin.
- Not doing enough physical activity to stay at a healthy body weight.
- Taking an antidepressant called paroxetine.

Childhood cancer survivors who get enough exercise and have a normal amount of anxiety have a lower risk of obesity.

Being underweight, overweight, or obese may be measured by weight, body mass index, percent of body fat, or size of the abdomen (belly fat).

Immune System

Surgery to remove the spleen increases the risk of immune system late effects. The risk of health problems that affect the immune system increases after treatment with the following:

- Surgery to remove the spleen.

- High-dose radiation therapy to the spleen which causes the spleen to stop working.

- Stem cell transplant followed by graft-versus-host disease which causes the spleen to stop working.

Late effects that affect the immune system may cause infection. Late effects that affect the immune system may increase the risk of very serious bacterial infections. This risk is higher in younger children than in older children and may be greater in the early years after the spleen stops working or is removed by surgery.

In addition, children with an increased risk of infection should be vaccinated on a schedule through adolescence against the following:

- Pneumococcal disease

- Meningococcal disease

- Haemophilus influenzae type b (Hib) disease

- Diphtheria-tetanus-pertussis (DTaP)

- Hepatitis B

Talk to your child's doctor about whether other childhood vaccinations given before cancer treatment need to be repeated.

Musculoskeletal System

Bone and Joint

Bone and joint late effects are more likely to occur after treatment for certain childhood cancers. Treatment for these and other childhood cancers may cause bone and joint late effects:

- Acute lymphoblastic leukemia (ALL)

- Bone cancer

- Brain and spinal cord tumors

- Ewing sarcoma

- Head and neck cancers

- Neuroblastoma

- Non-Hodgkin lymphoma

- Osteosarcoma

- Retinoblastoma

- Soft tissue sarcoma

- Wilms tumor

- Cancers treated with a stem cell transplant

Poor nutrition and not enough exercise may also cause bone late effects.

Surgery, chemotherapy, radiation therapy, and other treatments increase the risk of bone and joint late effects.

- **Radiation therapy.** Radiation therapy can stop or slow the growth of bone. The type of bone and joint late effect depends on the part of the body that received radiation therapy. Radiation therapy may cause any of the following:

  - Changes in the way the face or skull form, especially when treatment is given to children before age 5 or when high-dose radiation is given.

  - Short stature (being shorter than normal).

  - Scoliosis (curving of the spine) or kyphosis (rounding of the spine).

  - One arm or leg is shorter than the other arm or leg.

  - Osteoporosis (weak or thin bones that can break easily).

  - Osteoradionecrosis (parts of the jaw bone die from a lack of blood flow).

  - Osteochondroma (a benign tumor of the bone).

- **Surgery.** Amputation or limb-sparing surgery to remove the cancer and prevent it from coming back may cause late effects depending on where the tumor was, age of the patient, and type of surgery. Health problems after amputation or limb-sparing surgery may include:

  - Having problems with activities of daily living.

  - Not being able to be as active as normal.

  - Chronic pain or infection.

  - Problems with the way prosthetics fit or work.

  - Broken bone.

- The bone may not heal well after surgery.

- One arm or leg is shorter than the other.

- Studies show no difference in quality of life in childhood cancer survivors who had amputation compared to those who had limb-sparing surgery.

- **Chemotherapy and other drug therapy.** Risk may be increased in childhood cancer survivors who receive anticancer therapy that includes methotrexate or corticosteroids or glucocorticoids such as dexamethasone. Drug therapy may cause any of the following:

  - Osteoporosis (weak or thin bones that can break easily).

  - Osteonecrosis (one or more parts of a bone die from a lack of blood flow), especially in the hip or knee.

- **Stem cell transplant.** A stem cell transplant can affect the bone and joints in different ways:

  - Total-body irradiation (TBI) given as part of a stem cell transplant may affect the body's ability to make growth hormone and cause short stature (being shorter than normal). It may also cause osteoporosis (weak or thin bones that can break easily).

  - Osteochondroma (a benign tumor of the long bones, such as the arm or leg bones) may form.

  - Chronic graft-versus-host disease may occur after a stem cell transplant and cause joint contractures (tightening of the muscles that causes the joint to shorten and become very stiff). It may also cause osteonecrosis (one or more parts of a bone die from a lack of blood flow).

Reproductive System

Testicles

Testicular late effects are more likely to occur after treatment for certain childhood cancers. Treatment for these and other childhood cancers may cause testicular late effects:

- Acute lymphoblastic leukemia (ALL)

- Germ cell tumors

- Hodgkin lymphoma

- Non-Hodgkin lymphoma

- Sarcoma

- Testicular cancer

- Cancers treated with total-body irradiation (TBI) before a stem cell transplant

Surgery, radiation therapy, and certain types of chemotherapy increase the risk of late effects that affect the testicles. The risk of health problems that affect the testicles increases after treatment with one or more of the following:

- Surgery, such as the removal of a testicle, part of the prostate, or lymph nodes in the abdomen.

- Chemotherapy with alkylating agents, such as cyclophosphamide, dacarbazine, procarbazine, and ifosfamide.

- Radiation therapy to the abdomen, pelvis, or in the area of the hypothalamus in the brain.

- Total-body irradiation (TBI) before a stem cell transplant.

Late effects that affect the testicles may cause certain health problems. Late effects of the testicles and related health problems include the following:

- **Low sperm count:** A zero sperm count or a low sperm count may be temporary or permanent. This depends on the radiation dose and schedule, the area of the body treated, and the age when treated.

- **Infertility:** The inability to father a child.

- **Retrograde ejaculation:** Very little or no semen comes out of the penis during orgasm.

After treatment with chemotherapy or radiation, the body's ability to make sperm may come back over time.

Ovaries

Ovarian late effects are more likely to occur after treatment for certain childhood cancers. Treatment for these and other childhood cancers may cause ovarian late effects:

- Acute lymphoblastic leukemia (ALL)

- Germ cell tumors

- Hodgkin lymphoma

- Ovarian cancer

- Wilms tumor

- Cancers treated with total-body irradiation (TBI) before a stem cell transplant

Radiation therapy to the abdomen and certain types of chemotherapy increase the risk of ovarian late effects. The risk of ovarian late effects may be increased after treatment with any of the following:

- Surgery to remove one or both ovaries.

- Chemotherapy with alkylating agents, such as cyclophosphamide, mechlorethamine, cisplatin, ifosfamide, lomustine, busulfan, and especially procarbazine.

- Radiation therapy to the abdomen, pelvis, or lower back. In survivors who had radiation to the abdomen, the damage to the ovaries depends on the radiation dose, age at the time of treatment, and whether all or part of the abdomen received radiation.

- Radiation therapy to the abdomen or pelvis together with alkylating agents.

- Radiation therapy to the area near the hypothalamus in the brain.

- Total-body irradiation (TBI) before a stem cell transplant.

Late effects that affect the ovaries may cause certain health problems. Ovarian late effects and other health related problems include the following:

- Early menopause, especially in women who had their ovaries removed or were treated with both an alkylating agent and radiation therapy to the abdomen.

- Changes in menstrual periods.

- Infertility (inability to conceive a child).

- Puberty does not begin.

After treatment with chemotherapy, the ovaries may begin to work over time.

351

Fertility and Reproduction

Treatment for cancer may cause infertility in childhood cancer survivors. The risk of infertility increases after treatment with the following:

* In boys, treatment with radiation therapy to the testicles.

* In girls, treatment with radiation therapy to the pelvis, including the ovaries and uterus.

* Radiation therapy to an area near the hypothalamus in the brain or lower back.

* Total-body irradiation (TBI) before a stem cell transplant.

* Chemotherapy with alkylating agents, such as cisplatin, cyclophosphamide, busulfan, lomustine, and procarbazine.

* Surgery, such as the removal of a testicle or an ovary or lymph nodes in the abdomen.

Childhood cancer survivors may have late effects that affect pregnancy. Late effects on pregnancy include increased risk of the following:

* High blood pressure.

* Miscarriage or stillbirth.

* Low birth-weight babies.

* Early labor and/or delivery.

* Delivery by Cesarean section.

* The fetus is not in the right position for birth (for example, the foot or buttock is in position to come out before the head).

Children of childhood cancer survivors are not affected by the parent's previous treatment for cancer. The children of childhood cancer survivors do not appear to have an increased risk of birth defects, genetic disease, or cancer.

Respiratory System

Lung late effects are more likely to occur after treatment for certain childhood cancers. Treatment for these and other childhood cancers may cause lung late effects:

* Hodgkin lymphoma

- Wilms tumor

- Cancers treated with a stem cell transplant

Certain types of chemotherapy and radiation to the lungs increase the risk of lung late effects. The risk of health problems that affect the lungs increases after treatment with the following:

- Surgery to remove all or part of the lung or chest wall.

- Chemotherapy. In survivors treated with chemotherapy, such as bleomycin, busulfan, carmustine, or lomustine, and radiation therapy to the chest, there is a high risk of lung damage.

- Radiation therapy to the chest. In survivors who had radiation to the chest, the damage to the lungs and chest wall depends on the radiation dose, whether all or part of the lungs and chest wall received radiation, whether the radiation was given in small, divided daily doses, and the child's age at treatment.

- Total-body irradiation (TBI) or certain types of chemotherapy before a stem cell transplant.

The risk of lung late effects is greater in childhood cancer survivors who are treated with a combination of surgery, chemotherapy, and/or radiation therapy. The risk is also increased in survivors who have a history of the following:

- Infections or graft-versus-host disease after a stem cell transplant.

- Lung or airway disease, such as asthma, before cancer treatment.

- Smoking cigarettes or other substances.

Late effects that affect the lungs may cause certain health problems. Lung late effects and related health problems include the following:

- Radiation pneumonitis (inflamed lung caused by radiation therapy).

- Pulmonary fibrosis (the build-up of scar tissue in the lung).

- Other lung and airway problems such as chronic obstructive pulmonary disease (COPD), pneumonia, cough that does not go away, and asthma.

353

Senses

Hearing

Hearing problems are a late effect that is more likely to occur after treatment for certain childhood cancers. Treatment for these and other childhood cancers may cause hearing late effects:

- Brain tumors

- Head and neck cancers

- Neuroblastoma

- Retinoblastoma

Radiation therapy to the brain and certain types of chemotherapy increase the risk of hearing loss. The risk of hearing loss is increased in childhood cancer survivors after treatment with the following:

- Certain types of chemotherapy, such as cisplatin or high-dose carboplatin

- Radiation therapy to the brain

The risk of hearing loss is greater in childhood cancer survivors who were young at the time of treatment (the younger the child, the greater the risk), were treated for a brain tumor, or received radiation therapy to the brain and chemotherapy at the same time.

Seeing

Eye and vision problems are a late effect that is more likely to occur after treatment for certain childhood cancers. Treatment for these and other childhood cancers may cause eye and vision late effects:

- Retinoblastoma, rhabdomyosarcoma, and other tumors of the eye

- Brain tumors

- Head and neck cancers

- Acute lymphoblastic leukemia (ALL)

- Cancers treated with total-body irradiation (TBI) before a stem cell transplant

Radiation therapy to the brain or head increases the risk of eye problems or vision loss. The risk of eye problems or vision loss may be increased in childhood cancer survivors after treatment with any of the following:

- Radiation therapy to the brain, eye, or eye socket
- Surgery to remove the eye or a tumor near the optic nerve
- Certain types of chemotherapy, such as busulfan or corticosteroids
- Total-body irradiation (TBI) as part of a stem cell transplant
- Stem cell transplant (and a history of chronic graft-versus-host disease)

Late effects that affect the eye may cause certain health problems. Eye late effects and related health problems include the following:

- Having a small eye socket that affects the shape of the child's face as it grows
- Loss of vision
- Vision problems, such as cataracts or glaucoma
- Not being able to make tears
- Damage to the optic nerve and retina
- Eyelid tumors

Urinary System

Kidney

Certain types of chemotherapy increase the risk of kidney late effects. The risk of health problems that affect the kidney increases after treatment with the following:

- Chemotherapy including cisplatin, carboplatin, ifosfamide, and methotrexate
- Radiation therapy to the abdomen or middle of the back
- Surgery to remove part or all of a kidney
- Stem cell transplant

The risk of kidney late effects is greater in childhood cancer survivors who are treated with a combination of surgery, chemotherapy, and/or radiation therapy.

The following may also increase the risk of kidney late effects:

- Having cancer in both kidneys.

- Having a genetic syndrome that increases the risk of kidney problems, such as Denys-Drash syndrome or WAGR syndrome.

- Being treated with more than one type of treatment.

Late effects that affect the kidney may cause certain health problems. Kidney late effects or related health problems include the following:

- Damage to the parts of the kidney that filter and clean the blood

- Damage to the parts of the kidney that remove extra water from the blood

- Loss of electrolytes, such as magnesium, calcium, or potassium, from the body

- Hypertension (high blood pressure)

Bladder

Surgery to the pelvic area and certain types of chemotherapy increase the risk of bladder late effects. The risk of health problems that affect the bladder increases after treatment with the following:

- Surgery to remove all or part of the bladder

- Surgery to the pelvis, spine, or brain

- Certain types of chemotherapy, such as cyclophosphamide or ifosfamide

- Radiation therapy to areas near the bladder, pelvis, or urinary tract

- Stem cell transplant

Late effects that affect the bladder may cause certain health problems. Bladder late effects and related health problems include the following:

- Hemorrhagic cystitis (inflammation of the inside of the bladder wall, which leads to bleeding)

- Thickening of the bladder wall

- Trouble emptying the bladder
- Incontinence
- A blockage in the kidney, ureter, bladder, or urethra
- Urinary tract infection (chronic)

Part Five

Emotional, Cognitive, and Mental Health Issues in Cancer Care

Chapter 45

Dealing with Self-Image and Sexuality

Each of us has a mental picture of how we look, our "self-image." Although we may not always like how we look, we're used to our self-image and accept it. But cancer and its treatment can change how you look and feel about yourself. Know you aren't alone in how you feel. Many others have similar feelings.

Body Changes during and after Treatment

Some body changes are short-term while others will last forever. Either way, your looks may be a big concern during or after treatment. For example, people with ostomies after colon or rectal surgery are sometimes afraid to go out. They worry about carrying equipment around or fear that it may leak. Some may feel ashamed or afraid that others will reject them.

Every person changes in different ways. Some will be noticeable to other people, but some changes only you will notice. For some of these you may need time to adjust. Issues you may face include:

• Hair loss or skin changes

• Scars or changes in the way you look caused by surgery

This chapter includes text excerpted from "Self Image and Sexuality," National Cancer Institute (NCI), December 2, 2014.

- Weight changes

- Loss of limbs

- Loss of fertility, which means it can be hard to get pregnant or father a child

Even if others can't see them, your body changes may trouble you. Feelings of anger and grief about changes in your body are natural. Feeling bad about your body can also lower your sex drive. This loss may make you feel even worse about yourself.

Changes in the way you look can also be hard for your loved ones, which in turn, can be hard on you. For example, parents and grandparents often worry about how they look to a child or grandchild. They fear that changes in their appearance may scare the child or get in the way of their staying close.

Getting Help

How do you cope with body changes?

- Mourn your losses. They are real, and you have a right to grieve.

- Try to focus on the ways that coping with cancer has made you stronger, wiser, and more realistic.

- If you find that your skin has changed from radiation, ask your doctor about ways you can care for it.

- Look for new ways to enhance your appearance. A new haircut, hair color, makeup, or clothing may give you a lift. If you're wearing a wig, you can take it to a hairdresser to shape and style.

- If you choose to wear a breast form (prosthesis), make sure it fits you well. Don't be afraid to ask the clerk or someone close to you for help. And check your health insurance plan to see if it will pay for it.

Coping with these changes can be hard. But, over time, most people learn to accept them and move on. If you need to, ask your doctor to suggest a counselor who you can talk with about your feelings.

Staying Active

Many people find that staying active can help their self-image. Whether you swim, play a sport, or take an exercise class, you may find that being active helps you cope with changes. Talk with your doctor about ways you can stay active.

Hobbies and volunteer work can also help improve your self-image. You may like to read, listen to music, or knit for example. Or you could become a mentor or tutor, teach someone how to read or volunteer at a homeless shelter. You may find that you feel better about yourself when you get involved in helping others and doing things you enjoy.

Changes in Your Sex Life

It's common for people to have problems with sex because of cancer and its treatment. When your treatment is over, you may feel like having sex again. Until then, you and your spouse or partner may need to find new ways to show that you care about each other. This can include touching, holding, hugging, and cuddling.

Treatment-Related Problems

Sexual problems are often caused by changes to your body. Depending on the cancer you had, you may have short-term or long-term problems with sex after treatment. These changes result from chemotherapy, radiation surgery, or certain medicines. Sometimes emotional issues may cause problems with sex. Some examples include anxiety, depression, worry, and stress.

What types of problems occur? Common concerns are:

- **Worries about intimacy after treatment.** Some may struggle with their body image after treatment. Even thinking about being seen without clothes may be stressful. People may worry that having sex will hurt or that they won't be able to perform or will feel less attractive. Pain, loss of interest, depression, or cancer medicines can also affect sex drive.

- **Not being able to have sex as you did before.** Some cancer treatments cause changes in sex organs that also change your sex life.

- Some men can no longer get or keep an erection after treatment for prostate cancer, cancer of the penis, or cancer of the testes. Some treatments can also weaken a man's orgasm or make it dry.

- Some women find it harder, or even painful, to have sex after cancer treatment. Some cancer treatments can cause these problems, but there may be no clear cause. Some women also have a loss of sensation in their genital area.

- **Having menopause symptoms.** When women stop getting their periods, they can get hot flashes, dryness or tightness in the vagina, and/or other problems that can affect their desire to have sex.

- **Losing the ability to have children.** Some cancer treatments can cause infertility, making it impossible for cancer survivors to have children. Depending on the type of treatment, age, and length of time since treatment, you may still be able to have children.

Ask for Help

Even though you may feel awkward, let your doctor or nurse know if you're having problems. There may be treatments or other ways you and your loved one can give each other pleasure. If your doctor can't talk with you about sexual problems, ask for the name of a doctor who can. Some people also find it helpful to talk with other couples.

Sexual problems may not always get better on their own. Sometimes there can be an underlying medical problem that causes changes, such as:

- **Erection problems.** Medicine, assistive devices, counseling, surgery, or other approaches may help.

- **Vaginal dryness.** Dryness or tightness in the vagina can be caused by menopause. Ask whether using a water-based lubricant during sex, using vaginal dilators before sex, and/or taking hormones or using a hormone cream are options for you.

- **Muscle weakness.** You can help strengthen muscles in your genital area by doing Kegel exercises. This is when you practice controlling your muscles to stop the flow of urine. You can do these exercises even when you are not urinating. Just tighten and relax the muscles as you sit, stand, or go about your day.

Other issues you may want to talk about include:

- **Concerns about having children.** Discuss family planning concerns with your doctor. If you're a woman, ask if you still need to use birth control, even if you are not getting your period.

- **Talking with a counselor.** Some people find that sexual problems related to cancer start to strain their relationship with their partner. If this is the case, ask a nurse or social worker if you can talk to a counselor. Talking to someone alone, or with your partner, may help.

- **Seeing a specialist.** A sex therapist may be able to help you talk openly about your problems, work through your concerns, and come up with new ways to help you and your partner.

Tell Your Partner How You Feel

Talking to your loved one and sharing your feelings and concerns is very important. Even for a couple that has been together a long time, it can be hard to stay connected.

Let your partner know if you want to have sex or would rather just hug, kiss, and cuddle. He or she may be afraid to have sex with you. Or your partner may be worried about hurting you or think that you're not feeling well. Talk to your partner about any concerns you have about your sex life. Be open about your feelings and stay positive to avoid blame.

Finding Ways to Be Intimate

You can still have an intimate relationship in spite of cancer. Intimacy isn't just physical. It also involves feelings. Here are some ways to improve your intimate relationship:

- Focus on just talking and renewing your connection.

- Protect your time together. Turn off the phone and TV. If needed, find someone to take care of the kids for a few hours.

- Take it slow. Plan an hour or so to be together without being physical. For example, you may want to listen to music or take a walk.

- Try new touch. Cancer treatment or surgery can change a patient's body. Areas where touch used to feel good may now be numb or painful. Some of these changes will go away. Some will stay. For now, you can figure out together what kinds of touch feel good, such as holding, hugging, and cuddling.

Feeling Intimate after Treatment

Although cancer treatment may be over, sexual problems may remain for a while. But you can find other ways to show that you care about each other. Feeling close to your partner is important.

- Be proud of your body. It got you through treatment!

- Think of things that help you feel more attractive and confident.

- Focus on the positive. Try to be aware of your thoughts, since they can affect your sex life.

- Be open to change. You may find new ways to enjoy intimacy.

Dating

If you're single, body changes and concerns about sex can affect how you feel about dating. As you struggle to accept the changes yourself, you may also worry about how others will feel. For example, you may wonder how someone will react to physical things, such as hair loss, scars or ostomies. Or it can feel awkward to bring up sexual problems or loss of fertility, which can make feeling close even harder.

You may wonder how and when to tell a new person in your life about your cancer and body changes. For some cancer survivors, the fear of being rejected keeps them from seeking the social life they would like to have. Others who choose not to date may face pressure from friends or family to be more sociable. Here are some ideas that can make it easier to get back into social situations:

- Focus on activities that you have time to enjoy, such as taking a class or joining a club.

- Try not to let cancer be an excuse for not dating and trying to meet people.

- Wait until you feel a sense of trust and friendship before telling a new date about your cancer.

Think about dating as a learning process with the goal of having a social life you enjoy. Not every date has to be perfect. If some people reject you (which can happen with or without cancer), you have not failed. Try to remember that not all dates worked out before you had cancer.

Chapter 46

Spirituality in Cancer Care

Religious and spiritual values are important to patients coping with cancer. Studies have shown that religious and spiritual values are important to Americans. Most American adults say that they believe in God and that their religious beliefs affect how they live their lives. However, people have different ideas about life after death, belief in miracles, and other religious beliefs. Such beliefs may be based on gender, education, and ethnic background.

Many patients with cancer rely on spiritual or religious beliefs and practices to help them cope with their disease. This is called spiritual coping. Many caregivers also rely on spiritual coping. Each person may have different spiritual needs, depending on cultural and religious traditions. For some seriously ill patients, spiritual well-being may affect how much anxiety they feel about death. For others, it may affect what they decide about end-of-life treatments. Some patients and their family caregivers may want doctors to talk about spiritual concerns, but may feel unsure about how to bring up the subject.

Some studies show that doctors' support of spiritual well-being in very ill patients helps improve their quality of life. Healthcare providers who treat patients coping with cancer are looking at new ways to help them with religious and spiritual concerns. Doctors may ask patients which spiritual issues are important to them during treatment as well as near the end of life. When patients with advanced

This chapter includes text excerpted from "Spirituality in Cancer Care (PDQ®)– Patient Version," National Cancer Institute (NCI), May 18, 2015.

cancer receive spiritual support from the medical team, they may be more likely to choose hospice care and less aggressive treatment at the end of life.

Definition of Spirituality and Religion

Spirituality and religion may have different meanings. The terms spirituality and religion are often used in place of each other, but for many people they have different meanings. Religion may be defined as a specific set of beliefs and practices, usually within an organized group. Spirituality may be defined as an individual's sense of peace, purpose, and connection to others, and beliefs about the meaning of life. Spirituality may be found and expressed through an organized religion or in other ways. Patients may think of themselves as spiritual or religious or both.

Serious illness, such as cancer, may cause spiritual distress. Serious illnesses like cancer may cause patients or family caregivers to have doubts about their beliefs or religious values and cause much spiritual distress. Some studies show that patients with cancer may feel that they are being punished by God or may have a loss of faith after being diagnosed. Other patients may have mild feelings of spiritual distress when coping with cancer.

Spirituality and Quality of Life

Spiritual and religious well-being may help improve quality of life. It is not known for sure how spirituality and religion are related to health. Some studies show that spiritual or religious beliefs and practices create a positive mental attitude that may help a patient feel better and improve the well-being of family caregivers. Spiritual and religious well-being may help improve health and quality of life in the following ways:

- Decrease anxiety, depression, anger, and discomfort

- Decrease the sense of isolation (feeling alone) and the risk of suicide

- Decrease alcohol and drug abuse

- Lower blood pressure and the risk of heart disease

- Help the patient adjust to the effects of cancer and its treatment

- Increase the ability to enjoy life during cancer treatment

- Give a feeling of personal growth as a result of living with cancer

- Increase positive feelings, including:

  - Hope and optimism

  - Freedom from regret

  - Satisfaction with life

  - A sense of inner peace

Spiritual and religious well-being may also help a patient live longer.

Spiritual distress may also affect health. Spiritual distress may make it harder for patients to cope with cancer and cancer treatment. Healthcare providers may encourage patients to meet with experienced spiritual or religious leaders to help deal with their spiritual issues. This may improve their health, quality of life, and ability to cope.

Spiritual Assessment

A spiritual assessment may help the doctor understand how religious or spiritual beliefs will affect the way a patient copes with cancer.

A spiritual assessment is a method or tool used by doctors to understand the role that religious and spiritual beliefs have in the patient's life. This may help the doctor understand how these beliefs affect the way the patient responds to the cancer diagnosis and decisions about cancer treatment. Some doctors or caregivers may wait for the patient to bring up spiritual concerns. Others may use an interview or a questionnaire.

A spiritual assessment explores religious beliefs and spiritual practices. A spiritual assessment may include questions about the following:

- Religious denomination, if any

- Beliefs or philosophy of life

- Important spiritual practices or rituals

- Using spirituality or religion as a source of strength

- Being part of a community of support

- Using prayer or meditation

- Loss of faith

- Conflicts between spiritual or religious beliefs and cancer treatments

- Ways that healthcare providers and caregivers may help with the patient's spiritual needs

- Concerns about death and afterlife

- Planning for the end of life

The healthcare team may not ask about every issue the patient feels is important. Patients should bring up other spiritual or religious issues that they think may affect their cancer care.

Meeting the Patient's Spiritual and Religious Needs

To help patients with spiritual needs during cancer care, medical staff will listen to the wishes of the patient. Spirituality and religion are very personal issues. Patients should expect doctors and caregivers to respect their religious and spiritual beliefs and concerns. Patients with cancer who rely on spirituality to cope with the disease should be able to count on the healthcare team to give them support. This may include giving patients information about people or groups that can help with spiritual or religious needs. Most hospitals have chaplains, but not all outpatient settings do. Patients who do not want to discuss spirituality during cancer care should also be able to count on the healthcare team to respect their wishes.

Doctors and caregivers will try to respond to their patients' concerns, but may not take part in patients' religious practices or discuss specific religious beliefs.

The healthcare team may help with a patient's spiritual needs in the following ways:

- Suggest goals and options for care that honor the patient's spiritual and/or religious views.

- Support the patient's use of spiritual coping during the illness.

- Encourage the patient to speak with his/her religious or spiritual leader.

- Refer the patient to a hospital chaplain or support group that can help with spiritual issues during illness.

- Refer the patient to other therapies that have been shown to increase spiritual well-being. These include mindfulness relaxation, such as yoga or meditation, or creative arts programs, such as writing, drawing, or music therapy.

Chapter 47

Family Issues after Treatment

When cancer treatment ends, families are often unprepared for the fact that recovery takes time. In general, your recovery will take much longer than your treatment did. Survivors often say that they didn't realize how much time they needed to recover. This can lead to disappointment, worry, and frustration for everyone.

Families also may not realize that the way their family works may have changed permanently as a result of cancer. They may need help dealing with the changes and keeping the "new" family strong.

Some survivors say they would not have been able to cope without the help and love of their family members. And even though treatment has ended, they still receive a lot of support. For other families, problems that were present before the cancer diagnosis may still exist, or new ones may develop. You may receive less support than you had hoped.

Common problems with loved ones:

- People expect you to do what you did before your cancer. For instance, if you used to take care of the house or yard before your treatment, you may find that these jobs are still too much for you to handle. Yet family members who took over for you

This chapter includes text excerpted from "Family Issues after Treatment," National Cancer Institute (NCI), December 2, 2014.

may want life to go back to normal. They may expect you to do what you used to do around the house.

- You may expect more from your family than you receive. They may disappoint you, which might make you angry or frustrated. For example you may get less attention and concern than you did during treatment.

- You may still need to depend on others during this time. Even though you want to get back to the role you had in your family before, it may take a while to get into a routine.

At the same time you're going through these things, your family is still adjusting too. It may be hard for all of you to express feelings or know how to talk about your cancer.

Getting Help with Family Issues

After treatment, you may want to consider getting help from someone to help you and your family adjust. Ask your doctor or social worker to refer you to a counselor. An expert on family roles and concerns after cancer treatment may help your family work on your problems.

How do you cope with family issues? Here are some ideas that have helped others deal with family concerns:

- Let others know what you're able to do as you heal—and what not to expect. For example, don't feel like you have to keep the house or yard in perfect order because you always did in the past.

- Know that this is a new time in your life so it may take time to adjust. Roles in the family may change again and different emotions may get triggered. This is normal.

Give yourself time. You and your family will be able to adjust over time to the changes cancer brings. Just being open with each other can help ensure that each person's needs are met. Good communication is still very important.

Talking with Children and Teens

Help the children in your family understand that it may take a while for you to have the energy you used to have now that you are finished with treatment. Be open about what you can and can't do.

You don't have to tell your kids about every checkup or every symptom that occurs. But do tell them if you still have side effects that make certain things hard for you to do. If you're not able to do an activity or go to an event, the children may think that you're unhappy or mad at them.

Children of cancer survivors have said that these things are important once their parent has finished treatment. That you:

- Be honest with them.

- Speak as directly and openly as possible.

- Keep them informed about your cancer and involved in your recovery.

- Spend extra time with them.

With your permission, other family members should also be open with your children about your cancer and its treatment.

Chapter 48

Delirium

Delirium is a confused mental state that can occur in patients who have cancer, especially advanced cancer. Patients with delirium have problems with the following:

- Attention
- Thinking
- Awareness
- Behavior
- Emotions
- Judgment
- Memory
- Muscle control
- Sleeping and waking

There are three types of delirium:

- **Hypoactive:** The patient is not active and seems sleepy, tired, or depressed.
- **Hyperactive:** The patient is restless or agitated.

This chapter includes text excerpted from "Delirium (PDQ®)–Patient Version," National Cancer Institute (NCI), March 9, 2016.

- **Mixed:** The patient changes back and forth between being hypoactive and hyperactive.

The symptoms of delirium usually occur suddenly. They often occur within hours or days and may come and go. Delirium is often temporary and can be treated. However, in the last 24 to 48 hours of life, delirium may be permanent because of problems like organ failure. Most advanced cancer patients have delirium that occurs in the last hours to days before death.

Causes of Delirium

There is often more than one cause of delirium in a cancer patient, especially when the cancer is advanced and the patient has many medical conditions. Causes of delirium include the following:

- Organ failure, such as liver or kidney failure.

- Electrolyte imbalances: Electrolytes are important minerals (including salt, potassium, calcium, and phosphorous) in blood and body fluids. These electrolytes are needed to keep the heart, kidneys, nerves, and muscles working the way they should.

- Infections.

- Paraneoplastic syndromes: Symptoms that occur when cancer-fighting antibodies or white blood cells attack normal cells in the nervous system by mistake.

- Side effects of medicines and treatments: Patients with cancer may take medicines with side effects that include delirium and confusion. The effects usually go away after the medicine is stopped.

- Withdrawal from medicines that depress (slow down) the central nervous system (brain and spinal cord).

Risk Factors for Delirium

Patients with cancer are likely to have more than one risk factor for delirium. Identifying risk factors early may help prevent delirium or decrease the time it takes to treat it. Risk factors include the following:

- Serious illness

- Having more than one disease

- Older age

- Dementia
- Low level of albumin (protein) in the blood, which is often caused by liver problems
- Infection
- High level of nitrogen waste products in the blood, which is often caused by kidney problems
- Taking medicines that affect the mind or behavior
- Taking high doses of pain medicines, such as opioids

The risk increases when the patient has more than one risk factor. Older patients with advanced cancer who are hospitalized often have more than one risk factor for delirium.

Effects of Delirium

Delirium Causes Changes in the Patient That Can Upset the Family and Caregivers

Delirium may be dangerous to the patient if his or her judgment is affected. Delirium can cause the patient to behave in unusual ways. Even a quiet or calm patient can have a sudden change in mood or become agitated and need more care.

Delirium can be upsetting to the family and caregivers. When the patient becomes agitated, family members often think the patient is in pain, but this may not be the case. Learning about differences between the symptoms of delirium and pain may help the family and caregivers understand how much pain medicine is needed. Healthcare providers can help the family and caregivers learn about these differences.

Delirium May Affect Physical Health and Communication

Patients with delirium are:

- More likely to fall.
- Sometimes unable to control bladder and/or bowels.
- More likely to become dehydrated (drink too little water to stay healthy).

They often need a longer hospital stay than patients without delirium.

The confused mental state of these patients may make them:

- Unable to talk with family members and caregivers about their needs and feelings.

- Unable to make decisions about care.

This makes it harder for healthcare providers to assess the patient's symptoms. The family may need to make decisions for the patient.

Signs of Delirium

Possible signs of delirium include sudden personality changes, problems thinking, and unusual anxiety or depression. When the following symptoms occur suddenly, they may be signs of delirium:

- Agitation

- Not cooperating

- Changes in personality or behavior

- Problems thinking

- Problems paying attention

- Unusual anxiety or depression

Symptoms of Delirium

Early symptoms of delirium are like symptoms of depression and dementia. Delirium that causes the patient to be inactive may appear to be depression. Delirium and dementia both cause problems with memory, thinking, and judgment. Dementia may be caused by a number of medical conditions, including Alzheimer disease. Differences in the symptoms of delirium and dementia include the following:

- Patients with delirium often show changes in how alert or aware they are. Patients who have dementia usually stay alert and aware until the dementia becomes very advanced.

- Delirium occurs suddenly (within hours or days). Dementia appears gradually (over months to years) and gets worse over time.

Older patients with cancer may have both dementia and delirium. This can make it hard for the doctor to diagnose the problem. If treatment for delirium is given and the symptoms continue, then the diagnosis is more likely dementia. Checking the patient's health and symptoms over time can help diagnose delirium and dementia.

Diagnosis of Delirium

Doctors will try to find the causes of delirium.

- **Physical exam and history:** An exam of the body to check general signs of health, including checking for signs of disease, such as lumps or anything else that seems unusual. A history of the patient's health habits, past illnesses including depression, and treatments will also be taken. A physical exam can help rule out a physical condition that may be causing symptoms.

- **Laboratory tests:** Medical procedures that test samples of tissue, blood, urine, or other substances in the body. These tests help to diagnose disease, plan and check treatment, or monitor the disease over time.

Treatment of Delirium

Treatment includes looking at the causes and symptoms of delirium. Both the causes and the symptoms of delirium may be treated. Treatment depends on the following:

- Where the patient is living, such as home, hospital, or nursing home

- How advanced the cancer is

- How the delirium symptoms are affecting the patient

- The wishes of the patient and family

Treating the causes of delirium usually includes the following:

- Stopping or lowering the dose of medicines that cause delirium

- Giving fluids to treat dehydration

- Giving drugs to treat hypercalcemia (too much calcium in the blood)

- Giving antibiotics for infections

In a terminally ill patient with delirium, the doctor may treat just the symptoms. The doctor will continue to watch the patient closely during treatment.

Treatment without medicines can also help relieve symptoms. Controlling the patient's surroundings may help with mild symptoms of delirium. The following may help:

- Keep the patient's room quiet and well-lit, and put familiar objects in it

- Put a clock or calendar where the patient can see it

- Have family members around

- Keep the same caregivers as much as possible

Patients who may hurt themselves or others may need to have physical restraints.

Treatment May Include Medicines

Medicines may be used to treat the symptoms of delirium depending on the patient's condition and heart health. These medicines have serious side effects and the patient will be watched closely by a doctor. These medicines include the following:

- Haloperidol

- Olanzapine

- Risperidone

- Lorazepam

- Midazolam

Sedation may be used for delirium at the end of life or when delirium does not get better with treatment. When the symptoms of delirium are not relieved with standard treatments and the patient is near death, in pain, or has trouble breathing, other treatment may be needed. Sometimes medicines that will sedate (calm) the patient will be used. The family and the healthcare team will make this decision together.

The decision to use sedation for delirium may be guided by the following:

- The patient will have repeated assessments by experts before the delirium is considered to be refractory (doesn't respond to treatment).

- The decision to sedate the patient is reviewed by a team of healthcare professionals and not made by one doctor.

- Temporary sedation, for short periods of time such as overnight, is considered before continuous sedation is used.

- The team of healthcare professionals will work with the family to make sure the team understands the family's views and that the family understands palliative sedation.

Chapter 49

Cancer Survivors: Physical and Mental Health Concerns

Improving Health and Quality of Life after Cancer

While cancer survivors are living longer after their treatment, at least one-third of the more than 14 million survivors in the United States face physical, mental, social, job, or financial problems related to their cancer experience. These effects are also felt by family members, friends, and others who provide comfort and care to survivors.

Physical Health Concerns

Cancer survivors have a higher risk of having their first cancer come back, getting a new cancer, and having other health problems due to:

- The side effects of treatment.

- Genetic factors, such as those that can cause hereditary breast and ovarian cancer and Lynch syndrome.

- Behaviors like smoking, obesity, and lack of physical activity that can raise cancer risk.

This chapter includes text excerpted from "Improving Health and Quality of Life after Cancer," Centers for Disease Control and Prevention (CDC), October 25, 2016.

- Other risk factors, like health disparities, that contributed to the first cancer.

What Can Be Done?

After treatment ends, cancer survivors should get follow-up care—routine checkups and other cancer screenings. Follow-up care can help find new or returning cancers early and look for side effects of cancer treatment.

Survivors also can lower their risk of getting a new or second cancer by living a healthy lifestyle by:

- Avoiding tobacco.

- Limiting alcohol use.

- Avoiding too much exposure to ultraviolet rays from the sun and tanning beds.

- Eating a diet rich in fruits and vegetables.

- Keeping a healthy weight.

- Being physically active.

Mental Health Concerns

Cancer survivors report concerns with depression, anxiety about their cancer returning, and trouble with memory and concentration after cancer treatment. Recent research found that 10 percent of cancer survivors have mental health concerns, compared with only 6 percent of adults without a history of cancer. Cancer survivors who have other chronic illnesses are more likely to have mental health problems and poorer quality of life.

Fewer than one-third of survivors who have mental health concerns talk to their doctor about them, and many survivors don't use services like professional counseling or support groups.

What Can Be Done?

- Survivors should talk to their healthcare providers about their mental health status during and after treatment.

- Healthcare providers can offer cancer survivors mental health screening to check for and monitor changes in anxiety, depression, and other mental health concerns.

- Psychologists, social workers, and patient navigators can help survivors find appropriate and affordable mental health and social support services in both hospital and community settings.

- Physical activity has been linked to lower rates of depression among cancer survivors.

Chapter 50

Depression in Cancer Patients

Depression is not simply feeling sad. Depression is a disorder with specific symptoms that can be diagnosed and treated. About one-fourth of cancer patients become depressed. The numbers of men and women affected are about the same.

A person diagnosed with cancer faces many stressful issues. These may include:

- Fear of death
- Changes in life plans
- Changes in body image and self-esteem
- Changes in day to day living
- Money and legal concerns

Sadness and grief are normal reactions to a cancer diagnosis. A person with cancer may also have:

- Feelings of disbelief, denial, or despair
- Trouble sleeping
- Loss of appetite
- Anxiety or worry about the future

This chapter includes text excerpted from "Depression (PDQ®)–Patient Version," National Cancer Institute (NCI), March 30, 2016.

Not everyone who is diagnosed with cancer reacts in the same way. Some cancer patients may not have depression or anxiety, while others may have high levels of both.

Signs that you have adjusted to the cancer diagnosis and treatment include being able to stay active in daily life and continue in your roles such as:

• Spouse

• Parent

• Employee

Risk Factors

There are known risk factors for depression after a cancer diagnosis. Factors that increase the risk of depression are not always related to the cancer.

Risk factors related to cancer that may cause depression include the following:

• Learning you have cancer when you are already depressed for other reasons

• Having cancer pain that is not well controlled

• Having advanced cancer

• Being physically weakened by the cancer

• Being unmarried (for certain types of cancer)

• Having pancreatic cancer

• Taking certain medicines, such as:

  • Corticosteroids

  • Procarbazine

  • L-asparaginase

  • Interferon alfa

  • Interleukin-2

  • Amphotericin B

Risk factors not related to cancer that may cause depression include the following:

• A personal or family history of depression or suicide.

- A personal history of alcoholism or drug abuse.
- A personal history of mental problems.
- A weak social support system (not being married, having few family members or friends, having a job where you work alone).
- Stress caused by life events other than the cancer.
- Health problems that are known to cause depression (such as stroke or heart attack).

Medical Conditions That Can Cause Depression

Medical conditions that may cause depression include the following:

- Pain that doesn't go away with treatment
- Anemia
- Fever
- Abnormal levels of calcium, sodium, or potassium in the blood
- Not enough vitamin B12 or folate in your diet
- Too much or too little thyroid hormone
- Too little adrenal hormone
- Side effects of certain medicines

Depression and anxiety are common in patients whose cancer is advanced and can no longer be treated. Patients whose cancer can no longer be treated often feel depressed and anxious. These feelings can lower the quality of life. Terminally ill patients who are depressed report being troubled about:

- Symptoms
- Relationships
- Beliefs about life

Depressed terminally ill patients feel they are "being a burden" even when they don't depend very much on others.

Family members also have a risk of depression. Anxiety and depression are also common in family members caring for loved ones with cancer. Children are affected when a parent with cancer is depressed and may have emotional and behavioral problems themselves.

Good communication helps. Family members who talk about feelings and solve problems are more likely to have lower levels of anxiety and depression.

Symptoms of Depression

Major depression has specific symptoms that last longer than two weeks. It's normal to feel sad after learning you have cancer, but a diagnosis of depression depends on more than being unhappy. Symptoms of depression include the following:

- Feeling sad most of the time

- Loss of pleasure and interest in activities you used to enjoy

- Changes in eating and sleeping habits

- Nervousness

- Slow physical and mental responses

- Unexplained tiredness

- Feeling worthless

- Feeling guilt for no reason

- Not being able to pay attention

- Frequent thoughts of death or suicide

Your doctor will talk with you to find out if you have symptoms of depression. Your doctor wants to know how you are feeling and may want to discuss the following:

- The normal feelings cancer patients have. Talking with your doctor about this may help you see if your feelings are normal sadness or more serious.

- Your moods. You may be asked to rate your mood on a scale.

- How long the symptoms have lasted.

- How the symptoms affect your daily life, such as your relationships, your work, and your ability to enjoy your usual activities.

- All the medicines you are taking and other treatments you are receiving. Sometimes, side effects of medicines or the cancer can look like symptoms of depression. This is more likely during active cancer treatment or advanced cancer.

This information will help you and your doctor find out if you are feeling normal sadness or have a depressive disorder.

Checking for depression may be repeated at times when stress increases, such as when cancer gets worse or comes back after treatment.

Diagnosis of Depression

Physical exams, mental exams, and lab tests are used to diagnose depression. In addition to talking with you, your doctor may do the following to check for depression:

- **Physical exam and history:** An exam of the body to check general signs of health, including checking for signs of disease, such as lumps or anything else that seems unusual. A history of your health habits, past illnesses including depression, and treatments will also be taken. A physical exam can help rule out a physical condition that may be causing your symptoms.

- **Laboratory tests:** Medical procedures that test samples of tissue, blood, urine, or other substances in the body. These tests help to diagnose disease, plan and check treatment, or monitor the disease over time. Lab tests are done to rule out a medical condition that may be causing symptoms of depression.

- **Mental status exam:** An exam done to get a general idea of your mental state by checking the following:

  - How you look and act

  - Your mood

  - Your speech

  - Your memory

  - How well you pay attention and understand simple concepts

Treatment of Depression

The decision to treat depression depends on how long it has lasted and how much it affects your life. If you cannot adjust to the cancer diagnosis after a long time and you have lost interest in your usual activities, you may have depression that needs to be treated. Treatment of depression may include medicines, talk therapy, or both.

Treatment of Major Depression

Antidepressants help relieve depression and its symptoms. When you are taking antidepressants, it's important that they are used under the care of a doctor. You may be treated with a number of medicines during your cancer care. Some anticancer medicines may not mix safely with certain antidepressants or with certain foods, herbals, or nutritional supplements. It's important to tell your healthcare providers about all the medicines, herbals, and nutritional supplements you are taking, including medicines used as patches on the skin. This can help prevent unwanted reactions.

Many antidepressants take from 3 to 6 weeks to work. Usually, you begin at a low dose that is slowly increased to find the right dose for you. This helps to avoid side effects.

Check with your doctor before you stop taking an antidepressant. You may need to slowly reduce the dose of some types of antidepressants. This is to prevent side effects you may have if you suddenly stop taking the medicine.

Different Types of Antidepressants

Most antidepressants help treat depression by changing the levels of chemicals called neurotransmitters in the brain. Nerves use these chemicals to send messages to one another. Increasing the amount of these chemicals helps to improve mood. The different types of antidepressants act on these chemicals in different ways and have different side effects.

Three types of antidepressants are commonly used to treat depression in patients with cancer:

- SSRIs (selective serotonin reuptake inhibitors): Medicines that increase the brain chemical serotonin.

- Tricyclic antidepressants: Medicines that increase the brain chemicals serotonin and norepinephrine.

- Central nervous system (CNS) stimulants: Medicines that increase the brain chemicals dopamine and norepinephrine.

There are other types of antidepressants that may be used:

- Bupropion
- Venlafaxine
- Trazodone

- Mirtazapine

- Benzodiazepines

- Psychostimulants

- Monoamine oxidase inhibitors (MAOIs).

The antidepressant that is best for you depends on the following:

- Your symptoms

- Your medical problems

- Possible side effects of the antidepressant

- The form of medicine you are able to take (such as a pill or a liquid)

- Other medicines you are taking

- How you responded to antidepressants in the past

Counseling or talk therapy helps some cancer patients with depression. Your doctor may suggest you see a psychologist or psychiatrist for the following reasons:

- Your depression is getting worse

- The depression keeps you from continuing with your cancer treatment

- The antidepressants you are taking are causing unwanted side effects

- Your symptoms have been treated for 2 to 4 weeks and are not getting better

Most counseling or talk therapy programs for depression are offered in both individual and small-group settings. Some of these include:

- Crisis intervention

- Psychotherapy

- Cognitive-behavioral therapy

More than one type of therapy program may be right for you. Therapy programs for cancer patients teach about the following:

- Cancer and its treatment

- Relaxation skills and ways to lower stress

- Coping and problem-solving skills

- Getting rid of negative thoughts

- Social support

Patients in therapy often form a close personal bond with an understanding healthcare provider. Talking with a clergy member may also be helpful for some people.

Suicide Risk in Patients with Cancer

It's Common for Cancer Patients to Feel Hopeless at Times

Cancer patients sometimes feel hopeless. Although few cancer patients are reported to die by suicide, talk with your doctor if you feel hopeless or have thoughts of suicide. There are ways your doctor can help you. Getting treatment for major depression has been shown to lower the risk of suicide in cancer patients.

Risk Factors for Suicide May Be Related to the Cancer or Other Conditions

General risk factors for suicide include the following:

- A history of mental problems, especially those that cause you to act without thinking

- A family history of suicide

- A history of suicide attempts

- Depression or feeling hopeless

- Drug or alcohol abuse

- Recent death of a friend or spouse

- Few friends or little family support

Risk factors that are related to cancer include the following:

- A diagnosis of oral, throat, or lung cancer

- Advanced stage cancer and poor prognosis

- Confusion or being unable to think clearly

- Pain that is not relieved with treatment

- Physical changes such as the following:

  - Being unable to walk and move around on your own

  - Loss of bowel and bladder control

  - Loss of a limb (amputation)

  - Loss of eyesight or hearing

  - Paralysis

  - Being unable to eat or swallow

  - Extreme tiredness

Talking about thoughts of suicide with your doctor gives you a chance to describe your feelings and fears, and may help you feel more in control. Your doctor will try to find out what is causing your hopeless feelings, such as:

- Symptoms that are not well controlled

- Fear of having a painful death

- Fear of being alone during your cancer experience

You can find out what may be done to help relieve your emotional and physical pain

Controlling symptoms caused by cancer and cancer treatment is an important goal in preventing suicide. Having constant discomfort or pain can cause you to feel desperate. Keeping pain and other symptoms under control will help to:

- Relieve distress

- Make you feel more comfortable

- Prevent thoughts of suicide

Treatment may include antidepressants. Some antidepressants take a few weeks to work. The doctor may prescribe other medicines that work quickly to relieve distress until the antidepressant begins to work. Patients usually are given only a small number of doses at a time. For your safety, it's important to have frequent contact with a healthcare professional and avoid being alone until your symptoms are controlled. Your healthcare team can help you find social support.

Losing a loved one to suicide is especially hard for the family and friends. The shock and grief felt after the loss of a loved one to suicide is very difficult. Family members and others who loved the patient may feel like they have been left or rejected. They may feel guilty or angry or they may feel responsible for the suicide. Talking with a professional or a support group can be very helpful for family members and others who loved the patient. Support groups can:

- Offer friendship

- Give you time to talk about feelings

- Help you find ways to cope with the loss

    It may help just to know that these feelings are felt by others

Palliative Sedation

    Patients with advanced cancer or near the end of life may have:

- A lot of emotional distress and physical pain.

- Difficult and painful breathing.

- Confusion (especially when body systems begin to fail).

    Sedation can be given to ease these conditions. This is called palliative sedation. Deciding to use palliative sedation may be difficult for the family as well as the patient. The patient and family can get support from the healthcare team and mental health professionals when palliative sedation is used.

    Choices about care and treatment at the end of life should be made while you are still able to make them. Your thoughts and feelings about end-of-life sedation may depend on your own culture and beliefs. Some patients who become anxious facing the end of life may want to be sedated. Other patients may wish to have no procedures, including sedation, just before death. It is important for you to tell family members and healthcare providers of your wishes about sedation at the end of life. When you make your wishes about sedation known ahead of time, doctors and family members can be sure they're doing what you would want.

Depression in Children

    Most children cope well with cancer. A small number of children may have:

- Depression

- Anxiety

- Trouble sleeping

- Problems getting along with family or friends

- Problems staying on treatment

These problems can affect the child's cancer treatment and enjoyment of life. Children with severe late effects from cancer treatment may be more likely to have symptoms of depression. A mental health specialist can help children with depression.

Assessment for depression includes looking at the child's symptoms, behavior, and health history. As in adults, normal sadness in children is not depression. Depression lasts longer and has specific symptoms. The doctor may assess the child for depression if a behavior problem goes on for a long time. To assess for depression, the doctor will need the following information about the child:

- Home life with family

- How the child faces illness and treatment

- Age and stage of development

- Past illnesses and how the child responded to them

- Sense of self-worth

- Behavior, as seen by the parents, teachers, or others

The doctor will talk with the child and may use a set of questions or a checklist that helps to diagnose depression in children.

A diagnosis of depression depends on the symptoms and how long they have lasted. Children who are depressed have an unhappy mood and at least 4 of the following symptoms every day for 2 weeks or longer:

- Appetite changes

- Not sleeping or sleeping too much

- Being unable to relax and be still (such as pacing, fidgeting, and pulling at clothing)

- Frequent crying

- Loss of interest or pleasure in usual activities

- Lack of emotion in children younger than 6 years

- Feeling very tired or having little energy

- Feelings of worthlessness, blame, or guilt
- Unable to think or pay attention and frequent daydreaming
- Refusing to go to school
- Trouble learning and getting along with others
- Aggressive behavior
- Anger towards self, parents, and teachers
- Frequent thoughts of death or suicide

Treatment May Be Therapy or Medicine

Talk therapy is the main treatment for depression in children. Individual and group talk therapy are the main treatments for depression in children. This may include play therapy for younger children. Therapy will help the child cope with feelings of depression and also understand the cancer and its treatment.

Medicines for depression may be used with care. The doctor may prescribe antidepressants for children with severe depression and anxiety. Children taking antidepressants must be watched closely. SSRIs (selective serotonin reuptake inhibitors) are a type of antidepressant that usually have few side effects. However, in some children, teenagers, and young adults, SSRIs make depression worse or cause thoughts of suicide. The U.S. Food and Drug Administration (FDA) has warned that patients younger than age 25 who are taking SSRIs should be watched closely for signs that the depression is getting worse and for suicidal thinking or behavior. This is especially important during the first 4 to 8 weeks of treatment.

Chapter 51

Anxiety Disorders and Distress in Cancer Patients

Anxiety and distress can affect the quality of life of patients with cancer and their families. Patients living with cancer feel many different emotions, including anxiety and distress.

- Anxiety is fear, dread, and uneasiness caused by stress.

- Distress is emotional, mental, social, or spiritual suffering. Patients who are distressed may have a range of feelings from vulnerability and sadness to depression, anxiety, panic, and isolation.

Patients may have feelings of anxiety and distress while being screened for a cancer, waiting for the results of tests, receiving a cancer diagnosis, being treated for cancer, or worrying that cancer will recur (come back).

Anxiety and distress may affect a patient's ability to cope with a cancer diagnosis or treatment. It may cause patients to miss checkups or delay treatment. Anxiety may increase pain, affect sleep, and cause nausea and vomiting. Even mild anxiety can affect the quality of life for cancer patients and their families and may need to be treated.

This chapter includes text excerpted from "Adjustment to Cancer: Anxiety and Distress (PDQ®)–Patient Version," National Cancer Institute (NCI), January 7, 2015.

Levels of Distress

Some patients living with cancer have a low level of distress and others have higher levels of distress. The level of distress ranges from being able to adjust to living with cancer to having a serious mental health problem, such as major depression. However, most patients with cancer do not have signs or symptoms of any specific mental health problem. This chapter describes the less severe levels of distress in patients living with cancer, including:

- **Normal adjustment:** A condition in which a person makes changes in his or her life to manage a stressful event such as a cancer diagnosis. In normal adjustment, a person learns to cope well with emotional distress and solve problems related to cancer.

- **Psychological and social distress:** A condition in which a person has some trouble making changes in their life to manage a stressful event such as a cancer diagnosis. Help from a professional to learn new coping skills may be needed.

- **Adjustment disorder:** A condition in which a person has a lot of trouble making changes in his or her life to manage a stressful event such as a cancer diagnosis. Symptoms such as depression, anxiety, or other emotional, social, or behavioral problems occur and worsen the person's quality of life. Medicine and help from a professional to make these changes may be needed.

- **Anxiety disorder:** A condition in which a person has extreme anxiety. It may be because of a stressful event like a cancer diagnosis or for no known reason. Symptoms of anxiety disorder include worry, fear, and dread. When the symptoms are severe, it affects a person's ability to lead a normal life. There are many types of anxiety disorders:

  - Generalized anxiety disorder

  - Panic disorder (a condition that causes sudden feelings of panic)

  - Agoraphobia (fear of open places or situations in which it might be hard to get help if needed)

  - Social anxiety disorder (fear of social situations)

  - Specific phobia (fear of a specific object or situation)

  - Obsessive-compulsive disorder

  - Posttraumatic stress disorder

Risk Factors

Nearly half of cancer patients report having a lot of distress. Patients with lung, pancreatic, and brain cancers may be more likely to report distress, but in general, the type of cancer does not make a difference. Factors that increase the risk of anxiety and distress are not always related to the cancer. The following may be risk factors for high levels of distress in patients with cancer:

- Trouble doing the usual activities of daily living
- Physical symptoms and side effects (such as fatigue, nausea, or pain)
- Problems at home
- Depression or other mental or emotional problems
- Being younger, nonwhite, or female
- Having a lower level of education

Screening

Screening is usually done by asking the patient questions, either in an interview or on paper. Patients who show a high level of distress usually find it helpful to talk about their concerns with a social worker, mental health professional, palliative care specialist, or pastoral counselor.

Normal Adjustment

Patients living with cancer need to make adjustments in their lives to cope with the disease and changes in treatment. Living with a diagnosis of cancer involves many life adjustments. Normal adjustment involves learning to cope with emotional distress and solve problems caused by having cancer. Patients with cancer do not make these adjustments all at once, but over a period of time as their disease and treatment change. Patients may need to make adjustments when they:

- Learn the diagnosis
- Are being treated for cancer
- Finish treatment
- Learn that the cancer is in remission

- Learn that the cancer has come back

- Become a cancer survivor

Coping Methods

Patients find it easier to adjust if they can carry on with their usual routines and work, keep doing activities that matter to them, and cope with the stress in their lives.

Coping is the use of thoughts and behaviors to adjust to life situations. The way people cope is usually linked to their personality traits (such as whether they usually expect the best or worst, or are shy or outgoing).

Coping methods include the use of thoughts and behaviors in special situations. For example, changing a daily routine or work schedule to manage the side effects of cancer treatment is a coping method. Using coping methods can help a patient deal with certain problems, emotional distress, and cancer in his or her daily life.

Patients who adjust well are usually very involved in coping with cancer. They also continue to find meaning and importance in their lives. Patients who do not adjust well may withdraw from relationships or situations and feel hopeless. Studies are being done to find out how different types of coping methods affect the quality of life for cancer survivors.

Patients who are adjusting to the changes caused by cancer may have distress. Distress can occur when patients feel they are unable to manage or control changes caused by cancer. Patients with the same diagnosis or treatment can have very different levels of distress. Patients have less distress when they feel the demands of the diagnosis and treatment are low or the amount of support they get is high. For example, a healthcare professional can help the patient adjust to the side effects of chemotherapy by giving medicine for nausea.

The way each patient copes with cancer depends on many physical and emotional factors. The following factors affect how a patient copes with the stress of cancer:

- The type of cancer, cancer stage, and chance of recovery.

- Whether the patient is newly diagnosed, being treated, in remission, or having a recurrence.

- The patient's age.

- Whether the patient is able to get treatment.

- How well the patient usually copes with stress.

- The number of stressful life events the patient has had in the last year, such as starting a new job or moving.

- Whether the patient gets support from friends and family.

- Social pressures caused by other people's beliefs and fears about cancer.

Cancer patients need different coping skills at different points in time. The coping skills needed will change at important points in time. These include the following:

Learning the diagnosis: The process of adjusting to cancer begins before learning the diagnosis. Patients may feel worried and afraid when they have unexplained symptoms or are having tests done to find out if they have cancer.

A diagnosis of cancer can cause expected and normal emotional distress. Some patients may not believe it and ask, "Are you sure you have the right test results?" They may feel numb or in shock, or as if "This can't be happening to me." Many patients wonder, "Could I die from this?"

Many patients feel they are not able to think clearly and may not understand or remember important information that the doctor gives them about the diagnosis and treatment options. Patients should have a way to go over this information later. It helps to have someone with them at appointments, bring a tape recorder, or make a second appointment to ask the doctor questions and go over the treatment plan.

As patients accept the diagnosis, they begin to feel symptoms of distress, including:

- Depression

- Anxiety

- Loss of appetite

- Trouble sleeping

- Not being able to focus

- Trouble with the activities of daily life

- Not being able to stop thinking about cancer or death

When patients receive and understand information about cancer and their treatment options, they may begin to feel more hopeful.

Over time, by using ways to cope that have worked in the past and learning new ways to cope, patients usually adjust to having cancer. Extra professional help to deal with problems such as fatigue, trouble sleeping, and depression can be helpful during this time.

Being treated for cancer: As patients go through treatment for cancer, they use coping strategies to adjust to the stress of treatment. Patients may have anxiety or fears about:

- Procedures that may be painful

- Side effects such as hair loss, nausea and vomiting, fatigue, or pain

- Changes to daily routines at work or home

Patients usually adjust well when they can compare short-term discomfort to long-term benefit (for example living longer) and decide, "It's worth it." Questions that patients may ask during treatment include, "Will I survive this?"; "Will they be able to remove all the cancer?" or "What side effects will I have?" Finding ways to cope with problems caused by cancer such as feeling tired, getting to and from treatment, and changes in work schedule is helpful.

Finishing treatment: Finishing cancer treatment can cause mixed feelings. It may be a time of celebration and relief that treatment has ended. But it may also be a time of worry that the cancer could come back. Many patients are glad that treatment has ended but feel increased anxiety as they see their doctors less often. Other concerns include returning to work and family life and being very worried about any change in their health.

During remission, patients may become stressed before follow-up medical appointments because they worry that the cancer has come back. Waiting for test results can be very stressful.

Patients who are able to express both positive and negative emotions are more likely to adjust well. Patients are more able to cope with the emotional stress of finishing treatment and being in remission when they:

- Are honest about their emotions.

- Are aware of their own feelings and are able to share them with others.

- Are able to accept their feelings without thinking of them as right or wrong or good or bad and are willing to work through their emotions.

- Have support from others who are willing to listen and accept their feelings.

Learning that the cancer has come back: Sometimes cancer comes back and does not get better with treatment. The treatment plan then changes from one that is meant to cure the cancer to one that gives comfort and relieves symptoms. This may cause great anxiety for the patient. The patient may feel shock and be unable to believe it at first. This may be followed by a period of distress such as depression, trouble focusing, and being unable to stop thinking about death. Signs of normal adjustment include:

- Times of sadness and crying

- Feelings of anger at God or other higher power

- Times of pulling away from others and wanting to be alone

- Thoughts of giving up

Patients slowly adjust to the return of cancer. They stop expecting to be cured of cancer and begin a different kind of healing. This healing is a process of becoming whole again by changing one's life in many ways when faced with the possibility of death. It is very important that patients keep up hope while they adjust to the return of cancer. Some patients keep up hope through their spirituality or religious beliefs.

Becoming a Cancer Survivor

Patients adjust to finishing cancer treatment and being long-term cancer survivors over many years. As treatments for cancer have gotten better, cancer has become a chronic disease for some patients. Some common problems reported by cancer survivors as they face the future include:

- Feeling anxious that the cancer will come back.

- Feeling a loss of control.

- Reminders of chemotherapy (such as smells or sights) that cause anxiety and nausea.

- Symptoms of posttraumatic stress, such as being unable to stop thinking about cancer or its treatment or feeling separate from others and alone.

- Concerns about body image and sexuality.

Most patients adjust well and some even say that surviving cancer has given them a greater appreciation of life, helped them understand what is most important in their life, and stronger spiritual or religious beliefs.

Some patients may have more trouble adjusting because of medical problems, fewer friends and family members to give support, money problems, or mental health problems not related to the cancer.

Psychological and Social Distress

Feelings of emotional, social, or spiritual distress can make it hard to cope with cancer treatment. Almost all patients living with cancer have feelings of distress. Feelings of distress range from sadness and fears to more serious problems such as depression, panic, feeling uncertain about spiritual beliefs, or feeling alone or separate from friends and family.

Patients who are in distress during any phase of cancer need treatment and support for their distress. Patients are more likely to need to be checked and treated for distress during the following periods:

- Soon after diagnosis

- At the start of treatment

- At the end of treatment

- From time to time after finishing treatment and during remission

- If the cancer comes back

- If the goal of treatment changes from curing or controlling cancer to palliative therapy to relieve symptoms and improve quality of life

Patients who are having trouble coping with cancer may find it helpful to talk with a professional about their concerns and worries. These specialists include:

- Mental health professionals, including psychologists and psychiatrists

- Social workers

- Palliative care specialists

- Religious counselors

Patients who are in distress can be helped by different kinds of emotional and social support. Studies have shown that patients who are having trouble adjusting to cancer are helped by treatments that give them emotional and social support, including:

- Relaxation training

- Counseling or talk therapy

- Cancer education sessions

- Social support in a group setting

These types of treatment may be combined in different ways for one or more sessions. Studies have shown that patients with cancer who receive such therapies receive benefits compared to those who do not receive these therapies. Benefits include having lower levels of depression, anxiety, and disease- and treatment-related symptoms, as well as feeling more optimistic. Patients who have the most distress seem to get the most help from these therapies. However, patients who received these therapies did not live longer than those who did not receive them.

Adjustment Disorders

Adjustment disorders may cause serious problems in daily life. An adjustment disorder occurs when the patient's reaction to a stressful event:

- Is more severe than the expected amount of distress

- Affects relationships or causes problems at home or work

- Includes symptoms of depression and anxiety or other emotional, social, or behavioral problems

Causes of adjustment disorders in cancer patients include the following:

- Diagnosis

- Treatment

- Recurrence

- Side effects of treatment

An adjustment disorder usually begins within three months of a stressful event and lasts no longer than six months after the event is over. Some patients may have a chronic adjustment disorder because they have many causes of distress, one right after another.

An adjustment disorder may become a more serious mental disorder such as major depression. This is more common in children and adolescents than in adults.

Counseling

Individual (one-to-one) and group counseling have been shown to help cancer patients with adjustment disorders. Counseling may include treatment that focuses on the patient's thoughts, feelings, and behaviors. The following may help patients cope:

- Relaxation training
- Biofeedback
- Mental imagery exercises
- Problem-solving
- Plan for events that may happen in the future
- Change beliefs that are not true
- Distraction
- Thought stopping
- Positive thoughts

Counseling may be combined with antianxiety medicine or antidepressants. Counseling should be tried before medicine. Some patients are not helped by counseling or have a more severe mental health problem, such as severe anxiety or depression. These patients may be helped by an antianxiety or antidepressant medicine along with counseling.

Anxiety Disorders

Anxiety disorders are very strong fears that may be caused by physical or psychological stress. Studies show that almost half of all patients with cancer say they feel some anxiety and about one-fourth of all patients with cancer say they feel a great deal of anxiety. Patients living with cancer find that they feel more or less anxiety at different times. A patient may become more anxious as cancer spreads or treatment becomes more intense.

For some patients feelings of anxiety may become overwhelming and affect cancer treatment. This is especially true for patients who had periods of intense anxiety before their cancer diagnosis. Most patients who did not have an anxiety condition before their cancer diagnosis will not have an anxiety disorder related to the cancer.

Patients are more likely to have anxiety disorders during cancer treatment if they have any of the following:

- A history of an anxiety disorder

- A history of physical or emotional trauma

- Anxiety at the time of diagnosis

- Few family members or friends to give them emotional support

- Pain that is not controlled well

- Cancer that is not getting better with treatment

- Trouble taking care of their personal needs such as bathing or eating

Diagnosis of Anxiety Disorders

It may be hard to tell the difference between normal fears related to cancer and abnormally severe fears that can be described as an anxiety disorder. The diagnosis is based on how symptoms of anxiety affect the patient's quality of life, what kinds of symptoms began since the cancer diagnosis or treatment, when the symptoms occur, and how long they last.

Anxiety disorders cause serious symptoms that affect day-to-day life, including:

- Feeling worried all the time

- Not being able to focus

- Not being able to "turn off thoughts" most of the time

- Trouble sleeping most nights

- Frequent crying spells

- Feeling afraid most of the time

- Having symptoms such as fast heartbeat, dry mouth, shaky hands, restlessness, or feeling on edge

- Anxiety that is not relieved by the usual ways to lessen anxiety such as distraction by staying busy

Causes of Anxiety Disorders in Cancer Patients

In addition to anxiety caused by a cancer diagnosis, the following may cause anxiety in patients with cancer:

- **Pain:** Patients whose pain is not well controlled with medicine feel anxious, and anxiety can increase pain.

- **Other medical problems:** Anxiety may be a warning sign of a change in metabolism (such as low blood sugar), a heart attack, severe infection, pneumonia, or a blood clot in the lung. Sepsis and electrolyte imbalances can also cause anxiety.

- **Certain types of tumors:** Certain hormone-releasing tumors can cause symptoms of anxiety and panic attacks. Tumors that have spread to the brain and spinal cord and tumors in the lungs can cause other health problems with symptoms of anxiety.

- **Taking certain drugs:** Certain types of drugs, including corticosteroids, thyroxine, bronchodilators, and antihistamines, can cause restlessness, agitation, or anxiety.

- **Withdrawing from habit-forming drugs:** Withdrawal from alcohol, nicotine, opioids, or antidepressant medicine can cause agitation or anxiety.

Anxiety from these causes is usually managed by treating the cause itself.

A cancer diagnosis may cause anxiety disorders to come back in patients with a history of them. When patients who had an anxiety disorder in the past are diagnosed with cancer, then the anxiety disorder may come back. These patients may feel extreme fear, be unable to remember information given to them by caregivers, or be unable to follow through with medical tests and procedures. They may have symptoms including:

- Shortness of breath
- Sweating
- Feeling faint
- Fast heartbeat

Patients with cancer may have the following types of anxiety disorders:

Phobia: Phobias are fears about a situation or an object that lasts over time. People with phobias usually feel intense anxiety and avoid the situation or object they are afraid of. For example, patients with a phobia of small spaces may avoid having tests in small spaces, such as magnetic resonance imaging (MRI) scans.

Phobias may make it hard for patients to follow through with tests and procedures or treatment. Phobias are treated by professionals and include different kinds of therapy.

Panic disorder: Patients with panic disorder feel sudden intense anxiety, known as panic attacks. Symptoms of panic disorder include the following:

- Shortness of breath

- Feeling dizzy

- Fast heart beat

- Shaking

- Heavy sweating

- Feeling sick to the stomach

- Tingling of the skin

- Being afraid they are having a heart attack

- Being afraid they are "going crazy."

A panic attack may last for several minutes or longer. There may be feelings of discomfort that last for several hours after the attack. Panic attacks are treated with medicine and talk therapy.

Obsessive-compulsive disorder: Obsessive-compulsive disorder is rare in patients with cancer who did not have the disorder before being diagnosed with cancer.

Obsessive-compulsive disorder is diagnosed when a person uses persistent (obsessive) thoughts, ideas, or images and compulsions (repetitive behaviors) to manage feelings of distress. The obsessions and compulsions affect the person's ability to work, go to school, or be in social situations. Examples of compulsions include frequent hand washing or constantly checking to make sure a door is locked. Patients with obsessive-compulsive disorder may be unable to follow through with cancer treatment because of these thoughts and behaviors. Obsessive-compulsive disorder is treated with medicine and individual (one-to-one) counseling.

Generalized anxiety disorder: Patients with generalized anxiety disorder may feel extreme and constant anxiety or worry. For example, patients with supportive family and friends may fear that no one will care for them. Patients may worry that they cannot pay for their treatment, even though they have enough money and insurance.

A person who has generalized anxiety may feel irritable, restless, or dizzy, have tense muscles, shortness of breath, fast heartbeat, sweating, or get tired quickly. Generalized anxiety disorder sometimes begins after a patient has been very depressed.

Treatment for Anxiety Disorders

There are different types of treatment for patients with anxiety disorders, including methods to manage stress. Ways to manage stress include the following:

- Deal with the problem directly
- See the situation as a problem to solve or a challenge
- Get all of the information and support needed to solve the problem
- Break big problems or events into smaller problems or tasks
- Be flexible. Take situations as they come

Patients with anxiety disorders need information and support to understand their cancer and treatment choices. Psychological treatments for anxiety can also be helpful. These include the following:

- Individual (one-to-one) counseling
- Couple and family counseling
- Crisis counseling
- Group therapy
- Self-help groups

Other treatments used to lessen the symptoms of anxiety include the following:

- Hypnosis
- Meditation
- Relaxation training
- Guided imagery
- Biofeedback

Using different methods together may be helpful for some patients. Medicine may be used alone or combined with other types of treatment for anxiety disorders. Antianxiety medicines may be used if the patient doesn't want counseling or if it's not available. These medicines relieve symptoms of anxiety, such as feelings of fear, dread, uneasiness, and muscle tightness. They may relieve daytime distress and reduce insomnia. These medicines may be used alone or combined with other therapies.

Although some patients are afraid they may become addicted to antianxiety medicines, this is not a common problem in cancer patients. Enough medicine is given to relieve symptoms and then the dose is slowly lowered as symptoms begin to get better.

Studies show that antidepressants are useful in treating anxiety disorders. Children and teenagers being treated with antidepressants have an increased risk of suicidal thinking and behavior and must be watched closely.

Chapter 52

Cancer-Related Posttraumatic Stress (PTS)

Cancer-related posttraumatic stress (PTS) is a lot like posttraumatic stress disorder (PTSD) but not as severe. Patients have a range of normal reactions when they hear they have cancer. These include:

- Repeated frightening thoughts

- Being distracted or overexcited

- Trouble sleeping

- Feeling detached from oneself or reality

Patients may also have feelings of shock, fear, helplessness, or horror. These feelings may lead to cancer-related posttraumatic stress (PTS), which is a lot like posttraumatic stress disorder (PTSD). PTSD is a specific group of symptoms that affect many survivors of stressful events. These events usually involve the threat of death or serious injury to oneself or others. People who have survived military combat, natural disasters, violent personal attack (such as rape), or other life-threatening stress may suffer from PTSD. The symptoms for PTS and PTSD are a lot alike, but most cancer patients are able to cope and don't develop full PTSD. The symptoms of cancer-related PTS are not as severe and don't last as long as PTSD.

This chapter includes text excerpted from "Cancer-Related Posttraumatic Stress (PDQ®)–Patient Version," National Cancer Institute (NCI), July 7, 2015.

Cancer-Related Posttraumatic Stress (PTS)

Patients dealing with cancer may have symptoms of posttraumatic stress at any point from diagnosis through treatment, after treatment is complete, or during possible recurrence of the cancer. Parents of childhood cancer survivors may also have posttraumatic stress.

This chapter is about cancer-related posttraumatic stress in adults, its symptoms, and its treatment.

Factors That Affect the Risk of Cancer-Related PTS

Certain factors may make it more likely that a patient will have posttraumatic stress. It is not completely clear who has an increased risk of cancer-related posttraumatic stress. Certain physical and mental factors that are linked to PTS or PTSD have been reported in some studies:

Physical Factors

- Cancer that recurs (comes back) was shown to increase stress symptoms in patients.

- Breast cancer survivors who had more advanced cancer or lengthy surgeries, or a history of trauma or anxiety disorders, were more likely to be diagnosed with PTSD.

- In survivors of childhood cancer, symptoms of posttraumatic stress occurred more often when there was a longer treatment time.

Psychological, Mental, and Social Factors

- Previous trauma

- High level of general stress

- Genetic factors and biological factors (such as a hormone disorder) that affect memory and learning

- The amount of social support available

- Threat to life and body

- Having PTSD or other psychological problems before being diagnosed with cancer

- The use of avoidance to cope with stress

Certain protective factors may make it less likely that a patient will develop posttraumatic stress. Cancer patients may have a lower risk of posttraumatic stress if they have the following:

- Good social support

- Clear information about the stage of their cancer

- An open relationship with their healthcare providers

Symptoms of Cancer-Related PTS

Posttraumatic stress symptoms develop by conditioning. Conditioning occurs when certain triggers become linked with an upsetting event. Neutral triggers (such as smells, sounds, and sights) that occurred at the same time as upsetting triggers (such as chemotherapy or painful treatments) later cause anxiety, stress, and fear even when they occur alone after the trauma has ended.

Screening for Cancer-Related Posttraumatic Stress (PTS)

Cancer may involve stressful events that repeat or continue over time. The patient may suffer symptoms of posttraumatic stress anytime from diagnosis through completion of treatment and possible cancer recurrence, so screening may be needed more than once. Different screening methods may be used to find out if the patient is having symptoms of PTS or PTSD.

In patients who have a history of PTSD from a previous trauma, symptoms may start again by certain triggers during their cancer treatment (for example, being inside MRI or CT scanners). These patients also may have problems adjusting to cancer and cancer treatment.

Cancer survivors and their families need long-term monitoring for posttraumatic stress. Symptoms of posttraumatic stress usually begin within the first 3 months after the trauma, but sometimes they do not appear for months or even years afterwards. Therefore, cancer survivors and their families need long-term monitoring.

Some people who have had an upsetting event may show early symptoms but do not have full PTSD. However, patients with these early symptoms often develop PTSD later. These patients and their family members should receive repeated screening and long-term follow-up.

Triggers for Cancer-Related PTS

For a patient coping with cancer, the specific trauma that triggers cancer-related posttraumatic stress isn't always known. Because the cancer experience involves so many upsetting events, it is much harder to know the exact cause of stress than it is for other traumas, such as natural disasters or rape.

Triggers during the cancer experience may include the following:

- Being diagnosed with a life-threatening illness

- Receiving treatment

- Waiting for test results

- Learning the cancer has recurred

- It is important to know the triggers in order to get treatment

Symptoms of cancer-related posttraumatic stress (pts) are a lot like symptoms of other stress-related disorders. PTS has many of the same symptoms as depression, anxiety disorders, phobias, and panic disorder.

Some of the symptoms that may be seen in posttraumatic stress and in other conditions include:

- Feeling defensive, irritable, or fearful

- Being unable to think clearly

- Sleeping problems

- Avoiding other people

- Loss of interest in life

Treatment of Cancer-Related Posttraumatic Stress (PTS)

Although there are no specific treatments for posttraumatic stress in patients with cancer, treatments used for people with PTSD can be useful in relieving distress in cancer patients and survivors.

Cancer survivors with posttraumatic stress need early treatment with methods that are used to treat other trauma victims. Effects of posttraumatic stress are long-lasting and serious. It may affect the patient's ability to have a normal lifestyle and may affect personal relationships, education, and employment. Because avoiding places and persons linked with cancer is part of posttraumatic stress, the patient may avoid getting professional care.

It is important that cancer survivors are aware of the possible mental distress of living with cancer and the need for early treatment of posttraumatic stress. More than one kind of treatment may be used.

Crisis intervention techniques, relaxation training, and support groups may help symptoms of posttraumatic stress. The crisis intervention method aims to relieve distress and help the patient return to normal activities. This method focuses on solving problems, teaching coping skills, and providing a supportive setting for the patient.

Some patients are helped by methods that teach them to change their behaviors by changing their thinking patterns. Through cognitive behavioral therapy (CBT), patients may be helped to:

- Understand their symptoms

- Learn ways to cope and to manage stress (such as relaxation training)

- Become aware of thinking patterns that cause distress and replace them with more balanced and useful ways of thinking

- Become less sensitive to upsetting triggers

Support groups may also help people who have posttraumatic stress symptoms. In the group setting, patients can get emotional support, meet others with similar experiences and symptoms, and learn coping and management skills.

Medicines for Posttraumatic Stress

For patients with severe symptoms of posttraumatic stress, medicines may be used. For example:

- Tricyclic and monoamine oxidase inhibitor (MOA) antidepressants are used, especially when posttraumatic stress occurs along with depression.

- Selective serotonin reuptake inhibitors (SSRIs) such as fluoxetine may reduce the stress that occurs in what is known as the "fight-or-flight syndrome."

- Antianxiety medicines may help reduce symptoms of anxiety. In certain cases, antipsychotic medicines may reduce severe flashbacks.

Part Six

Maintaining Wellness during and after Cancer Treatment

Chapter 53

Nutrition in Cancer Care

Chapter Contents

Section 53.1

Cancer Treatment and Nutrition

This section includes text excerpted from "Nutrition in
Cancer Care (PDQ®)–Patient Version," National
Cancer Institute (NCI), January 8, 2016.

Good nutrition is important for cancer patients. Nutrition is a process in which food is taken in and used by the body for growth, to keep the body healthy, and to replace tissue. Good nutrition is important for good health. Eating the right kinds of foods before, during, and after cancer treatment can help the patient feel better and stay stronger. A healthy diet includes eating and drinking enough of the foods and liquids that have the important nutrients (vitamins, minerals, protein, carbohydrates, fat, and water) the body needs.

When the body does not get or cannot absorb the nutrients needed for health, it causes a condition called malnutrition or malnourishment.

Eating Habits during Cancer Treatment

Nutrition therapy is used to help cancer patients get the nutrients they need to keep up their body weight and strength, keep body tissue healthy, and fight infection. Eating habits that are good for cancer patients can be very different from the usual healthy eating guidelines.

Healthy eating habits and good nutrition can help patients deal with the effects of cancer and its treatment. Some cancer treatments work better when the patient is well nourished and gets enough calories and protein in the diet. Patients who are well nourished may have a better prognosis (chance of recovery) and quality of life.

Cancer can change the way the body uses food. Some tumors make chemicals that change the way the body uses certain nutrients. The body's use of protein, carbohydrates, and fat may be affected, especially by tumors of the stomach or intestines. A patient may seem to be eating enough, but the body may not be able to absorb all the nutrients from the food.

Effects of Cancer Treatment on Nutrition

Surgery and Nutrition

Surgery increases the body's need for nutrients and energy. The body needs extra energy and nutrients to heal wounds, fight infection, and recover from surgery. If the patient is malnourished before surgery, it may cause problems during recovery, such as poor healing or infection. For these patients, nutrition care may begin before surgery.

Surgery to the head, neck, esophagus, stomach, or intestines may affect nutrition. Most cancer patients are treated with surgery. Surgery that removes all or part of certain organs can affect a patient's ability to eat and digest food. The following are nutrition problems caused by specific types of surgery:

- Surgery to the head and neck may cause problems with:

- Chewing

- Swallowing

- Tasting or smelling food

- Making saliva

- Seeing

- Surgery that affects the esophagus, stomach, or intestines may keep these organs from working as they should to digest food and absorb nutrients.

All of these can affect the patient's ability to eat normally. Emotional stress about the surgery itself also may affect appetite.

Nutrition therapy can help relieve nutrition problems caused by surgery. Nutrition therapy can relieve or decrease the side effects of surgery and help cancer patients get the nutrients they need. Nutrition therapy may include the following:

- Nutritional supplement drinks.

- Enteral nutrition (feeding liquid through a tube into the stomach or intestines).

- Parenteral nutrition (feeding through a catheter into the bloodstream).

- Medicines to increase appetite.

It is common for patients to have pain, tiredness, and/or loss of appetite after surgery. For a short time, some patients may not be able to eat what they usually do because of these symptoms. Following certain tips about food may help. These include:

- Stay away from carbonated drinks (such as sodas) and foods that cause gas, such as:

  - Beans

  - Peas

  - Broccoli

  - Cabbage

  - Brussels sprouts

  - Green peppers

  - Radishes

  - Cucumbers

- Increase calories by frying foods and using gravies, mayonnaise, and salad dressings. Supplements high in calories and protein can also be used.

- Choose high-protein and high-calorie foods to increase energy and help wounds heal. Good choices include:

  - Eggs

  - Cheese

  - Whole milk

  - Ice cream

  - Nuts

  - Peanut butter

  - Meat

  - Poultry

  - Fish

- If constipation is a problem, increase fiber by small amounts and drink lots of water. Good sources of fiber include:

  - Whole-grain cereals (such as oatmeal and bran)

  - Beans

- Vegetables

- Fruit

- Whole-grain breads

Chemotherapy and Nutrition

Chemotherapy affects cells all through the body. Chemotherapy affects fast-growing cells and is used to treat cancer because cancer cells grow and divide quickly. Healthy cells that normally grow and divide quickly may also be killed. These include cells in the mouth, digestive tract, and hair follicles.

Chemotherapy may affect nutrition. Chemotherapy may cause side effects that cause problems with eating and digestion. When more than one anticancer drug is given, more side effects may occur or they may be more severe. The following side effects are common:

- Loss of appetite

- Inflammation and sores in the mouth

- Changes in the way food tastes

- Feeling full after only a small amount of food

- Nausea

- Vomiting

- Diarrhea

- Constipation

Nutrition therapy can help relieve nutrition problems caused by chemotherapy. Patients who have side effects from chemotherapy may not be able to eat normally and get all the nutrients they need to restore healthy blood counts between treatments. Nutrition therapy can help relieve these side effects, help patients recover from chemotherapy, prevent delays in treatment, prevent weight loss, and maintain general health. Nutrition therapy may include the following:

- Nutrition supplement drinks between meals.

- Enteral nutrition (tube feedings).

- Changes in the diet, such as eating small meals throughout the day.

Radiation Therapy and Nutrition

Radiation therapy can affect cancer cells and healthy cells in the treatment area. Radiation therapy can kill cancer cells and healthy cells in the treatment area. The amount of damage depends on the following:

- The part of the body that is treated.

- The total dose of radiation and how it is given.

Radiation therapy to any part of the digestive system often has side effects that cause nutrition problems. Most of the side effects begin a few weeks after radiation therapy begins and go away a few weeks after it is finished. Some side effects can continue for months or years after treatment ends.

The following are some of the more common side effects:

- For radiation therapy to the head and neck

  - Loss of appetite.

  - Changes in the way food tastes.

  - Pain when swallowing.

  - Dry mouth or thick saliva.

  - Sore mouth and gums.

  - Narrowing of the upper esophagus, which can cause choking, breathing, and swallowing problems.

- For radiation therapy to the chest

  - Infection of the esophagus.

  - Trouble swallowing.

  - Esophageal reflux (a backward flow of the stomach contents into the esophagus).

- For radiation therapy to the abdomen or pelvis

  - Diarrhea.

  - Nausea.

  - Vomiting.

  - Inflamed intestines or rectum.

  - A decrease in the amount of nutrients absorbed by the intestines.

Radiation therapy may also cause tiredness, which can lead to a decrease in appetite.

Nutrition therapy during radiation treatment can help the patient get enough protein and calories to get through treatment, prevent weight loss, help wound and skin healing, and maintain general health. Nutrition therapy may include the following:

- Nutritional supplement drinks between meals.

- Enteral nutrition (tube feedings).

- Changes in the diet, such as eating small meals throughout the day.

Patients who receive high-dose radiation therapy to prepare for a bone marrow transplant may have many nutrition problems and should see a dietitian for nutrition support.

Biologic Therapy and Nutrition

The side effects of biologic therapy are different for each patient and each type of biologic agent. The following nutrition problems are common:

- Fever

- Nausea

- Vomiting

- Diarrhea

- Loss of appetite

- Tiredness

- Weight gain

The side effects of biologic therapy can cause weight loss and malnutrition if they are not treated. Nutrition therapy can help patients receiving biologic therapy get the nutrients they need to get through treatment, prevent weight loss, and maintain general health.

Stem Cell Transplant and Nutrition

Stem cell transplant patients have special nutrition needs. Chemotherapy, radiation therapy and medicines used for a stem cell transplant may cause side effects that keep a patient from eating and digesting food as usual. Common side effects include the following:

- Changes in the way food tastes

- Dry mouth or thick saliva

- Mouth and throat sores

- Nausea

- Vomiting

- Diarrhea

- Constipation

- Weight loss and loss of appetite

- Weight gain

Nutrition therapy is very important for patients who have a stem cell transplant. Transplant patients have a very high risk of infection. High doses of chemotherapy or radiation therapy decrease the number of white blood cells, which fight infection. It is especially important that transplant patients avoid getting infections.

Patients who have a transplant need plenty of protein and calories to get through and recover from the treatment, prevent weight loss, fight infection, and maintain general health. It is also important to avoid infection from bacteria in food. Nutrition therapy during transplant treatment may include the following:

- A diet of cooked and processed foods only, because raw vegetables and fresh fruit may carry harmful bacteria.

- Guidelines on safe food handling.

- A specific diet based on the type of transplant and the part of the body affected by cancer.

- Parenteral nutrition (feeding through the bloodstream) during the first few weeks after the transplant, to give the patient the calories, protein, vitamins, minerals, and fluids they need to recover.

Section 53.2

Nutrition in Treating Cancer Symptoms

This section includes text excerpted from "Nutrition in
Cancer Care (PDQ®)–Patient Version," National Cancer
Institute (NCI), January 8, 2016.

Anorexia

Anorexia (the loss of appetite or desire to eat) is one of the most
common problems for cancer patients. Eating in a calm, comfortable
place and getting regular exercise may improve appetite. The following
may help cancer patients who have a loss of appetite:

- Eat small high-protein and high-calorie meals every 1–2 hours
  instead of three large meals. The following are high-calorie,
  high-protein food choices:

  - Cheese and crackers.

  - Muffins.

  - Puddings.

  - Nutritional supplements.

  - Milkshakes.

  - Yogurt.

  - Ice cream.

- Powdered milk added to foods such as pudding, milkshakes, or
  any recipe using milk.

- Finger foods (handy for snacking) such as deviled eggs, deviled
  ham on crackers, or cream cheese or peanut butter on crackers
  or celery.

- Chocolate.

- Add extra calories and protein to food by using butter, skim milk
  powder, honey, or brown sugar.

431

- Drink liquid supplements (special drinks that have nutrients), soups, milk, juices, shakes, and smoothies, if eating solid food is a problem.

- Eat breakfasts that have one-third of the calories and protein needed for the day.

- Eat snacks that have plenty of calories and protein.

- Eat foods that smell good. Strong odors can be avoided in the following ways:

  - Use boiling bags or microwave steaming bags.

  - Cook outdoors on the grill.

  - Use a kitchen fan when cooking.

  - Serve cold food instead of hot (since odors are in the rising steam).

  - Take off any food covers to release the odors before going into a patient's room.

  - Use a small fan to blow food odors away from patients.

  - Order take-out food.

- Try new foods and new recipes, flavorings, spices, and foods with a different texture or thickness. Food likes and dislikes may change from day to day.

- Plan menus ahead of time and get help preparing meals.

- Make and store small amounts of favorite foods so they are ready to eat when hungry.

Taste Changes

Changes in how foods taste may be caused by radiation treatment, dental problems, mouth sores and infections, or some medicines. Many cancer patients who receive chemotherapy notice a bitter taste or other changes in their sense of taste. A sudden dislike for certain foods may occur. This can cause a loss of appetite, weight loss, and a decreased quality of life. Some or all of a normal sense of taste may return, but it may take up to a year after treatment ends. The following may help cancer patients who have taste changes:

- Eat small meals and healthy snacks several times a day.

- Eat meals when hungry rather than at set mealtimes.

- Eat favorite foods and try new foods when feeling best.

- Eat poultry, fish, eggs, and cheese instead of red meat.

- Eat citrus fruits (oranges, tangerines, lemons, grapefruit) unless mouth sores are present.

- Add spices and sauces to foods.

- Eat meat with something sweet, such as cranberry sauce, jelly, or applesauce.

- Find non-meat, high-protein recipes in a vegetarian or Chinese cookbook.

- Use sugar-free lemon drops, gum, or mints if there is a metallic or bitter taste in the mouth.

- Rinse mouth with water before eating.

- Eat with family and friends.

- Have others prepare the meal.

- Use plastic utensils if foods have a metal taste.

Taking zinc sulfate tablets during radiation therapy to the head and neck may help a normal sense of taste come back faster after treatment.

Dry Mouth

Dry mouth is often caused by radiation therapy to the head and neck and by certain medicines. Dry mouth may affect speech, taste, and the ability to swallow or to use dentures or braces. There is also an increased risk of cavities and gum disease because less saliva is made to wash the teeth and gums.

The main treatment for dry mouth is drinking plenty of liquids. Other ways to help relieve dry mouth include the following:

- Keep water handy at all times to moisten the mouth.

- Eat moist foods with extra sauces, gravies, butter, or margarine.

- Eat foods and drinks that are very sweet or tart (to increase saliva).

- Eat ice chips or frozen desserts (such as frozen grapes and ice pops).

- Drink fruit nectar instead of juice.

- Suck on hard candy or chew gum.

- Use a straw to drink liquids.

- Clean teeth (including dentures) and rinse mouth at least four times a day (after eating and at bedtime). Don't use mouth rinses that contain alcohol.

Mouth Sores and Infections

Mouth sores can be caused by chemotherapy and radiation therapy. These treatments affect fast-growing cells, such as cancer cells. Normal cells inside the mouth also grow quickly and may be damaged by these cancer treatments. Mouth sores can be painful and become infected or bleed and make it hard to eat. By choosing certain foods and taking good care of their mouths, patients can usually make eating easier. The following can help patients who have mouth sores and infections:

- Eat soft foods that are easy to chew and swallow, such as the following:

  - Soft fruits, including bananas, applesauce, and watermelon.

  - Peach, pear, and apricot nectars.

  - Cottage cheese.

  - Mashed potatoes.

  - Macaroni and cheese.

  - Custards and puddings.

  - Gelatin.

  - Milkshakes.

  - Scrambled eggs.

  - Oatmeal or other cooked cereals.

- Stay away from the following:

  - Citrus fruits and juices, (such as oranges, tangerines, lemons, and grapefruit).

  - Spicy or salty foods.

  - Rough, coarse, or dry foods, including raw vegetables, granola, toast, and crackers.

- Use a blender to make vegetables (such as potatoes, peas, and carrots) and meats smooth.

- Add gravy, broth, or sauces to food.

- Drink high-calorie, high-protein drinks in addition to meals.

- Cook foods until soft and tender.

- Eat foods cold or at room temperature. Hot and warm foods can irritate a tender mouth.

- Cut foods into small pieces.

- Use a straw to drink liquids.

- Numb the mouth with ice chips or flavored ice pops before eating.

- Clean teeth (including dentures) and rinse mouth at least four times a day (after eating and at bedtime).

Nausea

Nausea caused by cancer treatment can affect the amount and kinds of food eaten. The following may help cancer patients control nausea:

- Eat before cancer treatments.

- Rinse out the mouth before and after eating.

- Eat foods that are bland, soft, and easy-to-digest, rather than heavy meals. Eat small meals several times a day.

- Eat dry foods such as crackers, bread sticks, or toast throughout the day.

- Slowly sip fluids throughout the day.

- Suck on hard candies such as peppermints or lemon drops if the mouth has a bad taste.

- Stay away from foods that are likely to cause nausea. For some patients, this includes spicy foods, greasy foods, and foods that have strong odors.

- Sit up or lie with the upper body raised for one hour after eating.

- Don't eat in a room that has cooking odors or that is very warm. Keep the living space at a comfortable temperature with plenty of fresh air.

Diarrhea

Diarrhea may be caused by cancer treatments, surgery on the stomach or intestines, or by emotional stress. Long-term diarrhea may lead to dehydration (lack of water in the body) or low levels of salt and potassium, which are important minerals needed by the body.

The following may help cancer patients control diarrhea:

- Eat broth, soups, bananas, and canned fruits to help replace salt and potassium lost by diarrhea. Sports drinks can also help.

- Drink plenty of fluids during the day. Liquids at room temperature may cause fewer problems than hot or cold liquids.

- Drink at least one cup of liquid after each loose bowel movement.

- Stay away from the following:

  - Greasy foods, hot or cold liquids, or caffeine.

  - High-fiber foods—especially dried beans and cruciferous vegetables (such as broccoli, cauliflower, and cabbage).

  - Milk and milk products, until the cause of the diarrhea is known.

  - Foods and beverages that cause gas (such as peas, lentils, cruciferous vegetables, chewing gum, and soda).

  - Sugar-free candies or gum made with sorbitol (sugar alcohol).

Low White Blood Cell Counts and Infections

A low white blood cell count may be caused by radiation therapy, chemotherapy, or the cancer itself. Patients who have a low white blood cell count have an increased risk of infection. The following may help cancer patients prevent infections when white blood cell counts are low:

- Stay away from:

  - Raw eggs or raw fish.

  - Old, moldy, or damaged fruits and vegetables.

  - Food sold in open bins or containers.

  - Salad bars and buffets when eating out.

- Wash hands often to prevent the spread of bacteria.

- Thaw foods in the refrigerator or microwave. Never thaw foods at room temperature. Cook foods immediately after thawing.

- Keep hot foods hot and cold foods cold.

- Cook all meat, poultry, and fish until well done.

- Refrigerate all leftovers within 2 hours of cooking and eat them within 24 hours.

- Buy foods packed as single servings, to avoid leftovers.

- Do not buy or eat food that is out of date.

- Do not buy or eat food in cans that are swollen, dented, or damaged.

Dehydration (Lack of Fluid)

The body needs plenty of water to replace the fluids lost every day. Nausea, vomiting, and pain may keep the patient from drinking and eating enough to get the amount of water the body needs. Long-term diarrhea causes a loss of fluid from the body. One of the first signs of dehydration (lack of water in the body) is feeling very tired. The following may help cancer patients prevent dehydration:

- Drink 8 to 12 cups of liquids a day. This can be water, juice, milk, or foods that have a lot of liquid in them, such as ice pops, flavored ices, and gelatins.

- Stay away from drinks that have caffeine in them, such as sodas, coffee, and tea (both hot and cold).

- Take a water bottle whenever leaving home. It is important to drink even if not thirsty.

- Drink most liquids between meals.

- Use medicines that help prevent and treat nausea and vomiting.

Constipation

It is very common for cancer patients to have constipation (fewer than three bowel movements a week). Constipation may be caused by the following:

- Too little water or fiber in the diet.

- Not being active.

- Cancer treatment, such as chemotherapy.

- Certain medicines used to treat the side effects of chemotherapy, such as nausea and pain.

  Preventing and treating constipation is a part of cancer care. To prevent constipation:

- Eat more fiber-containing foods. Twenty-five to 35 grams of fiber a day is best. Food labels show the amount of fiber in a serving. (Some sources of fiber are listed below.) Add a little more fiber each day and drink plenty of fluids at the same time to keep the fiber moving through the intestines.

- Drink 8 to 12 cups of fluid each day. Water, prune juice, warm juices, lemonade, and teas without caffeine can be very helpful.

- Take walks and exercise regularly. Wear shoes made for exercise.

  To treat constipation:

- Continue to eat high-fiber foods and drink plenty of fluids. Try adding wheat bran to the diet; begin with 2 heaping tablespoons each day for 3 days, then increase by 1 tablespoon each day until constipation is relieved. Do not take more than 6 tablespoons a day.

- Stay physically active.

- Use over-the-counter constipation treatments, if needed. These include:

- Bulk-forming products (such as Citrucel, Metamucil, Fiberall, and Fiber-Lax).

- Stimulants (such as Dulcolax and Senokot).

- Stool softeners (such as Colace and Surfak).

- Osmotics (such as milk of magnesia).

- Cottonseed and aerosol enemas can also help. Do not use lubricants such as mineral oil because they may keep the body from using important nutrients the way it should.

  Good food sources of fiber include the following:

- Legumes (beans and lentils)

- Vegetables

- Cold cereals (whole grain or bran)

- Hot cereals

- Fruit

- Whole-grain breads

Section 53.3

Nutrition in Advanced Cancer

This section includes text excerpted from "Nutrition in
Cancer Care (PDQ®)–Patient Version," National
Cancer Institute (NCI), January 8, 2016.

Palliative care helps relieve symptoms that bother the patient and helps improve the patient's quality of life. The goal of palliative care is to improve the quality of life of patients who have a serious or life-threatening disease. Palliative care is meant to prevent or treat symptoms, side effects, and psychological, social, and spiritual problems caused by a disease or its treatment.

Palliative care for patients with advanced cancer includes nutrition therapy and/or drug therapy. Nutrition needs are different for patients with advanced cancer. It is common for patients with advanced cancer to want less food. Patients usually prefer soft foods and clear liquids. Those who have problems swallowing may do better with thick liquids than with thin liquids. Patients often do not feel much hunger at all and may need very little food.

In patients with advanced cancer, most foods are allowed. During this time, eating can be focused on pleasure rather than getting enough nutrients. Patients usually cannot eat enough of any food that might cause a problem. However, some patients may need to stay on a special diet. For example, patients with cancer that affects the abdomen may need a soft diet to keep the bowel from getting blocked.

Answering the following questions may help to make decisions about using nutrition support:

- What are the wishes and needs of the patient and family?

- Will the patient's quality of life be improved?

- Do the possible benefits outweigh the risks and costs?

- Is there an advance directive? An advance directive is a legal document that states the treatment or care a person wishes to receive or not receive if he or she becomes unable to make medical decisions. One type of advance directive is a living will.

Cancer patients and their caregivers have the right to make informed decisions. The healthcare team and a registered dietitian can explain the benefits and risks of using nutrition support for patients with advanced cancer. In most cases, there are more harms than benefits, especially with parenteral nutrition support. However, for someone who still has good quality of life but is unable to get enough food and water by mouth, enteral feedings may be best. The benefits and risks of enteral nutrition during advanced cancer include the following:

Benefits

- May make the patient more alert.

- May be a comfort to the family.

- May relieve nausea.

- May make the patient feel more hopeful.

Harms

- Surgery may be needed to place a tube through the abdomen.

- May increase the amount of saliva in the mouth and throat. This may cause choking or pneumonia.

- May cause diarrhea or constipation.

- May cause nausea.

- May cause infection.

- Makes patient care harder for caregiver.

Section 53.4

Drug-Nutrient Interactions

This section includes text excerpted from "Nutrition in
Cancer Care (PDQ®)–Patient Version," National
Cancer Institute (NCI), January 8, 2016.

Some foods do not mix safely with certain drugs. Cancer patients
may be treated with a number of drugs. Taking certain foods and drugs
together may decrease or change how well the drugs work or cause
life-threatening side effects. The following table lists some of the food
and drug interactions that may occur with certain anticancer drugs:

Table 53.1. Drug-Food Interactions

Brand Name	Generic Name	Food Interactions
Targretin	Bexarotene	Grapefruit juice may increase the drug's effects.
Folex	Methotrexate	Alcohol may cause liver damage.
Rheumatrex		
Mithracin	Plicamycin	Supplements of calcium andvitamin D may decrease the drug's effect.
Matulane	Procarbazine	Alcohol may cause headache, trouble breathing, flushed skin, nausea, or vomiting, Caffeine may raise blood pressure.
Temodar	Temozolomide	Food may slow or decrease the drug's effect.

Some herbal supplements do not mix safely with certain drugs or
foods. Taking some herbal supplements with certain foods and drugs
may change how well cancer treatment works or cause life-threatening
side effects. Talk with your doctor about how herbal supplements may
affect your cancer treatment. Talk with your doctor about possible food
and drug interactions.

Nutrition and Lifestyle in Cancer Survivors

Everyone needs a healthy diet and exercise for good health and
to help prevent disease. Cancer survivors have special health needs,

especially because of the risks of late effects and the cancer coming back. Studies have shown that a healthy diet helps to prevent late effects such as obesity, heart disease, and metabolic syndrome. Researchers are also studying whether certain diet and exercise habits in cancer survivors can keep cancer from coming back or keep new cancers from forming.

Surveys show that many cancer survivors do not follow cancer prevention guidelines and have lifestyle behaviors that may increase their risk for late effects or make late effects worse. Education programs can help cancer survivors learn how to make behavior changes that keep them healthier. Programs that cover diet, exercise and stress management are more likely to help cancer survivors make lasting changes.

The effects of diet and lifestyle on cancer continue to be studied.

Nutrition in Cancer Prevention

The American Cancer Society (ACS) and the American Institute for Cancer Research (AICR) both have dietary guidelines that may help prevent cancer. Their guidelines are a lot alike and include the following:

- Eat a plant-based diet with a large variety of fruits and vegetables.

- Eat foods low in fat.

- Eat foods low in salt.

- Get to and stay at a healthy weight.

- Be active for 30 minutes on most days of the week.

- Drink few alcoholic drinks or don't drink at all.

- Prepare and store food safely.

- Do not use tobacco in any form.

The effect of soy on breast cancer and breast cancer prevention is being studied. Study results include the following:

- Some studies show that eating soy may decrease the risk of having breast cancer.

- Taking soy supplements in the form of powders or pills has not been shown to prevent breast cancer.

- Adding soy foods to the diet after being diagnosed with breast cancer has not been shown to keep the breast cancer from coming back.

Soy has substances in it that act like estrogen in the body. Studies were done to find out how soy affects breast cancer in patients who have tumors that need estrogen to grow. Some studies have shown that soy foods are safe for women with breast cancer when eaten in moderate amounts as part of a healthy diet.

If you are a breast cancer survivor be sure to check the most up-to-date information when deciding whether to include soy in your diet.

Chapter 54

Physical Activity for Cancer Survivors

What Is Physical Activity?

Physical activity simply means movement of the body that uses energy. Walking, gardening, briskly pushing a baby stroller, climbing the stairs, playing soccer, or dancing the night away are all good examples of being active. For health benefits, physical activity should be moderate or vigorous intensity.

Why Is Physical Activity Important?

Regular physical activity can produce long term health benefits. People of all ages, shapes, sizes, and abilities can benefit from being physically active. The more physical activity you do, the greater the health benefits.

Being physically active can help you:

- Increase your chances of living longer

This chapter contains text excerpted from the following sources: Text beginning with the heading "What Is Physical Activity?" is excerpted from "Physical Activity," ChooseMyPlate.gov, U.S. Department of Agriculture (USDA), June 19, 2015; Text beginning with the heading "Physical Activity after Cancer Treatment" is excerpted from "Physical Activity for Cancer Patients," Office of Disease Prevention and Health Promotion (ODPHP), U.S. Department of Health and Human Services (HHS), January 30, 2014.

- Feel better about yourself
- Decrease your chances of becoming depressed
- Sleep well at night
- Move around more easily
- Have stronger muscles and bones
- Stay at or get to a healthy weight
- Be with friends or meet new people
- Enjoy yourself and have fun

Physical Activity after Cancer Treatment

Patients emerging from cancer treatment are accustomed to detailed instructions from doctors regarding medications, radiation, surgery, etc. Yet when they complete treatment the doctor often sends them along with a simple directive to eat right and be physically active. Patients often are frightened by no longer having a protocol to fight their disease and bewildered as to what to do next.

For years there were questions about whether cancer survivors should even attempt physical activity. In 2010, the American College of Sports Medicine (ACSM), convened an expert panel to review the scientific evidence. The group reached the consensus that, "although there are specific risks associated with cancer treatments that need to be considered when survivors exercise, there seems to be consistent evidence that exercise is safe during and after cancer treatment."

The National Comprehensive Cancer Network (NCCN) doesn't advise running marathons or climbing mountains, but the organization says "it's wise to add some form of regular exercise to your daily life—even during cancer therapy." The group advocates "moderate aerobic exercise, such as riding a stationary bicycle or taking a daily walk, coupled with the use of light weights for strength training" to enhance well-being and spur recovery.

So What Should Cancer Patients and Survivors Do?

The best advice is to start a new physical activity program with the help of a trained specialist. The Cancer Exercise Training Institute (CETI) provides scientifically based information on exercise therapy as a critical component of cancer recovery. Cancer exercise specialists, or CES, are specifically trained at the institute to treat the range of conditions common to those undergoing cancer treatment. Many cancer patients present with limited range of motion, poor posture, neck and back pain and with lymphedema (or at a high risk for developing it).

A cancer exercise specialist also is well versed in the specific problems caused by different kinds of cancer(and their treatment) and can help guide the patient back to his or her best normal.

What Should Someone Expect from a Cancer Exercise Specialist?

The first visit will begin with a health history review. Next, the CES will conduct an initial fitness assessment, as well as postural, range of motion, and lymphedema assessments. He / She will conduct an interest profile to learn the forms of activity the patient is interested in. Then, the CES will develop a stretching and strengthening program and a cardiovascular fitness program specifically tailored to the patient.

The goal will be to help the cancer survivor become symptom free and physically active as smoothly and quickly as possible.

A Study on Physical Activity

A new study has found that people who engage in three to five times the recommended minimum level of leisure-time physical activity derive the greatest benefit in terms of mortality reduction when compared with people who do not engage in leisure-time physical activity. The *2008 Physical Activity Guidelines for Americans*, developed by the U.S. Department of Health and Human Services (HHS)' Physical Activity Guidelines Advisory Committee, recommend a minimum of 2.5 hours of moderate-intensity exercise per week or 1.25 hours of vigorous aerobic activity, but more activity is encouraged for additional health benefits. Before this study, experts did not know how much additional health benefit might accrue for those doing more exercise. This study confirms that much of the mortality benefit is realized by meeting the minimum recommended levels of physical activity and describes the increased mortality benefit associated with higher levels of physical activity. The study appeared online April 6, 2015, in *JAMA Internal Medicine*.

Hannah Arem, Ph.D., Division of Cancer Epidemiology and Genetics, National Cancer Institute (NCI), and her colleagues studied data from over half a million men and women in the United States and Europe who reported on their leisure-time physical activities, which included walking for exercise, jogging/running, swimming, tennis/

racquetball, bicycling, aerobics, and dance. The investigators also factored in data such as race/ethnicity, education, smoking status, history of cancer, history of heart disease, alcohol consumption, marital status, and body mass index. Their findings, which will help inform healthcare professionals, included the following:

1. Engaging in one to two times the recommended minimum level of leisure-time physical activity (i.e., 2.5 to 5 hours of moderate-intensity activity, such as walking, or 1.25 to 2.5 hours of vigorous-intensity activity, such as running) provided much of the observed longevity benefits: a 31 percent lower risk of death compared with people who did no leisure-time physical activity.

2. At three to five times the recommended minimum level of leisure-time physical activity the benefit appeared to level off at a 39 percent lower risk of death, compared with those who did no leisure-time physical activity. This level of exercise could be achieved by:

- walking 7 hours per week

- biking leisurely 5 hours per week

- running at a 10 minute/mile pace for 2.25 hours per week

3. At 10 or more times the recommended minimum level of leisure-time physical activity there was no additional mortality benefit, but there was also no increased risk of death.

Chapter 55

The Effect of Smoking on Cancer Recurrence

Smoking is the leading cause of cancer in the United States. Lung cancer is the leading cause of cancer death in both men and women in the United States.

Cancers Are Linked to Tobacco Use

Cancer risks linked to tobacco use include the following:

- Lung cancer and head and neck cancers are linked to tobacco use.

- People who started smoking before age 30 and have been smoking for a long time have a high risk of colorectal cancer.

- In smokers diagnosed with cancer, the cancer is more likely to have already spread.

Quitting smoking is helpful after cancer is diagnosed. Studies have found that smokers who quit are more likely to recover from cancer than are patients who continue to smoke. If you keep smoking, you may not respond well to treatment.

If you continue to smoke during cancer treatment, you may not respond to treatment as well as patients who do not smoke. Also, you

---

This chapter includes text excerpted from "Smoking in Cancer Care (PDQ®)– Patient Version," National Cancer Institute (NCI), June 27, 2014.

may have worse side effects from treatment. For example, patients who are given radiation therapy for laryngeal cancer are less likely to get their voice back to normal if they keep smoking.

Wounds from surgery heal more slowly in patients who keep smoking. Studies have found that prostate cancer patients who keep smoking have a higher risk of the cancer coming back, and of death from prostate cancer. However, prostate cancer patients who quit smoking for 10 years or longer lower their risk of death to about the same as nonsmokers.

Cancer patients who keep smoking increase their risk of having a second cancer. You have a higher risk of a second cancer if you keep smoking, whether you have a cancer that is smoking-related or not smoking-related. The risk of a second cancer may last for up to 20 years, even if the first cancer has been treated and is in remission (signs and symptoms of cancer have disappeared). Patients with oral and pharyngeal cancer who smoke have a high risk of a second cancer, but the risk is much less after 5 years of not smoking.

Smoking Is Dangerous for Cancer Patients and Survivors*

Smoking not only causes cancer but also interferes with cancer treatment. Cancer patients and cancer survivors who smoke are at greater risk for their cancer to recur. They are also more likely to die from their primary cancer and from secondary cancer (a cancer that occurs in a different organ). They are more likely to have serious medical issues from their cancer treatment—a condition known as treatment toxicity. They are also at higher risk for death from all other causes, such as pneumonia and infection. Quitting smoking improves the prognosis of cancer patients.

Text excerpted from "Smoking and Cancer," Centers for Disease Control and Prevention (CDC), October 15, 2014.

Counseling to Help You Quit Smoking

It is not easy to quit smoking and research has shown that people are more likely to quit if they have help. Mood changes are common in cancer patients and in people who smoke or are trying to quit smoking. Talk with your doctor if you have feelings of depression. Your doctor can offer counseling or other ways to help you quit smoking and treat depression when needed.

Not all smokers are motivated to quit. If you are not motivated to quit smoking, your doctor may be able to help you become motivated.

Your doctor or other healthcare professional may take the following steps to help you quit:

- Ask you about your smoking habits at every visit.

- Advise you to quit smoking.

- Help you with a plan to quit smoking by:

  - Setting a date to quit smoking.

  - Giving you self-help materials.

  - Recommending drug treatment.

- Plan follow-up visits with you.

It may take more than one try to quit smoking completely. When you first quit smoking, it is common to start again. There will be many stressful times that will make you want to smoke. Counseling can help you find ways to handle the stress other than by smoking. It may take more than a year to quit smoking completely, even when you are motivated.

You can find help online.

The following websites may be helpful:

- Smokefree.gov: Information about quitting smoking.

- Clearing the Air: Quit Smoking Today (www.smokefree.gov): Tips and advice on how to start a smoke-free life.

- BeTobaccoFree.gov: Information about the harmful health effects of smoking and tools for quitting.

Chapter 56

Learning to Relax

Importance of Relaxing

Many people with cancer have found that doing relaxation or imagery exercises has helped them cope with pain and stress.

Take the time to learn helpful relaxation skills, such as the ones below, and practice them when you can. You can also take a class, buy a relaxation digital versatile disc (DVD) or Compact disc (CD), or find other exercises online.

Getting Started

For each exercise, find a quiet place where you can rest undisturbed. Let others know you need time for yourself. Make the setting peaceful for you. For example, dim the lights and find a comfortable chair or couch.

You may find that your mind wanders, which is normal. When you notice yourself thinking of something else, gently direct your attention back to your body. Be sure to maintain your deep breathing.

Some people like to listen to slow, familiar music while they practice these exercises.

This chapter includes text excerpted from "Learning to Relax," National Cancer Institute (NCI), February 29, 2016.

Breathing and Muscle Tensing

- Get into a comfortable position where you can relax your muscles. Close your eyes and clear your mind of distractions. You can sit up or lie down. If you're lying down, you may want to put a small pillow under your neck and knees.

- Breathe deeply, at a slow and relaxing pace. Concentrate on breathing deeply and slowly, raising your belly with each breath, rather than just your chest.

- Next, go through each of your major muscle groups, tensing (squeezing) them for a few seconds and then letting go. Start at the top of your head and work your way down. Tense and relax your face and jaws, then shoulders and arms.

- Continue tensing and relaxing each muscle group as you go down (chest, lower back, buttocks, legs), ending with your feet. Focus completely on releasing all the tension from your muscles and notice the differences you feel when they are relaxed.

- When you are done, focus on the pleasant feeling of relaxation for as long as you like.

Slow Rhythmic Breathing

- Stare at an object or shut your eyes and think of a peaceful scene. Take a slow, deep breath.

- As you breathe in, tense your muscles. As you breathe out, relax your muscles and feel the tension leaving.

- Remain relaxed and begin breathing slowly and comfortably, taking about 9 to 12 breaths a minute. To maintain a slow, even rhythm, you can silently say to yourself, "In, one, two. Out, one, two."

- If you ever feel out of breath, take a deep breath, and continue the slow breathing.

- Each time you breathe out, feel yourself relaxing and going limp. Continue the slow, rhythmic breathing for up to 10 minutes.

- To end the session, count silently and slowly from one to three. Open your eyes. Say to yourself, "I feel alert and relaxed." Begin moving slowly.

Imagery

Imagery usually works best with your eyes closed. To begin, create an image in your mind. For example, you may want to think of a place or activity that made you happy in the past. Explore this place or activity. Notice how calm you feel.

If you have severe pain, you may imagine yourself as a person without pain. In your image, cut the wires that send pain signals from one part of your body to another. Or you may want to imagine a ball of healing energy. Others have found the following exercise to be very helpful:

- Close your eyes and breathe slowly. As you breathe in, say silently and slowly to yourself, "In, one, two," and as you breathe out, say "Out, one, two." Do this for a few minutes.

- Imagine a ball of healing energy forming in your lungs or on your chest. Imagine it forming and taking shape.

- When you're ready, imagine that the air you breathe in blows this ball of energy to the area where you feel pain. Once there, the ball heals and relaxes you. You may imagine that the ball gets bigger and bigger as it takes away more of your discomfort.

- As you breathe out, imagine the air blowing the ball away from your body. As it floats away, all of your pain goes with it.

- Repeat the last two steps each time you breathe in and out.

To end the imagery, count slowly to three, breathe in deeply, open your eyes, and say silently to yourself, "I feel alert and relaxed."

Chapter 57

What Is Normal after Cancer Treatment?

The end of cancer treatment is often a time to rejoice. Most likely you're relieved to be finished with the demands of treatment. You may be ready to put the experience behind you and have life return to the way it used to be. Yet at the same time, you may feel sad and worried. It can take time to recover. And it's very common to be thinking about whether the cancer will come back and what happens now. Often this time is called adjusting to a "new normal." You will have many different feelings during this time.

One of the hardest things after treatment is not knowing what happens next. Those who have gone through cancer treatment describe the first few months as a time of change. It's not so much "getting back to normal" as it is finding out what's normal for you now. People often say that life has new meaning or that they look at things differently.

Your new normal may include:

• Making changes in the way you eat and the things you do

• New or different sources of support

• Permanent scars on your body

• Not be able to do some things you used to do more easily

• Emotional scars from going through so much

This chapter includes text excerpted from "A New Normal," National Cancer Institute (NCI), December 2, 2014.

You may see yourself in a different way, or find that others think of you differently now. Whatever your new normal may be, give yourself time to adapt to the changes. Take it one day at a time.

Coping with Fear of Cancer Recurrence

When cancer treatment is over, patients are often faced with mixed emotions. While there is happiness and relief that come with the end of treatment, survivors may also feel fear and anxiety. Probably the most common fear is that the cancer will come back (a cancer recurrence).

Fear of recurrence is normal and often lessens over time. However, even years after treatment, some events may cause you to become worried. Follow-up visits, certain symptoms, the illness of a loved one, or the anniversary date of the date you were diagnosed can all trigger concern.

One step you can take is to be informed. Understand what you can do for your health now, and find out about the services available to you. Doing so can give you a greater sense of control.

Even though you can't control whether or not your cancer recurs, there are steps you can take to help cope with your fears.

Talk to Your Healthcare Team

- **Let your healthcare team know your concerns.** Be honest about the fears of your cancer coming back so they can address your worries. The risk of recurrence differs in each patient. Your healthcare team can give you the facts about your type of cancer and the chances of recurrence. They can assure you that they're looking out for you.

- **Know that it's common for cancer survivors to have fears about every ache and pain.** Talk to your healthcare team if you're having a symptom that worries you. You can get advice about whether or not to schedule an appointment. Just having a conversation with them about your symptoms may help calm your fears. And, over time, you may start to recognize certain feelings in your body as normal.

- **Keep notes about any symptoms you have.** Also take notes about any anxiety you feel. Write down questions for your healthcare team before follow-up visits so you can be prepared to tell them what you've been going through since your last check-up or conversation.

- **Talk to a counselor.** If you find that your fears are more than you can handle, ask for a referral for someone to talk to. If thoughts about cancer recurrence interfere with your daily life, you might feel better seeing a counselor or therapist. A professional may help you put your concerns in perspective.

- **Make sure you have a follow-up care plan.** Having a plan may give you a sense of control and a way to feel proactive with your health after treatment. See the next section to learn about your plan.

Take Care of Your Mind and Body

Even though you can't control whether or not your cancer recurs, you can use your energy to focus on wellness and manage stress. Here are some things you can do to take care of your mind and body:

- **Find ways to help yourself relax.** Relaxation exercises have been proven to help people with stress and may help you relax when you feel worried. Meditation and yoga also help reduce stress.

- **Talk to others.** Sharing your feelings with friends and family may help you feel better and realize that you're not alone. You can also join a support group to talk to others who are having the same fears.

- **Exercise.** Moderate exercise (examples: walking, biking, swimming) can help reduce anxiety and depression. It also may improve your mood and boost your self-esteem.

- **Eat a healthy diet.** Talk to a dietician or nutritionist about the foods you should eat to stay healthy and maintain your strength.

- **Write your feelings down.** It may help you to express your feelings by writing in a journal or a notebook. Many people find that getting their thoughts on paper helps them to let go of worries and fears.

- **Seek comfort from spirituality.** Many survivors have found their faith, religion, or sense of spirituality to be a source of strength.

- **Give back.** Some people like to channel their energy by volunteering and helping others. Being productive in this way gives them a sense of meaning and lets them turn their attention on others.

- **Take part in clubs, classes, or social gatherings.** Getting out of the house may help you focus on other things besides cancer and the worries it brings.

Chapter 58

Cancer Survivorship: Follow-Up Care

All cancer survivors should have follow-up care. Knowing what to expect after cancer treatment can help you and your family make plans, lifestyle changes, and important decisions.

Some common questions you may have are:

- Should I tell the doctor about symptoms that worry me?

- Which doctors should I see after treatment?

- How often should I see my doctor?

- What tests do I need?

- What can be done to relieve pain, fatigue, or other problems after treatment?

- How long will it take for me to recover and feel more like myself?

- Is there anything I can or should be doing to keep cancer from coming back?

- Will I have trouble with health insurance?

- Are there any support groups I can go to?

Coping with these issues can be a challenge. Yet many say that getting involved in decisions about their medical care and lifestyle was

This chapter includes text excerpted from "Facing Forward: Life after Cancer Treatment," National Cancer Institute (NCI), May 2014.

a good way for them to regain some of the control they felt they lost during cancer treatment.

Research has shown that people who feel more in control feel and function better than those who do not. Being an active partner with your doctor and getting help from other members of your healthcare team is the first step.

What Is Follow-Up Care?

Once you have finished your cancer treatment, you should receive a follow-up cancer care plan. Follow-up care means seeing a doctor for regular medical checkups. Your follow-up care plan depends on the type of cancer and type of treatment you had, along with your overall health. It is usually different for each person who has been treated for cancer.

In general, survivors usually return to the doctor every 3 to 4 months during the first 2 to 3 years after treatment, and once or twice a year after that. At these visits, your doctor will look for side effects from treatment and check if your cancer has returned (recurred) or spread (metastasized) to another part of your body.

At these visits, your doctor will:

* Review your medical history

* Give you a physical exam

Your doctor may run follow-up tests such as:

* Blood tests

* MRI or CT scans. These scans take detailed pictures of areas inside the body at different angles.

* Endoscopy. This test uses a thin, lighted tube to examine the inside of the body.

At your first follow-up visit, talk with your doctor about your follow-up care plan.

Medical Records and Follow-Up Care

Be sure to ask your oncologist for a written summary of your treatment. In the summary, he or she can suggest what aspects of your health need to be followed. Then, share this summary with any new doctors you see, especially your primary care doctor, as you discuss your follow-up care plan.

Many people keep their medical records in a binder or folder and refer to them as they see new doctors. This keeps key facts about your cancer treatment in the same place. Other kinds of health information you should keep include:

- The date you were diagnosed

- The type of cancer you were treated for

- Pathology report(s) that describe the type and stage of cancer

- Places and dates of specific treatment, such as:

- Details of all surgeries

- Sites and total amounts of radiation therapy

- Names and doses of chemotherapy and all other drugs

- Key lab reports, X-ray reports, CT scans, and MRI reports

- List of signs to watch for and possible long-term effects of treatment

- Contact information for all health professionals involved in your treatment and follow-up care

- Any problems that occurred during or after treatment

- Information about supportive care you received (such as special medicines, emotional support, and nutritional supplements)

Which Doctor Should I See Now? How Often?

You will need to decide which doctor will provide your follow-up cancer care and which one(s) you will see for other medical care. For follow-up cancer care, this may be the same doctor who provided your cancer treatment. For regular medical care, you may decide to see your main provider, such as a family doctor. For specific concerns, you may want to see a specialist. This is a topic you can discuss with your doctors. They can help you decide how to make transitions in care.

Depending on where you live, it may make more sense to get follow-up cancer care from your family doctor, rather than your oncologist. It's important to note that some insurance plans pay for follow-up care only with certain doctors and for a set number of visits.

In coming up with your schedule, you may want to check your health insurance plan to see what follow-up care it allows. No matter what your health coverage situation is, try to find doctors you feel comfortable with.

Always tell any new doctors you see about your history of cancer. The type of cancer you had and your treatment can

A Survivor's Wellness Plan

After cancer treatment, many survivors want to find ways to reduce the chances of their cancer coming back. Some worry that the way they eat, the stress in their lives, or their exposure to chemicals may put them at risk.

Cancer survivors find that this is a time when they take a good look at how they take care of themselves. This is an important start to living a healthy life.

When you meet with your doctor about follow-up care, you should also ask about developing a wellness plan that includes ways you can take care of your physical, emotional, social, and spiritual needs. If you find that it's hard to talk with your doctor about these issues, it may be helpful to know that the more you do it, the easier it becomes. And your doctor may suggest other members of the healthcare team for you to talk with, such as a social worker, clergy member, or nurse.

Changes You May Want to Think about Making

- **Quit smoking.** Research shows that smoking can increase the chances of getting cancer at the same site or another site.

- **Cut down on how much alcohol you drink.** Research shows that drinking alcohol increases your chances of getting certain types of cancers.

- **Eat well.** Healthy food choices and physical activity may help reduce the risk of cancer or recurrence. Talk with your doctor or a nutritionist to find out about any special dietary needs that you may have. The American Cancer Society (ACS) and the American Institute for Cancer Research (AICR) have developed similar diet and fitness guidelines that may help reduce the risk of cancer:

  - Eat a plant-based diet and have at least 5–9 servings of fruit and vegetables daily. Try to include beans in your diet, and eat whole grains (such as cereals, breads, and pasta) several times daily.

- Choose foods low in fat and low in salt.

- Get to and stay at a healthy weight.

- **Exercise and stay active.** Several recent reports suggest that staying active after cancer can help lower the risk of recurrence and can lead to longer survival. Moderate exercise (walking, biking, swimming) for about 30 minutes every—or almost every—day can:

  - Reduce anxiety and depression

  - Improve mood and boost self-esteem

  - Reduce fatigue, nausea, pain, and diarrhea

It is important to start an exercise program slowly and increase activity over time, working with your doctor or a specialist (such as a physical therapist) if needed. If you need to stay in bed during your recovery, even small activities like stretching or moving your arms or legs can help you stay flexible, relieve muscle tension, and help you feel better. Some people may need to take special care in exercising. Talk with your doctor before you begin any exercise program.

Talking with Your Doctor

During cancer treatment, you had a lot of practice in getting the most out of every doctor's visit. These same skills now apply to you as a survivor and are especially helpful if you are changing doctors or going back to a family or primary care doctor you may not have seen for a while.

It is important to be able to talk openly with your doctor. Both of you need information to manage your care. Be sure to tell your doctor if you are having trouble doing everyday activities, and talk about new symptoms to watch for and what to do about them. If you are concerned that the treatment you had puts you at a higher risk for having health problems, be sure to discuss this with your doctor as you develop your follow-up plan.

At each visit, mention any health issues you are having, such as:

- New symptoms.

- Pain that troubles you.

- Physical problems that get in the way of your daily life or that bother you, such as fatigue, trouble sleeping, sexual problems, or weight gain or loss.

- Other health problems you have, such as heart disease, diabetes, or arthritis.

- Medicines, vitamins, or herbs you are taking and other treatments you are using.

- Emotional problems, such as anxiety or depression, that you may have now or that you've had in the past.

- Changes in your family's medical history, such as relatives with cancer.

- Things you want to know more about, such as new research or side effects.

Just because you have certain symptoms, it doesn't always mean the cancer has come back. Symptoms can be due to other problems that need to be addressed.

Questions about Your Follow-Up Plan

- How often should I see my doctors?

- What follow-up tests, should be done (for example, CT scan, RI, bone scan)? How often?

- Are there symptoms that I should watch for?

- If I develop any of these symptoms, whom should I call?

Guidelines for Follow-Up Care

The following programs or organizations provide helpful follow-up care guidelines for some cancers. You can use them as you talk with your doctor—they aren't meant to contradict or take the place of your doctor's knowledge or judgment. Ask your oncologist for a treatment summary and a survivorship care plan. Both documents are recommended by the National Cancer Institute (NCI) and other cancer organizations.

- **Cancer.Net.** The American Society of Clinical Oncology (ASCO) has a series of follow-up care guides focused on breast and colorectal cancer. They can be viewed at www.cancer.net/ survivorship.

- **Children's Oncology Group Long-Term Follow-up Guidelines.** The Children's Oncology Group (COG) offers long-term follow-up guidelines for survivors of childhood, adolescent, and young adult cancers at www.survivorshipguidelines.org.

- **Journey Forward.** The Journey Forward is a program centered on its Survivorship Care Plan. By using an online Care Plan Builder, the oncologist creates a full medical summary and recommendations for follow-up care to be shared with patients and their primary care providers. It was created by the National Coalition for Cancer Survivorship (NCCS), UCLA Cancer Survivorship Center, Genentech, and WellPoint, Inc.

- **Life after Cancer Care.** M.D. Anderson's Cancer Center website lists follow-up guidelines for 15 different disease sites at www.mdanderson.org/patients-family/life-after-cancer.

- **Livestrong Care Plan.** Developed by Livestrong and the University of Pennsylvania, the Livestrong Care Plan gives individuals a specific survivor care plan, based on the information they enter into the online program.

- **NCCN.** The National Comprehensive Cancer Network website includes information about follow-up care for cancer, along with guidance on making formal survivorship plans.

Services to Think About

Talk with your doctor to help you locate services such as these:

- **Couples counseling.** You and your partner work with trained specialists who can help you talk about problems, learn about each other's needs, and find ways to cope. Counseling may include issues related to sex and intimacy.

- **Faith or spiritual counseling.** Some members of the clergy are trained to help you cope with cancer concerns, such as feeling alone, fear of death, searching for meaning, and doubts about faith.

- **Family support programs.** Your whole family may be involved in the healing process. In these programs, you and your family members take part in therapy sessions with trained specialists who can help you talk about problems, learn about each other's needs, and find answers.

- **Genetic counseling.** Trained specialists can advise you on whether to have genetic testing for cancer and how to deal with the results. It can be helpful for you and for family members who have concerns about their own health.

- **Home care services.** State and local governments offer many services that you may find useful after cancer treatment. For example, a nurse or physical therapist may be able to come to your home. You may also be able to get help with housework or cooking. Check the phone book under the categories Social Services, Health Services, or Aging Services.

- **Individual counseling.** Trained mental health specialists can help you deal with your feelings, such as anger, sadness, and concern for your future.

- **Long-term follow-up clinics.** All doctors can offer follow-up care, but there are also clinics that specialize in long-term follow-up after cancer. These clinics most often see people who are no longer being treated by an oncologist and who are considered disease-free. Ask your doctor if there are any follow-up cancer clinics in your area.

- **Nutritionists/Dietitians.** They can help you with gaining or losing weight and with healthy eating.

- **Occupational therapists.** They can help you regain, develop, and build skills that are important for day-to-day living. They can help you relearn how to do daily activities, such as bathing, dressing, or feeding yourself, after cancer treatment.

- **Oncology social workers.** These professionals are trained to counsel you about ways to cope with treatment issues and family problems related to your cancer. They can tell you about resources and connect you with services in your area.

- **Ostomy information and support.** The United Ostomy Association of America (UOAA) provides education, information, and support for people with intestinal/urinary diversions. Call 1-800-826-0826, or visit online at www.ostomy.org.

- **Pain clinics (also called Pain and Palliative Care Services).** These are centers with professionals from many different fields who are specially trained in helping people get relief from pain.

- **Physical therapists.** Physical therapists are trained to understand how different parts of your body work together. They can teach you about proper exercises and body motions that can help you gain strength and move better after treatment. They can also advise you about proper postures that help prevent injuries.

- **Quitting smoking (Smoking Cessation Services).** Research shows that the more support you have in quitting smoking, the greater your chance for success. Ask your doctor, nurse, social worker, or hospital about available programs, or call NCI's Smoking Quitline at 1-877-44-U-QUIT (1-877-448-7848).

- **Speech therapists.** Speech therapists can evaluate and treat any speech, language, or swallowing problems you may have after treatment.

- **Stress management programs.** These programs teach ways to help you relax and take more control over stress. Hospitals, clinics, or local cancer organizations may offer these programs and classes.

- **Support groups for survivors.** In-person and online groups enable survivors to interact with others in similar situations.

- **Survivor wellness programs.** These types of programs are growing in number, and they are meant for people who have finished their cancer treatment and are interested in redefining their life beyond cancer.

- **Vocational rehabilitation specialists.** If you have disabilities or other special needs, these specialists can help you find suitable jobs. They offer services such as counseling, education and skills training, and help in obtaining and using assistive technology and tools.

Chapter 59

Recurrent Cancer: When Cancer Comes Back

When cancer comes back after treatment, doctors call it a recurrence or recurrent cancer. Finding out that cancer has come back can cause feelings of shock, anger, sadness, and fear. But you have something now that you didn't have before—experience. You've lived through cancer already and you know what to expect. Also, remember that treatments may have improved since you were first diagnosed. New drugs or methods may help with your treatment or in managing side effects. In some cases, improved treatments have helped turn cancer into a chronic disease that people can manage for many years.

Why Cancer Comes Back

Recurrent cancer starts with cancer cells that the first treatment didn't fully remove or destroy. This doesn't mean that the treatment you received was wrong. It just means that a small number of cancer cells survived the treatment and were too small to show up in follow-up tests. Over time, these cells grew into tumors or cancer that your doctor can now detect.

Sometimes, a new type of cancer will occur in people who have a history of cancer. When this happens, the new cancer is known as

This chapter contains text excerpted from the following sources: Text in this chapter begins with excerpts from "Recurrent Cancer: When Cancer Comes Back," National Cancer Institute (NCI), January 18, 2016; Text beginning with the heading "Recurrent Cancer and Your Feelings" is excerpted from "When Cancer Returns," National Cancer Institute (NCI), September 2014.

a second primary cancer. Second primary cancer is different from recurrent cancer.

Types of Recurrent Cancer

Doctors describe recurrent cancer by where it develops and how far it has spread. The different types of recurrence are:

- **Local recurrence** means that the cancer is in the same place as the original cancer or very close to it.

- **Regional recurrence** means that the tumor has grown into lymph nodes or tissues near the original cancer.

- **Distant recurrence** means the cancer has spread to organs or tissues far from the original cancer. When cancer spreads to a distant place in the body, it is called metastasis or metastatic cancer. When cancer spreads, it is still the same type of cancer. For example, if you had colon cancer, it may come back in your liver. But, the cancer is still called colon cancer.

Staging Recurrent Cancer

To figure out the type of recurrence you have, you will have many of the same tests you had when your cancer was first diagnosed, such as lab tests and imaging procedures. These tests help determine where the cancer has returned in your body, if it has spread, and how far. Your doctor may refer to this new assessment of your cancer as "restaging."

After these tests, the doctor may assign a new stage to the cancer. An "r" will be added to the beginning of the new stage to reflect the restaging. The original stage at diagnosis does not change.

Treatment for Recurrent Cancer

The type of treatment that you have for recurrent cancer will depend on your type of cancer and how far it has spread. To learn about the treatments that may be used to treat your recurrent cancer, find your type of cancer for adult and childhood cancers.

Recurrent Cancer and Your Feelings

People feel so many emotions when they find out that their cancer has come back. Shock, fear, anger, and denial are just a few. The new diagnosis hits them as hard as it did the first time, or even harder. Regardless of your first reaction, starting cancer treatment again can place even more demands on your mind and spirit. You'll have good days and bad days. So just remember that it's okay to feel a lot of different emotions.

Some of these emotions may be ones you have had at other times in your life. But you may be feeling them more intensely. If you have dealt with them in the past, you may be able to cope with them now, too. If some of the feelings are new, or are so strong that it is hard to get through everyday activities, you may want to ask for help.

There are many people who may be able to help you. These include health psychologists, oncology social workers, other mental health experts, and leaders in your faith or spiritual community. They know many ways to help you cope with your feelings.

Stress

Stress is a normal reaction to cancer. After all, you're dealing with a lot: treatment, family, your job, money, and day-to-day living. Sometimes, you may not even notice that you are stressed. But your family and friends probably see a change. Anything that makes you feel calm or relaxed may help. So try to think of things that relax you and that you enjoy doing. Some people try deep breathing, listening to tapes that have nature sounds, or listening to music.

Hope

While you may be sad or depressed about your cancer recurrence, you do have reasons to feel hopeful. Science has advanced and cancer treatments have improved. So more people are surviving cancer than ever before. Nearly 10 million people who have a history of cancer are alive today.

In other words, cancer is becoming a disease that doctors can manage. To help build your sense of hope:

- Plan your days as you have always done.

- Don't limit the things you like to do just because you have cancer.

- Look for your own reasons to have hope.

Gratitude

Some people see their cancer coming back as a "wake-up call." They may realize the importance of enjoying the little things in life. They go places they've never been. They finish projects they had started but put aside. They spend more time with friends and family. They mend broken relationships.

It may be hard at first, but you can find joy in your life. Take note of what makes you smile. Pay attention to the things you do each day that you enjoy. They can be as simple as drinking your morning coffee, sitting with a pet, or talking to a friend. These small, day-to-day activities can give you comfort and pleasure.

You can also do things that are more meaningful to you. Everyone has special things, both large and small, that bring meaning to their life. For you, it may be visiting a garden in your city or town. It may be praying in a certain chapel. Or it could be playing golf or some other sport that you love. Whatever you choose, embrace the things that bring you joy when you can.

Anxiety

Cancer takes a toll on both your body and your mind. You are coping with so much now. You may feel overwhelmed. Pain and medicines for pain can also make you feel anxious or depressed. And you may be more likely to feel this way if you have had these feelings before.

Here are some signs of anxiety:

- Feeling very tense and nervous
- Racing heartbeat
- Sweating a lot
- Trouble breathing or catching your breath
- Having a lump in your throat or a knot in your stomach
- Feeling fear.

Feeling anxious can be normal. But if it begins to disrupt your daily life, tell a member of your healthcare team. They can suggest someone for you to talk to. Or they can give you medicines that will help. Some of the nondrug choices for pain may work for your anxiety as well.

Fear

It's normal to feel scared and worried. You may be afraid of pain or other side effects, either from the cancer or the treatment. You may worry about looking different as a result of your treatment. You may worry about taking care of your family, paying your bills, and keeping your job. You may be afraid of dying.

It's hard to deal with the fear of so many unknowns. Some people say it helps if you know what to expect in the future. Ask your health-care team questions, so you can understand more about your cancer and treatment choices. Also, update your will and other legal papers, if you haven't already done so. Then you won't have to worry about them. Fear can be overwhelming. Remember that others have felt this way, too. It's okay to ask for help.

Sadness and Depression

Sadness is a normal response to any serious illness. You may feel sad that you have to go through treatment again. You may feel sad that life won't be quite the same from now on. It's okay to feel blue. You don't need to be upbeat all the time or pretend to be cheerful. Many people say that they want the freedom to just give in to their feelings sometimes. But others say that it helps to look for what is good in life, even in the bad times. Depression can happen when sadness or despair seems to take over your life. Some of the signs listed on the next page are normal at a time like this. But if they last more than two weeks, talk to your doctor. Some symptoms could be due to physical problems. This is why it's important to let your doctor know about them.

Anger

You may also feel angry or frustrated. It's normal to ask, "Why me?" You may be mad at the cancer, your doctors, or your loved ones. If you are religious, you might even be angry with God. If you feel angry, it's helpful to remember that you don't have to pretend that everything is okay. Try to figure out why you are angry. Anger sometimes comes from feelings that are hard to show. These might be fear, panic, frustration, worry, or helplessness. It's not always easy to look at what is causing your anger. But it's healthy to try. Being open and dealing with your anger may help you let go of it. It's also good to know that anger is a form of energy. You can express this energy through exercise, art, or even just hitting the bed with a pillow.

Guilt

It's normal for some people to wonder whether they did things that caused their cancer to recur. People feel guilty for a number of reasons:

- They worry about how their family and friends feel.

- They envy other people's good health and are ashamed of this feeling.

- They blame themselves for certain lifestyle choices.

- They feel guilty that their first treatment didn't work.

- They wonder if they waited too long to go back to the doctor. Or they fear that they didn't follow the doctor's instructions the right way.

But it's important to remember that the treatment failed you. You didn't fail the treatment. We can't know why cancer returns in some people and not others. So, it's important for you to try to:

- Focus on things worthy of your time and energy.

- Let go of any mistakes you think you may have made.

- Forgive yourself.

You may want to share these feelings with your loved ones. Some people blame themselves for upsetting the people they love or worry that they'll be a burden to others. If you feel this way, take comfort knowing that many family members say that it is an honor and a privilege to care for their loved one. Many consider it a time when they can share experiences and become closer to one another. Others say that caring for someone else makes them take life more seriously and causes them to reevaluate their priorities. If you don't feel that you can talk openly about these things with your loved ones, getting counseling or joining a support group may also help. Let your healthcare team know if you would like to talk with someone about your feelings.

Loneliness

You may feel lonely, even when lots of people support and care for you. Here are some common feelings:

- You feel like no one else understands what you're going through, even those you love and care about.

- You feel distant from others. Or you find that your family and friends have a hard time dealing with your cancer.

- You realize that you aren't able to take part in as many events and activities as you used to.

Although it may be harder some days than others, remember that you aren't alone. Continue to do the things you've always done as best you can. If you want to, tell people that you don't want to be alone and that you welcome their visits. More than likely, your loved ones have feelings like yours. They may feel isolated from you and lonely if they are unable to talk with you.

Denial

You may feel that this is not happening to you. It's tough to accept that the cancer has come back. Feeling that you need more time to absorb everything is natural. You may need more time to adjust to the news. But this can become a serious problem if it lasts longer than it should. It can keep you from getting the treatment you need or talking about your treatment choices. As time passes, try to keep an open mind. Listen to what others around you suggest for your care.

Ways You Can Cope

Your feelings will come and go, just like they always have. If you have some strategies to deal with them, you have already taken a step in the right direction. Know that many other people have been where you are. Some do better when they join a support group. It helps them to talk with others who are facing the same challenges. You may prefer to join an online support group. That way you can chat with people from home. Be sure to check the privacy issues before you join. If support groups don't appeal to you, there are many experts who are trained to give cancer support. These include oncology social workers, psychologists or health psychologists, counselors, or members of your faith or spiritual community.

You may be able to continue many of your regular activities even though some may be more difficult than before. Whatever you do, remember to conserve your strength for the things you really want to do. Don't plan too many things for one day. Also try to stagger them during the day. Here are some things other people with cancer say have helped them cope. As you can see, even the little things help!

Part Seven

Information for Friends, Family Members, and Caregivers

Chapter 60

When Someone You Love Has Been Treated for Cancer

Who Is a Caregiver?

This chapter is for you if you are someone who helped your friend or family member get through cancer treatment. You are that person's "caregiver." You may have helped with day-to-day activities, doctor visits, and medical decisions. You may have been caring from a distance or traveling to help with care.

During the course of treatment, you may have had many roles. You may have done a range of things, from helping to get a second opinion and deciding about treatment, to talking with visitors, or trying to keep your loved one's spirits up. You may have worked with the medical team, too, about issues and concerns regarding care.

As treatment ends, patients and caregivers enter a new phase. Until now, you've probably stayed focused on getting the patient through treatment. You may feel that you haven't had time to think on your own about things and come to terms with the many changes that have occurred. Did you put your own feelings and needs on hold until treatment was over? Most caregivers do.

Once treatment ends, most people want to put the cancer experience behind them. Still, many caregivers aren't sure what to do next. It can

This chapter includes text excerpted from "When Someone You Love Has Completed Cancer Treatment," National Cancer Institute (NCI), September 2014.

be a time of mixed emotions—you may be happy treatment is over. But at the same time, the full impact of what you've gone through with your loved one may start to hit you.

Finding a "New Normal"

The end of cancer treatment is often a time to rejoice. Most people expect to put their cancer experience behind them and pick up where they left off in their lives. People are eager to get back to their normal routines and activities.

It's important to remember during this time that each person involved tends to adjust at his or her own pace. Some people are able to resume their regular activities right away. Others may need some extra time to recover. There may be pressure for you or your loved one to get back to the way things were before cancer. Yet it's important to know that for some, this can still be an emotional period.

Your loved one needs time to come to terms with what has happened. She still may be coping with the effects of treatment and adjusting to all the changes. She needs to figure out a "new normal." This means getting back to her old life, but in a way that's probably different than before. This also applies to you. Taking time for yourself and finding a new sense of normal is a process you will be adjusting to as well.

During treatment, you took on many roles. You may have been in charge of many decisions. Your loved one may have stepped back from decisions to stay focused on getting through treatment. It's common for caregivers to feel confused once it's over. You may have questions such as: How do I help my loved one now? Should I go back to work, or stay at home? When will he be ready to take on former roles and responsibilities? The answers to these questions vary with each person. As you move forward, try to be patient and take things one day at a time.

Shifting Your Focus Away from Treatment

The day your loved one finishes treatment is the milestone you've both been waiting for. It is a time of celebration and reflection for making it through your experience. You can begin to start taking back control of your life and thinking about other things that are important to you.

You may be glad to have free time where you aren't going to doctor visits, tests, treatment, and running related errands. Your loved one may start to feel better and you are able to venture out together to enjoy the things that are part of your life. Or you may decide to take a vacation or plan a special event. You may also have time to focus more on things you may have had to put on hold such as work and family issues.

Even though this is what you've been waiting for, it's important to recognize that it's a time when you may still have strong feelings.

The end of treatment is a time to:

- Celebrate.

- See what things your loved one is ready to handle again.

- Focus on other family and work issues that were put on hold.

- Sort out your feelings on the experience.

- Spend more time with friends and family.

Helping with Follow-Up Medical Care

Many caregivers are surprised to find that their loved one's recovery takes longer than they thought it would. For some people, recovery can be an ongoing process, involving physical and emotional changes. A lot of emotional support, love, and patience from you and other family members may be needed.

After treatment ends, you may begin to worry about whether the cancer will come back. This is one of the most common fears people have, especially during the first year after treatment. As time goes by, fear of cancer returning may lessen for you, and you may find that you aren't thinking about it as much. Yet even years after treatment, you may find that certain occasions, such as follow-up visits, anniversary of the cancer diagnosis, or even symptoms that may seem similar to when your loved one had cancer, may trigger concern and worry.

This is the time to begin shifting your focus from cancer treatment to follow-up tests and care. Your loved one should ask for a follow-up care plan. During follow-up care, the patient continues to see the doctors and specialists he saw during cancer treatment. They might recommend certain tests to monitor his health. They will also want to manage side effects from treatment and look for new ones that appear later. You may need to help keep track of information and help with your loved one's choices for care. Being active partners in decision-making can help both you and your loved one regain a sense of control that may have been lost during treatment.

At the first follow-up visit, the doctor will suggest a follow-up schedule. In general, people who have been treated for cancer return to the doctor every 3 to 4 months during the first 2 to 3 years after treatment. They then go once or twice a year after that for follow-up visits.

Meeting with the Doctor

If your loved one wants you to continue to go to doctor visits, ask how you might be helpful. You may want to talk to your loved one about any changes you're seeing in her, no matter how small. These may be:

- Fatigue

- Pain

- Lymphedema (swelling)

- Mouth or teeth problems

- Weight changes

- Bowel and bladder control

- Menopause symptoms

- Sexual problems

If you need to learn more, or do not understand, be sure to ask the doctor to explain. It's normal to have questions. Other caregivers have found it helpful to:

- Talk about ways to follow a healthy diet and lifestyle, if this will be something new. You may even want to talk with the doctor about developing a wellness plan for your loved one and family.

- Ensure that the patient asks for copies of any new tests or medical records at the time of the visit. Keep these in a folder or notebook, along with a list of medicines she is taking, in case you need them later. In it, include a list of important names and numbers you may need. This may be members of the healthcare team, pharmacists, and insurance contacts.

- Help keep track of your loved one's medication schedule and prescriptions to be filled.

- Talk about whether counseling would be helpful. A counselor could help you and your loved one cope with what has happened.

- Encourage your loved one to keep a "health journal." This can help keep track of any symptoms or side effects that occur between checkups.

Side Effects to Watch for after Treatment

It may take time for the patient to get over the side effects from treatment. All people recover differently, based on the type of treatment they had and their overall health. If your loved one seems frustrated, upset, or angry, it may help to understand that she may still be coping with some of the same problems that she had during treatment. Some of the most common side effects people report are:

- **Fatigue.** Feeling tired or worn out after treatment is one of the most common side effects the first year after treatment. Rest or sleep does not "cure" this type of fatigue. For some, fatigue gets better with time, and for others it may last years.

- **Pain.** Your loved one's skin may feel sensitive where she received radiation, or she may have pain or numbness in the hands and feet due to damaged nerves, or she may have pain in a missing limb or breast.

- **Memory Problems.** Memory and concentration problems can begin during and after treatment. They do not always go away. If a person is older, it may be hard to tell if the problems are age-related or not. Either way, some people feel that they cannot focus as they once did.

- **Lymphedema.** The patient may have swelling caused by a build-up of fluid in the tissues. It can be quite painful. Some types don't last very long, and other types can occur months or years after treatment. Lymphedema can also develop after an insect bite, minor injury, or burn.

- **Mouth or Teeth Problems.** These problems include dry mouth, cavities, changes in taste, painful mouth and gums, infections, and jaw stiffness or jawbone changes. Some people also have trouble swallowing. Some of these problems may go away after treatment. Others last a long time, or never go away. Some may develop months or years after treatment.

- **Weight Changes.** Some people have problems with weight loss because they have no desire to eat. Others have problems with weight gain. Unfortunately, the usual ways people try to lose weight may not work for them.

- **Bowel and Bladder Control.** Some treatments or surgery may cause problems with bowel and bladder control. This may be a total loss of control for some, while others have some control, but have to make lots of sudden trips to the bathroom. These problems are very upsetting for people. People often feel ashamed or afraid to go out in public.

- **Menopause Symptoms.** Some women stop getting their periods every month, or stop getting them altogether. For some younger women, their periods may start again, but for others they may not. Common signs are changes in periods, hot flashes, problems with the vagina or bladder, lack of interest in sex, and fatigue and sleep problems. Memory problems, mood swings, depression, and feeling irritable may also occur.

- **Sexual Problems.** Sexual problems in the body can be caused by changes from cancer treatment or the effects of pain medicine. Sometimes these problems are caused by depression, guilt, changes in body image, and stress. Some patients lose interest in sex because they struggle with their body image, or because they are tired or in pain. Others are not able to have sex as they did before because of changes in sex organs. Other main concerns people have are symptoms of menopause, and not being able to have children.

These are all common side effects you may want to watch for in your loved one. If he or she is struggling with any of these, you may want to suggest talking to the doctor about ways to get relief.

Reflection

The end of treatment often comes as a time to look forward to the future. New rituals and new beginnings can bring a sense of relief and joy to caregivers and their loved ones. It can also be a time of physical and emotional change. This is true not only for your loved one, but also for you as a caregiver. During treatment, your focus was on the patient's needs. Now that treatment is over, try to take time to get back in tune with yourself. Allow healing time for you, your loved one, and your family. Try to plan what you and your loved one can do to begin living without cancer as a main focus.

Whether good or bad, life-changing situations often give people the chance to grow, learn, and appreciate what's important to them. Many people who care for their friends or family members describe the experience as a personal journey. This is much like the way people with cancer describe their experience. It's not necessarily a journey they would have chosen for themselves. But they can use their skills, strength, and talents to support their loved ones while finding out more about themselves along the way.

Chapter 61

When Your Child
Has Cancer

Helping Your Child to Cope

Treatment brings many changes to a child's life and outlook. Changes to your child's daily routine, appearance, and friendships may be especially challenging to deal with. Not being able to go to school or do other normal activities can make your child feel alone. Long hospital stays and time away from friends and family can also take their toll.

You can help your child by letting her live as normal a life as possible. Although many activities may need to be changed, new activities and people can be added in their place. Talking with other families who are going through similar events may also be beneficial. Here are some ways to help your child:

- **Learn what to expect.** Ask how the type of treatment your child is receiving has affected other children, so you can prepare your child.

- **Be open and ready.** Encourage, but don't push, your child to share his feelings. Be there when your child comes to you.

- **Check out activities at the hospital.** Learn about events and programs at your child's hospital.

This chapter includes text excerpted from "Children with Cancer: A Guide for Parents," National Cancer Institute (NCI), September 2015.

- **Take care of yourself.** Children sense when their parents are stressed. It helps them cope knowing that their parents and siblings are getting support.

Changes in Appearance

It helps to feel good on the outside, even—or perhaps especially—when your child feels down and tired on the inside. Children can be sensitive about how they look and how others respond to them. Here are some ways to help your child:

- **Prepare for hair loss.** If treatment will cause your child's hair to fall out, let your child pick out a fun cap, scarf, and/or wig ahead of time. Try to pick out a wig before the hair falls out, so you can match it to their hair color. Sometimes cutting your child's hair short before treatment helps make hair loss a bit less upsetting.

- **Be aware of weight changes.** Some treatments may cause weight loss and others may cause weight gain. Get advice from a dietician so you know what to expect and how you can help your child prepare for and cope with physical changes.

- **Be creative.** You and your child may shop for outfits that your child likes. Sometimes a cool t-shirt or fun hat helps to build self-esteem.

Changes in Friendships

Your child's friendships are tested and may change during a long and serious illness. Sometimes, it may seem as though your child's old friends are no longer "there for them" or that they don't care anymore. Your child's friends might not know what to say. Or they might be afraid of saying the wrong thing, so they say nothing at all. Unfortunately, some children speak before they think or before they have the facts. No matter the reason, it can hurt when classmates and friends seem uncaring. Sometimes, it may seem as though your child's friends are moving on with their lives, and your child is left out. It may help if your child takes the first step and reaches out to friends.

The good news is that your child may make new friends through this experience. Going to support groups is one way to connect with others. Some groups meet in person and others meet online. Your child's social worker and child life specialist are also sources of support and guidance. For example, they can role-play conversations with your child that may be helpful. Here are some steps you can take with your child:

- **Help your child stay in touch with friends.** You can encourage and help your child to connect with friends through texts, e-mails, online video chats, phone calls, and/or social media sites. Sometimes a social worker or child life specialist can help your child think through what they would like to share with friends. If possible and when your child is up to it, friends may be able to visit.

- **Help your child know how to respond.** Sometimes people will stare, mistake your child's gender, or ask personal questions. Talk with your child and come up with an approach that works. Your child may choose to respond or to ignore comments.

Changes in Feelings

Although over time many children cope well, it's common for your child to feel anxious, sad, stressed, scared, or become withdrawn, from time to time. Talk with your child about what they are feeling and help them find ways to cope. You and your child can also meet with a social worker, child life specialist, or psychologist about feelings that don't have easy solutions or seem to be getting worse over time. These specialists can help your child manage difficult feelings before they cause physical problems, such as changes to sleeping or eating habits, anxiety, or depression.

Reassure children that they can always come to you. Listen and be open to what your child has to say. Some children prefer to express their feelings through drawing, painting, writing, or playing music. Try these tips to help your child cope with difficult emotions:

- **Find ways to distract or entertain your child.** Playing video games or watching movies can help your child to relax. Practices such as muscle relaxation, guided imagery, and biofeedback may also help.

- **Stay calm.** Your child can feel your emotions. If you often feel sad or anxious, talk with your child's healthcare team and your doctor about the best way to manage these emotions. However, if you often hide your feelings, your child may also hide their feelings from you.

- **Get help if you see signs of depression in your child.** It is normal for your child to feel down or sad sometimes, but if these feelings last for too long and happen on most days, they may be a sign of depression. Depression is a medical illness that can be treated. Child life specialists, social workers, counselors, psychologists, psychiatrists and other specialists are all people who can give your child extra support during this difficult time.

Changes in Schedule (Hospital and School)

Your child may spend more time at the hospital and less time at school during treatment. Here are some ways to help your child cope with long stays at the hospital and time away from school.

Hospital Stays

Being in the hospital can be difficult for anyone, especially children. It is a different setting, with new people and routines, strange machines, and sometimes painful procedures. Try these tips to make your child's time away from home a bit easier:

- **Bring in comfort items.** Let your child choose favorite things from home, such as photos, games, and music. These items can comfort children and help them to relax.

- **Visit game rooms or play rooms.** Many hospitals have places where children can play, relax, and spend time with other children at the hospital. These rooms often have toys, games, crafts, music, and computers. Encourage your child to take part in social events and other activities that are offered at the hospital.

- **Decorate your child's room.** Ask if you can decorate your child's hospital room. Posters, pictures, and other decorations may brighten the room and help cheer up your child. Window markers are a fun way to decorate windows. Check to see what items can be brought into your child's room, since there are sometimes medical restrictions.

- **Explore new activities.** If sports are off-limits, learn about other activities that can help your child stay active and have fun. Your child may also enjoy listening to music, reading, playing games, or writing. Some children with cancer find new skills and interests they never knew they had.

Missing School

Most children with cancer miss school during treatment. Some children are able to attend from time to time, whereas others need to take a leave of absence. Here are some ways to get the academic support your child needs during treatment:

- **Meet with your child's doctor.** Find out from the doctor how treatment may affect your child's energy level and ability to do schoolwork. Get a letter from the doctor that describes your child's medical situation, limitations, and how much school your child is likely to miss.

- **Learn about assistance from the hospital and your child's school.** Some hospitals have education coordinators and others have nurses who will tell you about education-related resources and assistance. Ask about an individualized education plan (IEP) for your child. This is an education plan for children with certain health conditions or disabilities. It describes what special services are needed (such as special class placement, extra help with class assignments and tests, tutoring, and other services such as counseling, speech therapy, and physical therapy) and how these services will be provided to your child.

- **Keep your child's teachers updated.** Tell your child's teachers and principal about your child's medical situation. Share the letter from your child's doctor. Learn what schoolwork your child will miss and ways for your child to keep up, as they are able. Talk with people at the school and hospital to make a plan that meets your child's educational needs both during and after treatment.

Going Back to School

It's best for most children with cancer to return to school as soon as they are able. It helps to have a routine and to be with other children. Still, the adjustment may be challenging. Your child may have fallen behind and have low energy. Friendships may have changed. Children often feel self-conscious about changes in appearance and weight. Ways to help your child get back into the swing of things at school:

- **Learn about back-to-school programs offered by many hospitals.** These programs help classmates and teachers learn about cancer and make your child's return to school easier.

- **Talk with your child's school** so they can give your child any needed support. The teachers can also talk with your child's classmates and help them welcome your child back. School counselors and school nurses may also be a big help.

- **Talk with parents of classmates** to let them know your child is coming back to school. Plan times for your child to get together with classmates, to catch up and play.

- **Check out the in-depth information links** on educational issues and school for children with cancer.

Signs of Depression

If your child has any of these signs, talk with the doctor.

- no longer enjoying activities that your child used to enjoy

- changes in eating or sleeping habits (e.g., not sleeping well)

- feeling or acting sad, nervous, sluggish, or tired

- feeling worthless or guilty, even for things that are no one's fault

- having trouble paying attention

- talking about death or suicide

Chapter 62

When Your Parent Has Cancer

What Your Parent May Be Feeling

Knowing what your parent may be feeling could help you figure out how to help, or at least to understand where he or she is coming from. You may be surprised to learn that they are feeling a lot of the same things you are:

- **Sad or depressed.** People with cancer sometimes can't do things they used to do. They may miss these activities and their friends. Feeling sad or down can range from a mild case of the blues to depression, which a doctor can treat.

- **Afraid.** Your parent may be afraid of how cancer will change his or her life and the lives of family members. He or she may be scared about treatment. Your parent may even be scared that he or she will die.

- **Anxious.** Your parent may be worried about a lot of things. Your mom or dad may feel stressed about going to work or paying the bills. Or he or she may be concerned about looking different because of treatment. And your mom or dad is probably very

This chapter includes text excerpted from "When Your Parent Has Cancer: A Guide for Teens," National Cancer Institute (NCI), February 2012. Review February 2017.

concerned about how you are doing. All these worries may upset your parent.

- **Angry.** Cancer treatment and its side effects can be difficult to go through. Anger sometimes comes from feelings that are hard to show, such as fear or frustration. Chances are your parent is angry at the disease, not at you. Lonely. People with cancer often feel lonely or distant from others. They may find that their friends have a hard time dealing with their cancer and may not visit. They may be too sick to take part in activities they used to enjoy. They may feel that no one understands what they're going through.

- **Hopeful.** There are many reasons for your parent to feel hopeful. Millions of people who have had cancer are alive today. People with cancer can lead active lives, even during treatment. Your parent's chances of surviving cancer are better today than ever before.

Changes in Your Family

Families say that it helps to make time to talk together, even if it's only for a short time each week. Talking can help your family stay connected. Here are some things to consider when talking with:

Growing Stronger as a Family

Some families can grow apart for a while when a parent has cancer. But there are ways to help your family grow stronger and closer. Teens who saw their families grow closer say that it happened because people in their family:

- **Tried** to put themselves in the other person's shoes and thought about how they would feel if they were the other person.

- **Understood** that even though people reacted differently to situations, they were all hurting. Some cried a lot. Others showed little emotion. Some used humor to get by.

- **Learned** to respect and talk about differences. The more they asked about how others were feeling, the more they could help each other.

Brothers and sisters

- If you are the oldest child, your brothers or sisters may look to you for support. Help them as much as you can. It's okay to let them know that you're having a tough time, too.

- If you are looking to your older brother or sister for help, tell them how you are feeling. They can help, but won't have all the answers.

Your parent who is well

- Expect your parent to feel some stress, just as you do.

- Your parent may snap at you. He or she may not always do or say the right thing.

- Lend a hand when you can.

Your parent with cancer

- Your mom or dad may be sick from the treatment or just very tired. Or maybe your parent will feel okay and want your company.

- Try talking if your mom or dad feels up to it. Let your parent know how much you love them.

How You Can Help Your Parent

Here are some things that others have done to help their parent at home. Pick one or two things to try each week.

Help with Care

- **Spend time with your parent.** Watch a movie together. Read the paper to your parent. Ask for help with your homework. Give hugs. Say, "I love you." Or just hang out in silence.

- **Lend a hand.** Bring water or offer to make a snack or small meal.

Help by Being Thoughtful

- **Try to be upbeat, but be "real," too.** Being positive can be good for you and your whole family. But don't feel like you always have to act cheerful, especially if it's not how you really feel. It's okay to share your thoughts with your parent—and let them comfort you. Be yourself.

- **Be patient.** You are all under stress. If you find you are losing your cool, listen to music, read, or go outside to shoot hoops or go for a run.

- **Share a laugh.** You've probably heard that laughter is good medicine. Watch a comedy on TV with your parent or tell jokes if that's your thing. Also, remember that you're not responsible for making everyone happy. You can only do so much.

- **Buy your parent a new scarf or hat.** Your parent might enjoy a new hat or scarf if he or she has lost their hair during treatment.

Help by Staying Involved

- **Keep your parent in the loop.** Tell your parent what you did today. Try to share what is going on in your life. Ask your parent how his or her day was.

- **Talk about family history.** Ask your parent about the past. Look through pictures or photo albums. Talk about what you're both proud of, your best memories, and how you both have met challenges. Write, or make drawings, about what you and your parent share with each other.

- **Keep a journal together.** Write thoughts or poems, draw, or put photos in a notebook that the two of you share. This can help you share your feelings when it might be hard to speak them aloud.

- **Help with younger brothers and sisters.** Play with your brothers and sisters to give your parent a break. Pull out games or read a book with your siblings. This will help you stay close and also give your parent time to rest.

Chapter 63

When Your Brother or Sister Has Cancer

Your Feelings

As you deal with your **sibling's** cancer, you may feel lots of different emotions. Some of the emotions you may feel are listed below:

Feeling Scared

It's normal to feel scared. Some of your fears may be real. Others may be based on things that won't happen. And some fears may lessen over time.

Some of the reasons you feel scared are listed below:

- My world is falling apart.
- I'm afraid that my brother or sister might die.
- I'm afraid that someone else in my family might catch cancer. (They can't.)

Feeling Guilty

You might feel guilty about having fun when your sibling is sick. This shows how much you care about them. But you should know

---

This chapter includes text excerpted from "When Your Brother or Sister Has Cancer: A Guide for Teens," National Cancer Institute (NCI), November 2013. Reviewed February 2017.

that it is both okay and important for you to do things that make you happy.

Some of the reasons you feel guilty are listed below:

- I feel guilty because I'm healthy and my brother or sister is sick.

- I feel guilty when I laugh and have fun.

Feeling Angry

Anger often covers up other feelings that are harder to show. If having cancer in your family means that you can't do what you like to do and go where you used to go, it can be hard. Even if you understand why it's happening, you don't have to like it. But, don't let anger build up inside. Try to let it out. And when you get mad, remember that it doesn't mean you're a bad person or you don't love your sibling. It just means you're mad.

Some of the reasons you feel angry are listed below:

- I am mad that my brother or sister is sick.

- I am angry at God for letting this happen.

- I am angry at myself for feeling the way I do.

- I am mad because I have to do all the chores now.

Feeling Neglected

When your brother or sister has cancer, it's common for the family's focus to change. Your parents don't mean for you to feel left out. It just happens because so much is going on. You may want to tell your parents how you feel and what you think might help. Try to remember that you are important and loved and that you deserve to feel that way, even though you might not get as much attention from your parents right now.

Some of the reasons you feel neglected are listed below:

- I feel left out.

- I don't get any attention any more.

- No one ever tells me what's going on.

- My family never talks anymore.

Feeling Lonely

Some of the reasons you feel lonely are listed below:

- My friends don't come over anymore.

- My friends don't seem to know what to say to me anymore.

- I miss being with my brother or sister the way we used to be.

Feeling Embarrassed

It can help to know that other teens also feel embarrassed. So do their siblings. In time it gets easier, and you will find yourself feeling more comfortable.

Some of the reasons you feel embarrassed are listed below:

- I'm sometimes embarrassed to be out in public with my sibling because of how they look.

- I feel silly when I don't know how to answer people's questions.

Feeling Jealous

Even if you understand why you are getting less attention, it's still not easy. Others who have a brother or sister with cancer have felt the same way. Try to share your feelings with your parents and talk about what you think might help.

One of the reason you feel jealous is listed below:

- I'm feeling upset that my brother or sister is getting all the attention.

What You're Feeling Is Normal

There is no one "right" way to feel. And you're not alone—many other teens in your situation have felt the same way. Some have said that having a brother or sister with cancer changes the way they look at things in life. Some even said that it made them stronger.

Dealing with Your Feelings

A lot of people are uncomfortable sharing their feelings. They ignore them and hope they'll go away. Others choose to act cheerful when they're really not. They think that by acting upbeat they won't feel sad or angry anymore. This may help for a while, but not over the long run. Actually, holding your feelings inside can keep you from getting the help that you need.

Try these tips:

- **Talk** with family and friends that you feel close to. You owe it to yourself.

- **Write** your thoughts down in a journal.

- **Join a support group** to meet other kids who are facing some of the same things you are. Or meet with a counselor.

It is probably hard to imagine right now, but, if you let yourself, you can grow stronger as a person through this experience.

Helping Your Brother or Sister

Help by Just Being There

- **Hang out together.** Watch a movie together. Read or watch TV together. Decorate your brother's or sister's bedroom with pictures or drawings. Go to the activity room at the hospital and play a game or do a project together.

- **Comfort one another.** Just being in the same room as your brother or sister can be a big comfort. Do what feels best for the two of you. Give hugs or say "I love you." Laugh or cry together. Talk to one another. Or just hang out in silence.

Help by Being Thoughtful

- **Help your brother or sister stay in touch with friends.** Ask your sibling's friends to write notes, send pictures, or record messages. Help your brother or sister send messages to their friends. If your brother or sister is up for it, invite friends to hang out with them.

- **Share a laugh.** You've probably heard that laughter is good medicine. Watch a comedy or tell jokes together, if that is your thing.

- **Be patient.** Be patient with each other. Your brother or sister may be cranky or even mean. As bad as you feel, your brother or sister is probably feeling even worse. If you find you are losing your cool, go for a run, read, or listen to music.

- **Make a snack.** Make a snack for the two of you to share. Make a picnic by putting a blanket on the porch or in the bedroom.

- **Buy a new scarf or hat.** Your brother or sister might like a new hat or scarf if they have lost their hair during treatment. Get a matching hat or scarf for yourself, too.

- **Try to be upbeat, but be "real," too.** Being positive can be good for you and your whole family. But don't feel like you have to act cheerful all the time if that's not how you really feel. Try to be yourself.

Help by Staying Involved

- **Keep a journal together.** Write thoughts or poems, doodle, or put photos in a notebook. Take turns with your sibling writing in a journal. This can help you both share your thoughts when it might be hard to talk about them.

- **Go for a walk together.** If your brother or sister feels up to it, take a walk together. Or, open a window or sit on the front porch together.

The ideas above are for those times when you have extra energy to give. Don't forget to take care of yourself, too. You deserve it.

Changes in Your Family

Changing Routines and Responsibilities

Your family may be going through a lot of changes. You may be the oldest, youngest, or middle child in your family. You may live with one parent or two. Whatever your family situation, chances are that things have changed since your brother or sister got sick. This chapter looks at some of these changes and ways that others have dealt with them.

Your parents may ask you to take on more responsibility than others your age. Your parents may be spending more time with your brother or sister. You might resent it at first. Then again, you may grow and learn a lot from the experience. Families say that it helps to make time to talk together—even if it's only for a short time each week. Talking can help your family stay connected. Here are some things to consider when talking with:

Other brothers and sisters

- If you are the oldest child, your younger brothers or sisters may look to you for support. Help them as much as you can. It's okay to let them know that you are having a tough time, too.

503

- If you are looking to your older brother or sister for help, tell them how you are feeling. They can help, but they may not have all the answers.

Your parents

- Expect your parents to feel some stress, just like you may. Your parents may not always do or say the right thing.

- Try to make the most of the time you do have with your parents. Let them know how much it means to you. Maybe you can go out to dinner together, or they can come to your sports game, from time to time.

- Sometimes you may have to take the first step to start a conversation. You may feel guilty for wanting to have your needs met— but you shouldn't. You are important and loved, too.

- Keep talking with your parents, even though it may be hard.

Your brother or sister with cancer

- Your brother or sister may be sick from the treatment and want to be alone. Or maybe they feel okay and want your company.

Get Help When You Feel Down and Out

Many teens feel low or down when their brother or sister is sick. It's normal to feel sad or "blue" during difficult times. However, if these feelings last for 2 weeks or more and start to interfere with things you used to enjoy, you may be depressed. The good news is that there is hope and there is help. Often, talking with a counselor can help. Below are some signs that you may need to see a counselor.

Are you:

- Feeling helpless and hopeless? Thinking that life has no meaning?

- Losing interest in being with family or friends?

- Finding that everything or everyone seems to get on your nerves?

- Feeling really angry a lot of the time?

- Thinking of hurting yourself?

Do you find that you are:

- Losing interest in the activities you used to enjoy?

- Eating too little or a lot more than usual?

- Crying easily or many times each day?

- Using drugs or alcohol to help you forget?

- Sleeping more than you used to? Less than you used to?

- Feeling tired a lot?

If You Answered "Yes" to Any of These Questions

It's important to talk to someone you trust. Going to see a counselor doesn't mean that you are crazy. In fact, it means that you have the strength and courage to recognize that you are going through a difficult time and need help.

Part Eight

Additional Help and Information

Chapter 64

A Glossary of Cancer Care Terms

benign: A tumor or cells that are not cancerous.

biological therapy: A treatment that works with your body's immune system to help it fight cancer cells or to control side effects from other cancer treatments.

biopsy: A biopsy is a minor surgery to get body fluid or small pieces of body tissue to look at under a microscope to see if there are cancer cells. The removed cells or tissues are usually examined by a pathologist.

bone marrow transplant: Bone marrow transplants are often used to treat blood cancers. Bone marrow is a spongy tissue found inside bones. For a bone marrow transplant, cells are taken from the bone marrow of a donor and put inside a patient to make new blood cells.

bone marrow: The soft, sponge-like tissue in the center of most bones. Bone marrow makes all kinds of blood cells: white blood cells, red blood cells, and platelets (clotting cells).

cancer: A disease in which cells grow out of control. Cancer cells can invade nearby tissue and spread to other parts of the body.

cancer survivor: A person who has been diagnosed with cancer, from the time of diagnosis until the end of life.

This glossary contains terms excerpted from documents produced by several sources deemed reliable.

carcinoma: A cancer that starts in the skin or the tissues that line internal organs.

caregiver: A person who provides support and help to a cancer survivor.

cell: The basic unit that makes up the human body. Cells contain genetic information.

chemotherapy: Special medicines used to shrink or kill cancer cells. The drugs can be pills you take or medicines given in your veins, or sometimes both.

chronic disease: A disease that a person has for a long period of time. Cancer can be a chronic disease.

clinical trials: Studies that research drugs, medical plans, treatments, or devices to see if they are safe and effective for people who have cancer or other illnesses. Clinical trials can also study whether interventions that change health behaviors, such as diet, are effective.

complementary and alternative medicine (CAM): Medicines and health practices that are not standard cancer treatments. Meditation, yoga, and supplements like vitamins and herbs are some examples.

deoxyribonucleic acid (DNA): The chemicals that make up the genes in cells. Some cancers can be carried and passed along by families through their DNA.

depression: A mental condition marked by ongoing feelings of sadness, despair, loss of energy, and difficulty dealing with normal daily life. Other symptoms of depression include feeling worthless or hopeless, loss of pleasure in activities, changes in eating or sleeping habits, and thoughts of death or suicide. Depression can affect anyone, and can be successfully treated.

diagnosis: A person is found to have a disease or condition, such as cancer.

emotional distress: Feelings of depression, fear, and anxiety that can happen after being diagnosed with cancer.

false positive: A test result that indicates that a person may have cancer when he or she does not.

family history: A record of the current and past medical conditions of a person's parents, brothers, sisters, children, grandparents, aunts, uncles, and other family members to help understand a person's risk of cancer. Knowing a person's family history can help show a pattern of certain diseases that may be inherited or run in the family.

follow-up care: Getting routine checkups and other cancer screenings after cancer treatment ends. Follow-up care can help find new or returning cancers early and look for side effects of cancer treatment.

formal caregivers: People who are trained and paid to provide care, such as nurses, therapists, social workers, and home health aides. Formal caregivers may work for home care agencies, community or social service agencies, or for-profit providers.

genes: The instructions that tell cells how to behave and what type of cells to become. Genes are responsible for traits passed along in families, like eye color, height, and even cancer risk.

genetics: The study of genes and how they affect the human body.

hormone: A chemical made by glands in your body. Hormones move in the bloodstream. They control the actions of certain cells or organs. Some hormones can also be made in the laboratory.

hormone therapy: Treatment that adds, blocks, or removes hormones. To slow or stop the growth of certain cancers (such as prostate and breast cancer), synthetic hormones or other drugs may be given to block the body's natural hormones.

imaging test: Different tests that create images of parts of the body, such as X-rays, magnetic resonance imaging (MRI), computed tomography (CT), and positron emission tomography (PET).

immune system: The body's natural defense system against getting an infection and disease. White blood cells are the main part of your immune system that fight infections.

infection: When germs enter a person's body and multiply, causing disease. The germs may be bacteria, viruses, yeast, or fungi. When the body's natural defense system is strong, it can often fight the germs and prevent infection. Some cancer treatments can weaken the natural defense system.

informal caregivers: People who provide unpaid care for cancer patients and often are family members, friends, and neighbors.

inherited: Transmitted through genes that have been passed from parents to their offspring (children).

intravenous (IV): Into or within a vein. Intravenous usually refers to a way of giving a drug or other substance through a needle or tube inserted into a vein.

late effect: A health problem that occurs months or years after a disease is diagnosed or after treatment has ended. Late effects may be caused by cancer or cancer treatment. They may include physical, mental, psychosocial problems, and second cancers.

leukemia: Starts in blood-forming tissue such as the bone marrow. Large numbers of abnormal blood cells form and enter the bloodstream.

long-term side effect: A problem that is caused by a disease or treatment of a disease and may continue for months or years after treatment. Some long-term side effects of cancer treatment vary for patients and can include heart, lung, kidney, or gastrointestinal tract problems; pain, numbness, tingling, loss of feeling, or heat or cold sensitivity in the hands or feet; fatigue; hearing loss; cataracts; and dry eyes or dry mouth.

lymphoma and multiple myeloma: Begin in the cells of the immune system.

malignant: A tumor or cells that are cancerous.

metastasis: The spread of cancer from one part of the body to another, through the lymph system or bloodstream. A tumor formed by cells that have spread is called a "metastatic tumor" or a "metastasis." The metastatic tumor contains cells that are like those in the original (primary) tumor.

mutation: A change in the DNA of a cell. Most mutations do not cause cancer, though some are linked to higher risk for cancer.

neutropenia: When the body has very low levels of certain white blood cells called neutrophils (infection-fighting white blood cells). It is a common side effect of chemotherapy treatment.

oncology: The branch of medicine that focuses on the development, diagnosis, and treatment of cancer. A medical doctor who manages a person's care and treatment after a cancer diagnosis is called an oncologist.

patient navigator: A person who guides a cancer patient through tests, treatment, and follow-up care.

primary cancer: The original cancer that develops in one place in the body.

psychologist: An expert or specialist in psychology (the study of the mind and behavior).

psychosocial factors: A person's thoughts, emotions, behaviors, spirituality, and social interactions. Psychosocial factors contribute to the way people view themselves and the world around them and the way they view life situations and events. These factors are also related to well-being and how people feel about themselves and others in their life.

quality of life: A cancer survivor's overall enjoyment of life, including his or her sense of well-being and the physical, mental, emotional, and social ability to do the things he or she wants to do.

radiation therapy: Using high-energy rays (similar to X-rays) to kill cancer cells.

radiologist: Doctors who specialize in diagnosing and treating diseases and injuries using medical imaging techniques, such as X-rays, computed tomography (CT), magnetic resonance imaging (MRI), nuclear medicine, positron emission tomography (PET), and ultrasound.

recurrence: When a cancer comes back in the same place after treatment or after remission.

relapse: The return of cancer after a period of improvement.

remission: When the cancer has gotten smaller, is gone, or is under control. Partial remission means that the cancer is still there, but the tumor is smaller or there is less cancer throughout the body. Complete remission means doctors cannot find any signs of cancer in the body.

risk factor: Something that is linked with a person's chance of getting a disease. A risk factor is not necessarily a causal factor. These can include 1) behaviors such as smoking or exercise; 2) demographic characteristics such as sex, age, education, and income; 3) genetics; and 4) geographic location.

sarcoma: A cancer that develops in connective tissue like muscle or fat.

screening test: A test to look for cancer before symptoms appear.

screening: Checking for cancer before symptoms appear. Screening may find diseases at an early stage, when there may be a better chance of treatment. Examples of cancer screening tests include mammograms for breast cancer, colonoscopy for colorectal cancer, and the Pap test and HPV test for cervical cancer.

second opinion: When a person gets an opinion from more than one doctor or specialist.

secondary cancer: A cancer that has spread to another part of the body from the area where it started.

side effects: Unwanted reactions or effects from medication or therapy. In chemotherapy, common side effects include hair loss and nausea. Having a lowered number of white blood cells is also a side effect of chemotherapy treatment.

social worker: Social workers help individuals, families, and groups as part of a team of professionals who provide care to patients. Social workers can help cancer patients with financial and family problems, emotional support, health insurance questions, or understanding the medical system.

stage: A way to describe cancer, usually on the basis of the size of the tumor, whether lymph nodes contain cancer, and whether it has spread to other organs or tissues in the body.

stem cell: A cell from which other types of cells develop. For example, blood cells develop from blood-forming stem cells.

stem cell transplant: Stem cell transplants may be done after chemotherapy or radiation therapy. Stem cells are cells that live in the bone marrow and make new blood cells. Stem cell transplants take stem cells from the blood of a donor and put them into a cancer patient after treatment.

support group: A group of people with similar concerns who help each other by sharing experiences, knowledge, and information.

support network: A group of people who help a cancer survivor like caregivers, friends, family members, doctors, and therapists.

surgeon: A doctor who performs surgeries.

surgery: Medical treatment to remove damaged or diseased parts of the body, such as the removal of tissue with cancer cells.

surveillance (medical): Closely watching a patient's condition, but not treating it unless there are changes in test results. Surveillance is also used to find early signs that a disease has come back. Surveillance can be used to monitor a person's health by doing certain tests on a regular schedule. It may be done for individuals who are at increased risk of cancer, patients in early stages of cancer, or survivors who are in remission. The term also is used in the field of epidemiology to describe the continuous collection, analysis, and interpretation of data.

survivorship care plan: A complete record of a cancer patient's cancer history, treatments given, the need for future checkups and cancer tests, possible long-term effects of the treatment, and ideas for staying healthy. The plan needs to identify the healthcare providers that were responsible for care.

symptom: A sign of illness in the body. There are some symptoms that are associated different types of cancer. For example, breast cancer, gynecologic cancers, colorectal cancer, and prostate cancer have different symptoms.

tissue: A group or layer of cells that work together to perform a specific function.

tumor: A tumor is an abnormal growth of body tissue. Tumors can be cancerous (malignant) or noncancerous (benign). Cancerous tumors can have uncontrolled growth and may spread to other parts of the body. Noncancerous tumors do not grow or spread.

Chapter 65

Terms to Help You Understand Your Medical Bill and Health Insurance

allowed amount: Maximum amount on which payment is based for covered healthcare services. This may be called "eligible expense," "payment allowance" or "negotiated rate." If your provider charges more than the allowed amount, you may have to pay the difference.

appeal: A request for your health insurer or plan to review a decision or a grievance again.

balance billing: When a provider bills you for the difference between the provider's charge and the allowed amount.

claim: A request for a benefit (including reimbursement of a healthcare expense) made by you or your healthcare provider to your health insurer or plan for items or services you think are covered.

coinsurance: Your share of the costs of a covered healthcare service, calculated as a percent (for example, 20%) of the allowed amount for the service. You pay co-insurance plus any deductibles you owe.

complications of pregnancy: Conditions due to pregnancy, labor and delivery that require medical care to prevent serious harm to the health of the mother or the fetus. Morning sickness and a nonemergency caesarean section aren't complications of pregnancy.

Excerpted from "Glossary of Health Coverage and Medical Terms," Center for Medicare and Medicaid Services (CMS), February 25, 2016.

copayment: A fixed amount (for example, $15) you pay for a covered healthcare service, usually when you receive the service. The amount can vary by the type of covered healthcare service.

cost sharing: Your share of costs for services that a plan covers that you must pay out of your own pocket (sometimes called "out-of-pocket costs"). Some examples of cost sharing are copayments, deductibles, and coinsurance. Family cost sharing is the share of cost for deductibles and out-of-pocket costs you and your spouse and/or child(ren) must pay out of your own pocket. Other costs, including your premiums, penalties you may have to pay or the cost of care a plan doesn't cover usually are not considered cost sharing.

cost-sharing reductions: Discounts that reduce the amount you pay for certain services covered by an individual plan you purchase through the Marketplace. You may get a discount if your income is below a certain level, and you choose a Silver level health plan or if you're a member of a federally recognized tribe, which includes being a shareholder in an Alaska Native Claims Settlement Act corporation.

deductible: The amount you owe for healthcare services your health insurance or plan covers before your health insurance or plan begins to pay. For example, if your deductible is $1000, your plan won't pay anything until you've met your $1000 deductible for covered healthcare services subject to the deductible. The deductible may not apply to all services.

diagnostic test: Tests to figure out what your health problem is. For example, an X-ray can be a diagnostic test to see if you have a broken bone.

durable medical equipment (DME): Equipment and supplies ordered by a healthcare provider for everyday or extended use. Coverage for DME may include: oxygen equipment, wheelchairs, crutches or blood testing strips for diabetics.

emergency medical condition: An illness, injury, symptom or condition so serious that a reasonable person would seek care right away to avoid severe harm.

emergency medical transportation: Ambulance services for an emergency medical condition.

emergency room care: Emergency services you get in an emergency room.

emergency services: Evaluation of an emergency medical condition and treatment to keep the condition from getting worse.

excluded services: Healthcare services that your health insurance or plan doesn't pay for or cover.

formulary: A list of drugs your plan covers. A formulary may include how much your share of the cost is for each drug. Your plan may place drugs at different cost sharing levels or tiers. For example, a formulary may include generic drug and brand name drug tiers and different cost sharing amounts will apply to each tier.

grievance: A complaint that you communicate to your health insurer or plan.

habilitation services: Healthcare services that help a person keep, learn or improve skills and functioning for daily living.

health insurance: A contract that requires your health insurer to pay some or all of your healthcare costs in exchange for a premium.

home healthcare: Healthcare services a person receives at home.

hospice services: Services to provide comfort and support for persons in the last stages of a terminal illness and their families.

hospital outpatient care: Care in a hospital that usually doesn't require an overnight stay.

hospitalization: Care in a hospital that requires admission as an inpatient and usually requires an overnight stay. An overnight stay for observation could be outpatient care.

individual responsibility requirement: Sometimes called the "individual mandate," the duty you may have to be enrolled in health coverage that provides minimum essential coverage. If you don't have minimum essential coverage, you may have to pay a penalty when you file your federal income tax return unless you qualify for a health coverage exemption.

in-network co-insurance: The percent (for example, 20%) you pay of the allowed amount for covered healthcare services to providers who contract with your health insurance or plan. In-network co-insurance usually costs you less than out-of-network co-insurance.

in-network co-payment: A fixed amount (for example, $15) you pay for covered healthcare services to providers who contract with your health insurance or plan. In-network co-payments usually are less than out-of-network co-payments.

marketplace: A marketplace for health insurance where individuals, families and small businesses can learn about their plan options;

compare plans based on costs, benefits and other important features; apply for and receive financial help with premiums and cost sharing based on income; and choose a plan and enroll in coverage. Also known as an "Exchange." The Marketplace is run by the state in some states and by the federal government in others. In some states, the Marketplace also helps eligible consumers enroll in other programs, including Medicaid and the Children's Health Insurance Program (CHIP). Available online, by phone and in-person.

maximum out-of-pocket limit: Yearly amount the federal government sets as the most each individual or family can be required to pay in cost sharing during the plan year for covered, in-network services. Applies to most types of health plans and insurance. This amount may be higher than the out-of-pocket limits stated for your plan.

medically necessary: Healthcare services or supplies needed to prevent, diagnose or treat an illness, injury, condition, disease or its symptoms and that meet accepted standards of medicine.

minimum essential coverage: Health coverage that will meet the individual responsibility requirement. Minimum essential coverage generally includes plans, health insurance available through the Marketplace or other individual market policies, Medicare, Medicaid, CHIP, TRICARE, and certain other coverage.

minimum value standard: A basic standard for measuring the percentage of permitted costs covered by the plan. If you're offered an employer plan that pays for at least 60% of the total allowed costs of benefits, the plan offers minimum value and you may not qualify for premium tax credits and cost sharing reductions to buy a plan from the Marketplace.

network provider (preferred provider): A provider who has a contract with your health insurer or plan who has agreed to provide services to members of a plan. You will pay less if you see a provider in the network. Also called "preferred provider" or "participating provider."

network: The facilities, providers and suppliers your health insurer or plan has contracted with to provide healthcare services.

orthotics and prosthetics: Leg, arm, back and neck braces, and artificial legs, arms, and eyes, and external breast prostheses incident to mastectomy resulting from breast cancer. These services include: adjustment, repairs, and replacements required because of breakage, wear, loss or a change in the patient's physical condition.

out-of-network co-insurance: The percent (for example, 40%) you pay of the allowed amount for covered healthcare services to providers who do not contract with your health insurance or plan. Out-of-network co-insurance usually costs you more than in network coinsurance.

out-of-network co-payment: A fixed amount (for example, $30) you pay for covered healthcare services from providers who do not contract with your health insurance or plan. Out-of-network copayments usually are more than in-network co-payments.

out-of-network provider (non-preferred provider): A provider who doesn't have a contract with your plan to provide services. If your plan covers out-of-network services, you'll usually pay more to see an out-of-network provider than a preferred provider. Your policy will explain what those costs may be. May also be called "non-preferred" or "non-participating" instead of "out-of-network provider."

out-of-pocket limit: The most you pay during a policy period (usually a year) before your health insurance or plan begins to pay 100% of the allowed amount. This limit never includes your premium, balance-billed charges or healthcare your health insurance or plan doesn't cover. Some health insurance or plans don't count all of your co-payments, deductibles, co-insurance payments, out-of-network payments or other expenses toward this limit.

physician services: Healthcare services a licensed medical physician (M.D.- Medical Doctor or D.O.- Doctor of Osteopathic Medicine) provides or coordinates.

plan: A benefit your employer, union or other group sponsor provides to you to pay for your healthcare services.

preauthorization: A decision by your health insurer or plan that a healthcare service, treatment plan, prescription drug or durable medical equipment is medically necessary. Sometimes called prior authorization, prior approval or precertification.

preferred provider: A provider who has a contract with your health insurer or plan to provide services to you at a discount. Check your policy to see if you can see all preferred providers or if your health insurance or plan has a "tiered" network and you must pay extra to see some providers.

premium tax credits: Financial help that lowers your taxes to help you and your family pay for private health insurance. You can get this help if you get health insurance through the Marketplace and your income is below a certain level. Advance payments of the tax credit can be used right away to lower your monthly premium costs.

premium: The amount that must be paid for your health insurance or plan. You and/or your employer usually pay it monthly, quarterly or yearly.

prescription drug coverage: Health insurance or plan that helps pay for prescription drugs and medications.

prescription drugs: Drugs and medications that by law require a prescription.

preventive care: Routine healthcare, including screenings, check-ups, and patient counseling, to prevent or discover illness, disease, or other health problems.

primary care physician: A physician (M.D.- Medical Doctor or D.O.- Doctor of Osteopathic Medicine) who directly provides or coordinates a range of healthcare services for a patient.

primary care provider: A physician (M.D.- Medical Doctor or D.O.- Doctor of Osteopathic Medicine), nurse practitioner, clinical nurse specialist or physician assistant, as allowed under state law, who provides, coordinates or helps a patient access a range of healthcare services.

provider: A physician (M.D.- Medical Doctor or D.O.- Doctor of Osteopathic Medicine), healthcare professional or healthcare facility licensed, certified or accredited as required by state law.

reconstructive surgery: Surgery and follow-up treatment needed to correct or improve a part of the body because of birth defects, accidents, injuries or medical conditions.

referral: A written order from your primary care provider for you to see a specialist or get certain healthcare services. In many health maintenance organizations (HMOs), you need to get a referral before you can get healthcare services from anyone except your primary care provider. If you don't get a referral first, the plan may not pay for the services.

rehabilitation services: Healthcare services that help a person keep, get back or improve skills and functioning for daily living that have been lost or impaired because a person was sick, hurt or disabled. These services may include physical and occupational therapy, speech-language pathology and psychiatric rehabilitation services in a variety of inpatient and/or outpatient settings.

screening: A type of preventive care that includes tests or exams to detect the presence of something, usually performed when you have no symptoms, signs or prevailing medical history of a disease or condition.

skilled nursing care: Services from licensed nurses in your own home or in a nursing home. Skilled care services are from technicians and therapists in your own home or in a nursing home.

specialist: A physician specialist focuses on a specific area of medicine or a group of patients to diagnose, manage, prevent or treat certain types of symptoms and conditions. A non-physician specialist is a provider who has more training in a specific area of healthcare.

specialty drug: A type of prescription drug that, in general, requires special handling or ongoing monitoring and assessment by a healthcare professional, or is relatively difficult to dispense. Generally, specialty drugs are the most expensive drugs on a formulary.

urgent care: Care for an illness, injury or condition serious enough that a reasonable person would seek care right away, but not so severe as to require emergency room care.

usual, customary and reasonable (UCR): The amount paid for a medical service in a geographic area based on what providers in the area usually charge for the same or similar medical service. The UCR amount sometimes is used to determine the allowed amount.

Chapter 66

Resources for Cancer Patients

Resources for Finding and Evaluating Cancer Treatments and Healthcare Providers

Agency for Healthcare Research and Quality (AHRQ)
5600 Fishers Ln.
Seventh Fl.
Rockville, MD 20857
Toll-Free: 800-358-9295
Phone: 301-427-1104
Website: www.ahrq.gov

American Board of Medical Specialties (ABMS)
353 N. Clark St.
Ste. 1400
Chicago, IL 60654
Phone: 312-436-2600
Website: www.abms.org

American College of Surgeons (ACS)
633 N. Saint Clair St.
Chicago, IL 60611-3211
Toll-Free: 800-621-4111
Phone: 312-202-5000
Fax: 312-202-5001
Website: www.facs.org

American Society for Laser Medicine and Surgery (ASLMS)
2100 Stewart Ave., Ste. 240
Wausau, WI 54401
Toll-Free: 877-258-6028
Phone: 715-845-9283
Fax: 715-848-2493
Website: www.aslms.org
E-mail: information@aslms.org

Resources in this chapter were compiled from several sources deemed reliable; all contact information was verified and updated in February 2017.

American Society of Clinical Oncology (ASCO)
2318 Mill Rd.
Ste. 800
Alexandria, VA 22314
Toll-Free: 888-651-3038
Phone: 571-483-1300
Fax: 571-366-9537
Website: www.asco.org
E-mail: customerservice@asco.
org

Association of Community Cancer Centers (ACCC)
1801 Research Blvd.
Ste. 400
Rockville, MD 20850
Phone: 301-984-9496
Fax: 301-770-1949
Website: www.accc-cancer.org

Cancer Trials Support Unit (CTSU)
Toll-Free: 1-888-823-5923 /
1-866-651-2878
Phone: 763-406-8600
Fax: 1-888-691-8039
Website: www.ctsu.org
E-mail: ctsucontact@westat.com

Center for International Blood and Marrow Transplant Research (CIBMTR)
500 N. Fifth St.
Minneapolis, MN 55401-1206
Toll-Free: 888-597-7674
Fax: 763-406-5749
Website: www.cibmtr.org
E-mail: help@bmtinfonet.org

CureSearch
4600 East-West Hwy.
Ste. 600
Bethesda, MD 20814
Toll-Free: 800-458-6223
Fax: 301-718-0047
Website: www.curesearch.org
E-mail: info@curesearch.org

Dana Farber Cancer Institute (DFCI)
450 Brookline Ave.
Boston, MA 02215-5450
Toll-Free: 866-408-DFCI
(866-408-3324)
Phone: 617-632-6366
TDD: 857-215-0112
Website: www.dana-farber.org

Federal Trade Commission (FTC)
600 Pennsylvania Ave. N.W.
Washington, DC 20580
Toll-Free: 877-FTC-HELP
(877-382-4357)
Phone: 202-326-2222
TTY: 202-326-2502
Website: www.ftc.gov

Joint Commission on Accreditation of Healthcare Organizations (JCAHO)
1 Renaissance Blvd.
Oakbrook Terrace, IL 60181
Phone: 630-792-5000
Fax: 630-792-5005
Website: www.jointcommision.
org
E-mail: jciaccreditation@jcrinc.
com

The National Association for Proton Therapy (NAPT)
8400 Westpark Dr.
Second Fl.
McLean, VA 22102
Phone: 202-495-3133
Website: www.proton-therapy. org
E-mail: info@proton-therapy.org

National Cancer Institute (NCI)
BG 9609 MSC 9760
9609 Medical Center Dr.
Bethesda, MD 20892-9760
Toll-Free: 1-800-422-6237
Website: www.cancer.gov

National Center for Complementary and Integrative Health (NCCIH)
9000 Rockville Pike
Bethesda, MD 20892
Toll-Free: 1-888-644-6226
TTY: 1-866-464-3615
Website: www.nccih.nih.gov
E-mail: info@nccih.nih.gov

National Comprehensive Cancer Network (NCCN)
275 Commerce Dr.
Ste. 300
Fort Washington, PA 19034
Toll-Free: 888-909-6226
Phone: 215-690-0300
Fax: 215-690-0280
Website: www.nccn.org

Pediatric Oncology Branch (POB)
Bldg. 10 Rm. 1W-3750
Bethesda, MD 20892
Toll-Free: 877-624-4878
Phone: 301-496-4256
Website: www.ccr.cancer.gov/ Pediatric-Oncology-Branch
E-mail: ncipediatrics@mail.nih. gov

U.S. Food and Drug Administration (FDA)
10903 New Hampshire Ave.
Silver Spring, MD 20993
Toll-Free: 1-888-INFO-FDA (1-888-463-6332)
Website: www.fda.gov

Resources for Locating Clinical Trials for Cancer Care

CenterWatch
10 Winthrop Sq.
Fifth Fl.
Boston, MA 02110
Toll-Free: 866-219-3440
Phone: 617-948-5100
Website: www.centerwatch.com
E-mail: support@centerwatch. com

EmergingMed
2605 Meridian Pkwy
Ste. 115
Durham, NC 27713
Toll-Free: 1-877-601-8601
Website: www.emergingmed.com
E-mail: ContactUs@ EmergingMed.com

National Cancer Institute Cancer Trials
BG 9609 MSC 9760
9609 Medical Center Dr.
Bethesda, MD 20892-9760
Toll-Free: 1-800-422-6237
Website: www.cancer.gov/about-cancer/treatment/clinical-trials/search

U.S. National Library of Medicine (NLM)
8600 Rockville Pike
Bethesda, MD 20894
Phone: 888-FIND-NLM
(888-346-3656)
Website: www.nlm.nih.gov
E-mail: custserv@nlm.nih.gov

National Organizations That Offer Services to People with Cancer and Their Families

American Cancer Society (ACS)
250 Williams St. N.W.
Atlanta, GA 30303
Toll-Free: 800-227-2345
Phone: 404-320-3333
Website: www.cancer.org

Be The Match®
500 N. Fifth St.
Minneapolis, MN 55401-1206
Toll-Free: 800-507-5427
Phone: 763-406-5800
Website: www.bethematch.org
E-mail: foundation@nmdp.org

Bloch Cancer Foundation, Inc.
1 H&R Block Way
Kansas City, MO 64105
Toll-Free: 800-433-0464
Phone: 816-854-5050
Fax: 816-854-8024
Website: www.blochcancer.org
E-mail: hotline@blochcancer.org

Cancer Hope Network (CHN)
2 North Rd., Ste. A
Chester, NJ 07930
Toll-Free: 877-HOPENET
(877-467-3638)
Fax: 908-879-6518
Website: www.cancerhopenetwork.org

Cancer Information and Counseling Line (CICL)
American Society of Clinical Oncology (ASCO)
2318 Mill Rd.
Ste. 800
Alexandria, VA 22314
Toll-Free: 800-525-3777
Phone: 571-483-1780
Fax: 571-366-9537
Website: www.cancer.net
E-mail: contactus@cancer.net

Cancer Care
National Office
275 Seventh Ave., 22nd Fl.
New York, NY 10001
Toll-Free: 800-813-HOPE
(800-813-4673)
Phone: 212-712-8400
Fax: 212-712-8495
Website: www.cancercare.org
E-mail: info@cancercare.org

ENCOREPlus®
515 North St.
White Plains, NY 10605
Phone: 914-949-6227
Website: www.ywcawpcw.org

Gilda's Club Twin Cities
10560 Wayzata Blvd.
Minnetonka, MN 55305
Phone: 612–227–2147
Website: www.
gildasclubtwincities.org
E-mail: info@
GildasClubTwinCities.org

International Association of Laryngectomees (IAL)
925B Peachtree St. N.E.
Ste. 316
Atlanta, GA 30309
Toll-Free: 866-425-3678
Website: www.theial.com
E-mail: office@theial.com

KidsCope
2045 Peachtree Rd., Ste. 150
Atlanta, GA 30309
Website: www.kidscope.org

LIVESTRONG
2201 E. Sixth St.
Austin, TX 78702
Toll-Free: 855-220-7777
Phone: 877-236-8820
Website: www.livestrong.org

Living Beyond Breast Cancer (LBBC)
40 Monument Rd., Ste. 104
Bala Cynwyd, PA 19004
Toll-Free: 855-807-6386
Phone: 610-645-4567
Fax: 610-645-4567
Website: www.lbbc.org
E-mail: mail@lbbc.org

National Bone Marrow Transplant Link (nbmtLINK)
20411 W. 12 Mile Rd., Ste.108
Southfield, MI 48076
Toll-Free: 800-LINK-BMT
(800-546-5268)
Website: www.nbmtlink.org
E-mail: info@nbmtlink.org

National Coalition for Cancer Survivorship (NCCS)
8455 Colesville Rd., Ste. 930
Silver Spring, MD 20910
Toll-Free: 877-NCCS-YES
(877-622-7937)
Phone: 301-650-9127
Website: www.canceradvocacy.org
E-mail: info@canceradvocacy.org

National Lymphedema Network (NLN)
2288 Fulton St., Ste. 307
Berkeley, CA 94704
Toll-Free: 1-800-541-3259
Phone: 510-809-1660
Fax: 510-809-1699
Website: www.lymphnet.org
E-mail: nln@lymphnet.org

National Pediatric Cancer Foundation (NPCF)
5550 W. Executive Dr.
Ste. 300
Tampa, FL 33609
Toll-Free: 1-813-269-0955
Website: www.nationalpcf.org
E-mail: fundingresearch@
NationalPCF.org

Office of Cancer Survivorship (OCS)
Division of Cancer Control and
Population Sciences
9609 Medical Center Dr.
MSC 9764
Bethesda, MD 20892
Toll-Free: 1-800-422-6237
Phone: 240-276-6690
Website: www.cancercontrol.
cancer.gov/ocs

Patient Advocate Foundation (PAF)
421 Butler Farm Rd.
Hampton, VA 23666
Toll-Free: 1-866-512-3861
Phone: 800-532-5274
Fax: 757-873-8999
Website: www.patientadvocate.
org

Sisters Network®, Inc.
2922 Rosedale St.
Houston, TX 77004
Toll-Free: 866-781-1808
Phone: 713-781-0255
Fax: 713-780-8998
Website: www.
sistersnetworkinc.org
E-mail: infonet@
sisternetworkinc.org

Starlight Children's Foundation
2049 Century Park E.
Ste. 4320
Los Angeles, CA 90067
Phone: 310-479-1212
Website: www.starlight.org

Support for People with Oral and Head and Neck Cancer (SPOHNC)
P.O. Box 53
Locust Valley, NY 11560-0053
Toll-Free: 800-377-0928
Fax: 516-671-8794
Website: www.spohnc.org
E-mail: info@spohnc.org

13thirty Cancer Connect
1000 Elmwood Ave.
Rochester, NY 14620
Phone: 585-563-6221

United Ostomy Association of America (UOAA)
P.O. Box 525
Kennebunk, ME 04043-0525
Toll-Free: 800-826-0826
Website: www.ostomy.org

Us TOO International Prostate Cancer Education and Support Network
2720 S. River Rd., Ste. 112
Des Plaines, IL 60018-4106
Toll-Free: 800-80-Us TOO
(800-808-7866)
Phone: 630-795-1002
Fax: 630-795-1602
Website: www.ustoo.org
E-mail: ustoo@ustoo.org

Vital Options International (VOI)
Phone: 818-508-5657
Website: www.vitaloptions.org
E-mail: info@vitaloptions.org

Chapter 67

The National Cancer Institute Cancer Centers Program

Alabama

University of Alabama at Birmingham (UAB) Comprehensive Cancer Center
1824 Sixth Ave. S.
Wallace Tumor Institute 202
Birmingham, AL 35233
Toll-Free: 1-800-UAB-0933
(1-800-822-0933)
Phone: 205-934-5077
TTY: 205-975-9973
Website: www3.ccc.uab.edu

Arizona

University of Arizona Cancer Center (UACC)
3838 N. Campbell Ave.
Tucson, AZ 85719
Toll-Free: 520-694-CURE
(520-694-2873)
Phone: 520-626-2548
Website: www.uacc.arizona.edu

Excerpted from "Find a Cancer Center," National Cancer Institute (NCI), September 14, 2016. All contact information was verified and updated in February 2017.

California

Chao Family Comprehensive Cancer Center (CFCCC)
Bldg. 23 101 The City Dr. S.
Orange, CA 92868
Toll-Free: 877-827-8839
Phone: 714-456-8600
Website: www.cancer.uci.edu

City of Hope Comprehensive Cancer Center
1500 E. Duarte Rd.
Duarte, CA 91010
Toll-Free: 800-826-4673
Phone: 626-256-HOPE
(626-256-4673)
Website: www.cityofhope.org

Jonsson Comprehensive Cancer Center (JCCC)
8-684 Factor Bldg.
Box 951781
Los Angeles, CA 90095-1781
Toll-Free: 888-ONC-UCLA
(888-662-8252)
Phone: 310-825-5268
Fax: 310-206-5553
Website: www.cancer.ucla.edu

Salk Institute Cancer Center
10010 N. Torrey Pines Rd.
La Jolla, CA 92037
Phone: 858-453-4100
Website: www.salk.edu

Sanford Burnham Prebys Medical Discovery Institute (SBP)
10901 N. Torrey Pines Rd.
La Jolla, CA 92037
Phone: 858-646-3100
Fax: 858-646-3199
Website: www.sbpdiscovery.org
E-mail: info@SBPdiscovery.org

Stanford Cancer Institute
Lorry Lokey Bldg./SIM
1265 Campus Dr., Ste. G2103
Stanford, CA 94305-5456
Phone: 650-736-7716
Fax: 650-736-0607
Website: med.stanford.edu

UC Davis Comprehensive Cancer Center (UCDCCC)
2279 45th St.
Sacramento, CA 95817
Toll-Free: 800-770-9261
Phone: 916-734-5959
Website: www.ucdmc.ucdavis.edu/cancer
E-mail: cancer.center@ucdmc.ucdavis.edu

UC San Diego Health
200 W. Arbor Dr.
San Diego, CA 92103
Toll-Free: 800-926-8273
Phone: 858-657-7000
Website: health.ucsd.edu

UCSF (University of California San Francisco) Helen Diller Family Comprehensive Cancer Center
Box 0981, UCSF
San Francisco, CA 94143-0981
Toll-Free: 888-689-8273
Phone: 415-476-2557
Fax: 415-476-3541
Website: cancer.ucsf.edu
E-mail: communications@cc.ucsf.edu.

USC Norris Comprehensive Cancer Center
1441 Eastlake Ave.
Los Angeles, CA 90033
Phone: 323-865-0816
Fax: 323-865-0102
Website: uscnorriscancer.usc.edu

Colorado

University of Colorado Cancer Center
13001 E. 17th Pl.
Aurora, CO 80045
Phone: 720-848-0300
Website: www.ucdenver.edu

Connecticut

Yale Cancer Center (YCC)
333 Cedar St.
P.O. Box 208028
New Haven, CT 06520-8028
Phone: 203-785-4095
Fax: 203-785-4116
Website: yalecancercenter.org

District of Columbia

Georgetown Lombardi Comprehensive Cancer Center
3800 Reservoir Rd. N.W.
Washington, DC 20057
Phone: 202-444-4000
Website: www.lombardi.georgetown.edu

Florida

Moffitt Cancer Center
12902 USF Magnolia Dr.
Tampa, FL 33612
Toll-Free: 888-MOFFITT
(888-663-3488)
Phone: 813-745-4673
Website: www.moffitt.org

Georgia

Winship Cancer Institute (WCI)
1365-C Clifton Rd. N.E.
Atlanta, GA 30322
Toll-Free: 888-WINSHIP
(888-946-7447)
Phone: 404-778-1900
Website: www.winshipcancer.emory.edu

Hawaii

University of Hawaii Cancer Center (UH Cancer Center)
701 Ilalo St., Ste. 600
Honolulu, HI 96813
Phone: 808-586-3010
Fax: 808-586-3052
Website: www.uhcancercenter.org

Illinois

Robert H. Lurie Comprehensive Cancer Center
675 N. St. Clair, 21st Fl.
Chicago, IL 60611
Toll-Free: 866-LURIE-CC
(866-587-4322)
Phone: 312-908-5250
Fax: 312-908-1372
Website: cancer.northwestern.edu

The University of Chicago Comprehensive Cancer Center (UCCCC)
5841 S. Maryland Ave.
Chicago, IL 60637
Toll-Free: 855-702-8222
Phone: 773-702-6180
Website: cancer.uchicago.edu

Indiana

Indiana University Melvin and Bren Simon Cancer Center
535 Barnhill Dr.
Indianapolis, IN 46202
Toll-Free: 888-600-4822
Phone: 317-278-0070
Website: www.cancer.iu.edu

Purdue University Center for Cancer Research (PUCCR)
201 S. University St.
Hansen Life Sciences Bldg.
Rm. 141
West Lafayette, IN 47907-2064
Phone: 765-494-9129
Fax: 765-494-9193
Website: www.cancerresearch.purdue.edu
E-mail: cancerresearch@purdue.edu

Iowa

Holden Comprehensive Cancer Center
University of Iowa Hospitals and Clinics
200 Hawkins Dr.
Iowa City, IA 52242
Toll-Free: 800-777-8442
Phone: 319-356-1616
Website: uihc.org/medical-services/holden-comprehensive-cancer-center

Kansas

The University of Kansas Cancer Center (KUCC)
3901 Rainbow Blvd.
Kansas City, KS 66160-7220
Toll-Free: 844-323-1227
Phone: 913-588-1227
Website: www.kucancercenter.org

Kentucky

UK Markey Cancer Center
University of Kentucky
800 Rose St.
Lexington, KY 40536
Toll-Free: 866-340-4488
Phone: 859-257-4488
Fax: 859-323-2074
Website: www.ukhealthcare.uky.
edu

Maine

**The Jackson Laboratory
Cancer Center (JAXCC)**
600 Main St.
Bar Harbor, ME 04609
Phone: 207-288-6000
Fax: 207-288-6150
Website: www.jax.org

Maryland

**Sidney Kimmel
Comprehensive Cancer
Center**
The Johns Hopkins University
401 North Bdwy.
The Harry and Jeanette
Weinberg Bldg., Ste. 1100
Baltimore, MD 21287
Toll-Free: 410-464-6713
Phone: 410-502-1033
Website: www.hopkinsmedicine.
org

**University of Maryland
Marlene and Stewart
Greenebaum Comprehensive
Cancer Center (UMGCC)**
22 S. Greene St.
Baltimore, MD 21201
Toll-Free: 800-492-5538
Phone: 410-328-7904
TDD: 800-735-2258
Fax: 410-328-3018
Website: www.umm.edu

Massachusetts

**Dana-Farber / Harvard
Cancer Center**
450 Brookline Ave. BP332A
Boston, MA 02215
Toll-Free: 877-420-3951
Phone: 617-632-2100
Fax: 617-632-4452
Website: www.dfhcc.harvard.edu
E-mail: dfhcc@partners.org

**Koch Institute for Integrative
Cancer Research (KIICR)**
Massachusetts Institute of
Technology (MIT)
500 Main St., Bldg. 76
Cambridge, MA 02139-4307
Phone: 617-253-6403
Website: www.ki.mit.edu

Michigan

**Barbara Ann Karmanos
Cancer Institute (BAKCI)**
4100 John R
Detroit, MI 48201
Toll-Free: 800-KARMANOS
(800-527-6266)
Website: www.karmanos.org
E-mail: info@karmanos.org

University of Michigan Comprehensive Cancer Center (UMCCC)
1500 E. Medical Center Dr.
CCGC 6-303
Ann Arbor, MI 48109-0944
Toll-Free: 800-865-1125
Website: www.mcancer.org

Minnesota

Masonic Cancer Center (MCC)
University of Minnesota
420 Delaware St. S.E.
Minneapolis, MN 55455
Phone: 612-624-8484
Website: www.cancer.umn.edu
E-mail: mccadmin@umn.edu

Mayo Clinic Cancer Center (MCCC)
200 First St. S.W.
Rochester, MN 55905
Phone: 507-284-2511
Website: www.mayoclinic.org

Missouri

Alvin J. Siteman Cancer Center
4921 Parkview Pl.
St. Louis, MO 63110
Toll-Free: 800-600-3606
Phone: 314-362-5196
Website: siteman.wustl.edu

Nebraska

Fred and Pamela Buffett Cancer Center
985230 Nebraska Medical Center
Phone: 402-559-4696
Website: www.buffettcancercenter.com
E-mail: msommerfeld@nebraskamed.com

New Hampshire

Norris Cotton Cancer Center (NCCC)
Dartmouth-Hitchcock Medical Center
1 Medical Center Dr.
Lebanon, NH 03756
Toll-Free: 800-543-1624
Phone: 603-650-5000
TDD: 603-650-8034
Website: www.dartmouth-hitchcock.org
E-mail: answers@hitchcock.org

New Jersey

Rutgers Cancer Institute of New Jersey (RCINJ)
195 Little Albany St.
New Brunswick, NJ 08903-2681
Phone: 732-235-CINJ
(732-235-2465)
Website: www.cinj.org

New Mexico

University of New Mexico Cancer Center (UNM Cancer Center)
1201 Camino de Salud N.E.
Albuquerque, NM 87102
Toll-Free: 800-432-6806
Phone: 505-272-4946
Fax: 505-925-0100
Website: www.cancer.unm.edu

New York

Albert Einstein Cancer Center (AECC)
1300 Morris Park Ave.
Bronx, NY 10461
Phone: 718-430-2000
Website: www.einstein.yu.edu
E-mail: information@einstein.yu.edu

Cold Spring Harbor Laboratory Cancer Center (CSHL)
1 Bungtown Rd.
Cold Spring Harbor, NY 11724
Phone: 516-367-8800
Website: www.cshl.edu

Herbert Irving Comprehensive Cancer Center (HICCC)
1130 St., Nicholas Ave.
New York, NY 10032
Phone: 212-851-4680
Website: www.hiccc.columbia.edu

Laura and Isaac Perlmutter Cancer Center at NYU Langone
550 First Ave.
New York, NY 10016
Phone: 212-731-6000
Website: nyulangone.org

North Carolina

Duke Cancer Institute (DCI)
DUMC Box 3494
20 Duke Medicine Cir.
Durham, NC 27710
Toll-Free: 800-633-3853
Website: www.dukehealth.org

UNC Lineberger Comprehensive Cancer Center
450 West Dr.
Chapel Hill, NC 27514
Toll-Free: 866-869-1856
Phone: 919-966-3036
Fax: 919-966-3015
Website: www.unclineberger.org

The Comprehensive Cancer Center of Wake Forest University (CCCWFU)
Medical Center Blvd.
Winston-Salem, NC 27157
Toll-Free: 888-716-9253
Website: www.wakehealth.edu

Ohio

Case Comprehensive Cancer Center (Case CCC)
11100 Euclid Ave., Wearn 152
Cleveland, OH 44106-5065
Phone: 216-844-8797
Fax: 216-844-7832
Website: cancer.case.edu
E-mail: cancer@case.edu

The Ohio State University Comprehensive Cancer Center
460 W. 10th Ave.
Columbus, OH 43210
Toll-Free: 800-293-5066
Phone: 614-293-5066
Fax: 614-293-9449
Website: www.cancer.osu.edu
E-mail: jamesline@osumc.edu

Oregon

Knight Cancer Institute (KCI)
Oregon Health and Science University (OHSU)
3181 S.W. Sam Jackson Park Rd.
Portland, OR 97239-3098
Phone: 503-494-1617
Website: www.ohsu.edu

Pennsylvania

Abramson Cancer Center
The Hospital of the University of Pennsylvania
3400 Spruce St.
Philadelphia, PA 19104
Toll-Free: 800-789-7366
Phone: 215-615-5858
Website: www.pennmedicine.org/cancer

Fox Chase Cancer Center
333 Cottman Ave.
Philadelphia, PA 19111-2497
Toll-Free: 888-FOX-CHASE
(888-369-2427)
Phone: 215-728-2570
Fax: 215-728-5666
Website: www.foxchase.org

Sidney Kimmel Cancer Center (SKCC)
Bluemle Life Sciences Bldg.
233 S. 10th St.
Ste. 1050
Philadelphia, PA 19107
Phone: 215-503-5692
Website: www.
kimmelcancercenter.org

University of Pittsburgh Cancer Institute (UPCI)
5150 Centre Ave.
Pittsburgh, PA 15232
Phone: 412-647-2811
Website: www.upci.upmc.edu

The Wistar Institute Cancer Center
3601 Spruce St.
Philadelphia, PA 19104
Phone: 215-898-3700
Website: www.wistar.org

South Carolina

Hollings Cancer Center (HCC)
86 Jonathan Lucas St.
MSC 955
Charleston, SC 29425
Phone: 843-792-0700
Website: www.
hollingscancercenter.org

Tennessee

St. Jude Children's Research Hospital
262 Danny Thomas Pl.
Memphis, TN 38105
Toll-Free: 866-278-5833
TTY: 901-595-1040
Website: www.stjude.org

Vanderbilt-Ingram Cancer Center (VICC)
691 Preston Bldg.
Nashville, TN 37232
Toll-Free: 877-936-8422
Phone: 615-936-8422
Website: www.vicc.org

Texas

Cancer Therapy & Research Center (CTRC)
7979 Wurzbach Rd.
San Antonio, TX 78229
Toll-Free: 800-340-2872
(800-340-CTRC)
Phone: 210-450-1000
Website: www.uthscsa.edu

Dan L Duncan Comprehensive Cancer Center
Baylor College of Medicine
1 Baylor Plaza
Ste. 450A
Houston, TX 77030
Phone: 713-798-1354
Fax: 713-798-2716
Website: www.bcm.edu

Harold C. Simmons Comprehensive Cancer Center
The University of Texas
Southwestern Medical Center
5323 Harry Hines Blvd.
Dallas, TX 75390
Toll-Free: 866-460-HOPE
(866-460-4673)
Phone: 214-648-3111
Website: www.utsouthwestern.edu/simmons

The University of Texas MD Anderson Cancer Center
1515 Holcombe Blvd., Unit 91
Houston, TX 77030
Toll-Free: 888-512-7249
Website: www.mdanderson.org

Utah

Huntsman Cancer Institute (HCI)
2000 Circle of Hope
Salt Lake City, UT 84112
Toll-Free: 877-585-0303
Phone: 801-585-0303
Website: www.huntsmancancer.org

Virginia

Massey Cancer Center
Virginia Commonwealth
University (VCU)
401 College St.
P.O. Box 980037
Richmond, VA 23298-0037
Phone: 804-828-0450
Fax: 804-828-8453
Website: www.massey.vcu.edu
E-mail: AskMassey@vcu.edu

University of Virginia
Cancer Center
1240 Lee St.
Charlottesville, VA 22903
Toll-Free: 800-223-9173
Phone: 434-924-9333
Website: www.cancer.uvahealth.
com

Washington

Fred Hutchinson / University
of Washington Cancer
Consortium
1100 Fairview Ave. N.
Seattle, WA 98109
Phone: 206-667-4520
Fax: 206-667-6068
Website: www.cancerconsortium.
org

Wisconsin

University of Wisconsin
Carbone Cancer Center
(UWCCC)
600 Highland Ave.
Madison, WI 53792
Toll-Free: 800-323-8942
Phone: 608-263-6400
Website: www.uwhealth.org

Chapter 68

Financial Assistance for Cancer Care

American Childhood Cancer Organization (ACCO)
P.O. Box 498
Kensington, MD 20895-0498
Toll-Free: 1-855-858-2226
Phone: 301-962-3520
Fax: 301-962-3521
Website: www.acco.org
E-mail: staff@acco.org

Benefits.gov
Toll-Free: 1-800-FED-INFO
(1-800-333-4636)
Website: benefits.gov

Cancer Financial Assistance Coalition (CFAC)
Website: www.cancerfac.org
E-mail: contact@cancerfac.org

CancerCare
275 Seventh Ave.
22nd Fl.
New York, NY 10001
Toll-Free: 1-800-813-4673
Phone: 212-712-8400
Website: www.cancercare.org
E-mail: info@cancercare.org

Catholic Charities USA (CCUSA)
2050 Ballenger Ave., Ste. 400
Alexandria, VA 22314
Toll-Free: 1-800-919-9338
Phone: 703-549-1390
Fax: 703-549-1656
Website: www.
catholiccharitiesusa.org
E-mail: info@
catholiccharitiesusa.org

Excerpted from "General Living Expenses," National Cancer Institute (NCI). All contact information was verified and updated in February 2017.

Cleaning for a Reason Foundation
211 S. Stemmons
Ste. G
Lewisville,TX 75067
Phone: 877-337-3348
Fax: 972-316-4138
Website: www.
cleaningforareason.org
E-mail: info@cleaningforareason.
org

Eldercare Locator
Toll-Free: 1-800-677-1116
Website: www.eldercare.gov
E-mail: eldercarelocator@n4a.
org

Hospice Education Institute (HEI)
3 Unity Sq.
P.O. Box 98.
Machiasport, ME 04655-0098
Toll-Free: 1-800-331-1620
Phone: 207-255-8800
Fax: 207-255-8008
Website: www.hospiceworld.org
E-mail: info@hospiceworld.org

Leukemia and Lymphoma Society (LLS)
3 International Dr.
Ste. 200
Rye Brook, NY 10573
Phone: 914-949-5213
Fax: 914-949-6691
Website: www.lls.org
E-mail: infocenter@lls.org

Lymphoma Research Foundation (LRF)
115 Bdwy.
Ste. 1301
New York, NY 10006
Toll-Free: 1-800-500-9976
Phone: 212-349-2910
Fax: 212-349-2886
Website: www.lymphoma.org
E-mail: LRF@lymphoma.org

The National Children's Cancer Society (NCCS)
500 North Bdwy.
Ste.1850
St. Louis, MO 63102
Phone: 314-241-1600
Website: www.thenccs.org

The Salvation Army National Headquarters
615 Slaters Ln.
P.O. Box 269
Alexandria, VA 22313
Toll-Free: 1-800-SA-TRUCK
(1-800-728-7825)
Website: www.
salvationarmyusa.org

The SAMFund
89 South St.
Ste. LL02
Boston, MA 02111
Phone: 617-938-3484
Fax: 866-496-8070
Website: www.thesamfund.org

Sarcoma Alliance
775 E. Blithedale
Ste. 334
Mill Valley, CA 94941
Phone: 415-381-7236
Fax: 415-381-7235
Website: www.sarcomaalliance.
org
E-mail: info@sarcomaalliance.
org

Social Security
Administration (SSA)
Windsor Park Bldg.
6401 Security Blvd.
Baltimore, MD 21235
Toll-Free: 1-800-772-1213
TTY:1-800-325-0778
Website: www.ssa.gov

United Way Worldwide
701 N. Fairfax St.
Alexandria, VA 22314
Phone: 703-836-7112
Website: www.unitedway.org

Index

Index

GVHD *see* graft-versus-host disease

H

habilitation services, defined 519
hair loss
  cancer treatment and self-image
    361, 490
  chemotherapy side effects 71
  overview 257–60
"Hair Loss (Alopecia)" (NCI) 257n
haloperidol
  delirium medicines 380
  tabulated *210*
Harold C. Simmons Comprehensive
  Cancer Center, contact 541
Hb *see* hemoglobin
HBV *see* hepatitis B virus
HDR *see* high-dose radiation
health disparities, physical health
  concerns 384
health insurance
  body images 362
  cancer follow-up care 463
  cancer-related fatigue 266
  defined 519
  finding a doctor 6
  hospice services 128
  joining clinical trials 141
  off-label drugs 105
healthcare plan, second opinion 13
hearing problems, childhood
  cancers 354
heart
  CAM in cancer care 115
  electrolyte imbalances 376
  fatigue 266
  fecal impaction 223
  immunotherapy side effects 73
  late effects of cancer treatment 338
  polysomnogram 327
heart attack
  anxiety disorders 410
  depression 389
  late effects of cancer 338
heart disease
  cancer follow-up care 466
  cancer pain 281
  gastrointestinal complications 222

heart disease, *continued*
  late effects of cancer treatment 337
  nutrition care 442
  palliative care 123
  physical activity 448
  sexual and fertility problems 295
  spirituality 368
heart failure, late effects of cancer
  treatment 338
helper T cells, cancer vaccine 152
hematologist, finding a doctor 8
hemoglobin (Hb; Hgb)
  cancer-related fatigue 272
  lab tests 25
  pruritus 304
hepatitis B virus (HBV),
  vaccine 4, 153
herbal products, CAM in cancer
  care 110
herbal tea
  CAM in cancer care 108
  drug-nutrient interactions 441
  see also Essiac; Flor Essence
Herbert Irving Comprehensive Cancer
  Center (HICCC), contact 539
Hgb *see* hemoglobin
high-dose radiation
  immune system 347
  nutrition in cancer care 429
Hodgkin lymphoma
  cancer medications 90
  cardiovascular system 336
  digestive system 340
  endocrine system 345
  pruritus 308
  respiratory system 352
Holden Comprehensive Cancer Center
  (HCCC), contact 536
Hollings Cancer Center (HCC),
  contact 540
home healthcare
  defined 519
  transitional care planning 133
hormone
  defined 511
  tabulated *32*
  targeted therapy 76
hormone replacement therapy, hot
  flashes and night sweats 298

laser, cancer surgery 64
late effects
  childhood cancer treatments,
    overview 335–57
  defined 512
"Late Effects of Treatment for
  Childhood Cancer (PDQ®)–Patient
  Version" (NCI) 335n
LDH *see* lactate dehydrogenase
"Learning to Relax" (NCI) 453n
leukemia
  defined 512
  lab tests 25
  tabulated *31*
Leukemia and Lymphoma Society
  (LLS), contact 544
leukocytes, immune system 151
laxatives, gastrointestinal
  complications 221
liquid cancers *see* leukemias
liver, late cancer treatment effects 343
liver cancer, tumor marker 30
LIVESTRONG, contact 529
Living Beyond Breast Cancer (LBBC),
  contact 529
living will, end-of-life decisions 134
local anesthetic, cancer pain 285
lomustine, brain tumors 85
loneliness, recurrent cancer 476
long-term side effect, defined 512
lorazepam, delirium 380
loss of appetite, palliative care 122
loss of sensation, self-image and
  sexuality 364
loved ones, palliative care 124
lung cancer
  cancer medications 87
  cancer recurrence 449
  lab tests 25
  types of cancer treatments 65
lycopene, nutritional therapies 114
lymphangiosarcoma, defined 318
lymphedema, oral complications 254
"Lymphedema (PDQ®)–Patient
  Version" (NCI) 309n
lymphocytes, immune system 151
lymphoma, lab tests 25
Lymphoma Research Foundation
  (LRF), contact 544

lymphoma and multiple myeloma,
  defined 512
Lynch syndrome, physical health
  concerns 383

M

magnesium, electrolytes 356
magnetic resonance imaging (MRI)
  defined 312
  imaging 27
major depression, cancer patients 390
malignant, defined 512
malnutrition
  head and neck cancers 250
  oral complications 250
mammography, screening 4
manual lymphedema therapy,
  defined 113
marketplace, defined 519
marijuana, CAM in cancer care 110
Masonic Cancer Center (MCC),
  contact 538
massage therapy, lymphedema 317
Massey Cancer Center, contact 541
Matulane (procarbazine) *441*
maximum out-of-pocket limit,
  defined 520
Mayo Clinic Cancer Center (MCCC),
  contact 538
mechlorethamine, alkylating
  agents 351
medically necessary, defined 520
Medicare, palliative care 125
medications
  cancer treatment 446
  cancer-related fatigue 274
  delirium 379
  depression 246
  end-of-life decisions 134
  fever 158
  lymphedema 317
  nutrient interactions 441
  overview 84–103
  pain management 110
  posttraumatic stress disorder 419
  pruritus 306
  sexual dysfunction 363
  transitional care option 133

LONGWOOD PUBLIC LIBRARY
800 Middle Country Road
Middle Island, NY 11953
(631) 924-6400
longwoodlibrary.org

LIBRARY HOURS

Monday-Friday	9:30 a.m. - 9:00 p.m.
Saturday	9:30 a.m. - 5:00 p.m.
Sunday (Sept-June)	1:00 p.m. - 5:00 p.m.